Swine Diseases and Health Management

Swine Diseases and Health Management

Editor: Willow Adams

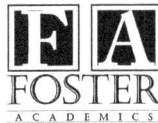

FOSTER
ACADEMICS

www.fosteracademics.com

www.fosteracademics.com

FA
FOSTER
ACADEMICS

Cataloging-in-Publication Data

Swine diseases and health management / edited by Willow Adams.
    p. cm.
Includes bibliographical references and index.
ISBN 978-1-63242-867-7
1. Swine--Diseases. 2. Swine--Health. 3. Swine--Diseases--Treatment.
4. Swine--Health--Management. 5. Veterinary medicine. I. Adams, Willow.
SF971 .S95 2019
636.408 96--dc23

Foster Academics,
118-35 Queens Blvd., Suite 400,
Forest Hills, NY 11375, USA

ISBN 978-1-63242-867-7 (Hardback)

Contents

Preface

The world is advancing at a fast pace like never before. Therefore, the need is to keep up with the latest developments. This book was an idea that came to fruition when the specialists in the area realized the need to coordinate together and document essential themes in the subject. That's when I was requested to be the editor. Editing this book has been an honour as it brings together diverse authors researching on different streams of the field. The book collates essential materials contributed by veterans in the area which can be utilized by students and researchers alike.

African swine fever, classical swine fever, pseudorabies, influenza A virus in swine, etc. are some of the common swine diseases. Classical swine fever (CSF) is a highly contagious disease of swine that causes skin lesions, fever and convulsions, and ultimately culminates in death. Artificial immunization procedures can confer immunity against this condition. Diagnostic tests, such as direct and indirect immunofluorescence, ELISA and histology of the brain can be used to detect the disease. Swine vesicular disease (SVD) is another acute and contagious viral disease that is caused by the swine vesicular disease virus. It is typically characterized by fever, ulcers in the mouth and snout, feet and teats. This disease can infect pigs by exposure to feed containing lethal meal scraps, or infected fecal matter. Since no vaccine exists for this condition, various eradication measures are adopted such as quarantining infected areas, disposal and depopulation of infected pigs and disinfecting contaminated premises. This book covers in detail some existing theories and innovative concepts revolving around swine health. Some of the diverse topics covered in this book address the varied swine diseases that fall under this category. It is a vital tool for all researching or studying swine diseases as it gives incredible insights into emerging trends and concepts.

Each chapter is a sole-standing publication that reflects each author's interpretation. Thus, the book displays a multi-facetted picture of our current understanding of application, resources and aspects of the field. I would like to thank the contributors of this book and my family for their endless support.

Editor

Factors affecting the daily feed intake and feed conversion ratio of pigs in grow-finishing units

C. R. Pierozan[1], P. S. Agostini[2*], J. Gasa[2], A. K. Novais[1], C. P. Dias[1], R. S. K. Santos[1], M. Pereira Jr[1], J. G. Nagi[1], J. B. Alves[1] and C. A. Silva[1]

Abstract

Background: The aim of this study was to use mathematical modeling to identify and quantify the main factors that affect daily feed intake (DFI) and feed conversion ratio (FCR) in grow-finishing (GF) pig units. We evaluated the production records of 93 GF farms between 2010 and 2013, linked to a company, working in a cooperative system, located in western Paraná State, Brazil. A total of 683 batches, consisting of approximately 495,000 animals, were used. Forty production factors related to the management, health, plant and equipment, nutrition, genetics and environment were considered. The number of pigs per pen, type of feeder, origin and sex (the last two variables were combined in the models) of the animals and initial and final body weights were included in the final models to predict DFI and FCR (dependent variables). Additionally, the duration of the GF phase was included for the parameter FCR. All factors included in the final models had significant effects for both dependent variables.

Results: There was a reduction in DFI (0.04 kg) ($P < 0.001$) and an improvement in FCR (6.0 points) ($P < 0.001$) in batches from pens with less than 20 animals compared with batches from pens with more than 20 animals. In barns with "other" feeder types (mostly the linear dump type) different of conical semiautomatic feeder, a reduction of DFI (0.03 kg) ($P < 0.05$) and improved FCR (3.0 points) ($P < 0.05$) were observed. Batches of barrows from units specialized for producing piglets (SPU) had higher DFI (approximately 0.02 kg) ($P < 0.01$) than batches of females and batches of mixed animals from SPU, and batches of mixed animals from farms not specialized for piglet production (farrow-to-finish farms). Batches of females from SPU and mixed batches from SPU had better FCR (5.0 and 3.0 points respectively) ($P < 0.001$ and $P < 0.001$, respectively) than batches of piglets originating from farrow-to-finish farms. The variables selected for the final models explained approximately 50 and 64 % of the total variance in DFI and FCR, respectively.

Conclusions: The models are tools for the interpretation of the factors related to the evaluated parameters, aiding in the identification of critical aspects of production. The main parameters affecting DFI and FCR in this company during the GF period were the number of pigs per pen, the type of feeder used and the combination origin-sex of the animals.

Keywords: Feed intake, Feed conversion ratio, Grow-finishing pigs, Production factors

* Correspondence: pieroagostini@hotmail.com
[2]Grup de Nutrició, Maneig i Benestar Animal, Department de Ciència Animal i dels Aliments, Universitat Autònoma de Barcelona, 08193 Bellaterra, Spain
Full list of author information is available at the end of the article

Background

Feed accounts by approximately 65–75 % of pig production cost and 75 % of that feed consumed in the grow-finishing (GF) phase [1]. Despite the economic importance of the GF phase, few studies of Brazilian farms have aimed to quantify the effect of the main production factors over the performance of GF pigs. Although the major factors affecting pig performance are known [2–4], such as genetics, nutrition and feeding, housing conditions and health, studies relating these variables with each other, especially genetics to nutrition and feeding [5, 6] and health [7] are scarce. Those that relate production parameters to the conditions of facilities and equipment involved [8] are even scarcer. Agostini et al. [9] have established a relationship among production factors and performance indexes from more than one million pigs in GF phase from eight different companies in Spain. From the results important recommendations were made, both for immediate changes in feeding, nutrition and management and for future action in genetics, construction and environmental issues. The same authors [10] also indicated that models within company are more reliable than models obtained among companies, since each company has its specific management, nutrition and facilities features across its farms.

When evaluating the effects of production factors upon a specific livestock parameter, mathematical models are a potentially effective tool. These models are primarily intended to represent a simplification of reality that from a mathematical point of view, describes a phenomenon based on factors of interest [11]. The use of modeling has allowed researchers in agricultural systems to develop concepts, methods and tools to direct the activity as a whole [12]. According to Dent et al. [13], the model construction process itself contributes to a better understanding and description of a given system.

The aim of this study was to use mathematical models to identify and quantify the impact of various intrinsic and extrinsic production factors on the daily feed intake (DFI) and the feed conversion ratio (FCR) in grow-finishing (GF) pig farms of a single company. The results may help company managers to predict the production rates and to focus their limited resources in the areas of higher profit.

Methods

Data collection

Animal Care and Use Committee approval was not necessary as this study used a database of a survey carried out in existing commercial farms.

Between 2010 and 2013, the historical production parameters of 683 batches of pigs in GF phase (totaling approximately 495,000 animals) from all the 93 farms (7.34 batches per farm) integrated to a company located in Western Paraná (Brazil) were used.

The workflow followed the study conducted by Agostini et al. [9] and was developed in two stages. In the first stage the variables of interest were chosen, representing the most important factors affecting the livestock production records of the company. Then a model that offers reliability, speed and efficiency in collecting the information was later established. Differently from the study of Agostini et al. [9], the data belong to all farms integrated in the company and with a greater number of batches per farm. All farms provided batches from different seasons.

The dependent and independent variables were selected by taking into account recent scientific work and the field experience of the company's staff. The dependent variables choose were the DFI and FCR. The total feed intake per animal was calculated as the total amount of feed in kilograms delivered to each batch during the GF period, minus the amount of feed remained in the silos when the animals were sent to slaughter, divided by the number of pigs marketed. Then the DFI was calculated as the total feed intake per animal divided by the average number of days that the animals remained in the GF unit. FCR was obtained by dividing the total feed intake of each batch by the difference between the total kilograms of pigs sent to slaughter and the total kilograms of pigs that entered at the GF batch. Mortality rate was not considered in the calculations of DFI and FCR since feed intake and body weight of dead animals were not registered.

Initially, four continuous independent variables were evaluated: number of pigs placed (NPP), initial weight (IW), final weight (FW), and duration of GF phase (DGF) as presented in Table 1. The NPP was the total number of pigs housed in the GF units. The IW corresponded to the pigs' live weight in kilograms when they

Table 1 Descriptive values of dependent and independent continuous variables selected for the final models

Variable	N° batches	Mean	SD	Minimum	1st quartile	Median	3rd quartile	Maximum
Number of pigs	683	726	430	200	499	608	919	2393
IW (kg)	683	22.7	1.2	18.9	22.2	22.8	23.4	27.6
FW (kg)	683	117	5	100	113	117	120	132
DGF (day)	683	107	4	96	104	107	110	120
DFI (kg/pig)	682	2.15	0.10	1.82	2.09	2.15	2.22	2.48
FCR (kg/kg)	682	2.45	0.12	2.15	2.36	2.45	2.54	2.86

SD standard deviation, *IW* initial weight, *FW* final weight; *DGF* duration of growing-finishing phase, *DFI* daily feed intake, *FCR* feed conversion ratio entered the GF units, and the FW to the average live weight of pigs at slaughter. The DGF was the period, in days, that animals remained in the GF unit. Because the data concerning the NPP were not normally distributed, this variable was considered as categorical.

Approximately forty categorical independent variables were also evaluated (Table 2) that represented factors of production related to facilities, herd health, and aspects of livestock management systems and nutrition. To obtain this information, questionnaires were given both as digital spreadsheets (Excel 12.0, Office 2007) and on paper.

Statistical analysis

The collected data were entered into an Excel spreadsheet before statistical analysis was carried out. The analysis was done in two phases: exploratory analysis and model development as previously carried out by Oliveira et al. [8], Agostini et al. [14] and Maes et al. [15]. In the exploratory analysis phase, a frequency study of the categorical variables was conducted using the SAS FREQ procedure (SAS Inst., Inc., Cary, NC, USA, version 9.2) (occurrence percentages in Table 2). Categorical variables with absence of variability among their categories (more than 90 % of the total batches included to a given category) were initially excluded for further statistical analysis (Table 2).

Measures of central tendency (mean and median) and dispersion (standard deviation, quartiles and amplitude) for the continuous variables were computed using the SAS MEANS procedure (Table 1). The distributions of continuous variables were evaluated using the SAS UNIVARIATE procedure. In all these analyses, the batch was considered the experimental unit, defined as a single group of piglets that came from the nursery phase and were housed in a GF unit until slaughter. All batches were managed as all-in all-out systems.

Mixed linear regression models were fit using the SAS MIXED procedure, using the variables that were coded in the first phase as predictors. The effect of farm and batch within the farm were considered as random factors, and the variance was estimated using the restricted maximum likelihood method. The comparison of the final models' goodness of fit was based on the proportion of variance explained by the different models, using the coefficient of determination (R^2) as a parameter.

In the second phase, a single regression model was used where each variable was included as a fixed effect for each single dependent variable. The independent variables with $P \leq 0.20$ were selected for use in the multivariate analysis.

Pearson and Spearman correlations were performed between independent variables to avoid multicollinearity between continuous variables and confounding problems between categorical variables. When two variables had high correlation coefficients (absolute value ≥ 0.60), only one was used in the multivariate analysis; the choice between them was made by comparing the P values in the univariate analysis, and additionally evaluating their biological relevance with respect to the dependent variable. In that case the variables "origin" and "sex" of the animals showed a relationship being used only in particular combinations and hence both were grouped as a single combined variable (ORIGSEX).

Subsequently, all independent variables selected in the univariate analysis were submitted to the procedure "stepwise", where all factors with $P < 0.05$ were kept in the final multivariate model. Fixed-effect testing was based on the F-test with denominator degrees of freedom approximated by the Satterthwaite's procedure. Significant interactions ($P < 0.05$) between the variables in the multivariate model were tested and included.

After obtaining the models for each dependent variable, the residuals were plotted against the predicted values to check the homogeneity of variances and the presence of outliers. All the factors with $P < 0.05$ in the final models for each of the two dependent variables (DFI and FCR) were considered statistically significant.

Results
Daily feed intake

The DFI per pig per batch was 2.15 ± 0.10 kg (ranging from 1.82 to 2.48 kg) (Table 1). Multivariate regression analysis indicated that DFI was influenced by the number of pigs per pen ($P < 0.001$), type of feeder ($P = 0.03$), ORIGSEX ($P = 0.01$), IW ($P < 0.001$) and FW ($P < 0.001$) (Table 3). The total variance of DFI in the model without predictors (the null model) was 0.009541, where 0.00346 (36.3 %) was observed between farms and 0.006081 (63.7 %) between batches from the same farm. After the variables were included in the multivariate model, the residual variance for the DFI was reduced to 0.004806, which indicated that approximately 50 % of the total variance of DFI was explained by the variables included in the final model (Table 4). The residual distribution of DFI is highlighted in Fig. 1. The percentages of the variance explained between farms and between batches within a farm, using the final model for DFI, were 60.8 and 43.3 %, respectively (Table 4).

In batches with less than 20 animals per pen, the DFI per pig was lower (0.04 ± 0.01 kg) than in batches with more than 20 animals. In pens where the feeder was not semiautomatic (of these, the most common type was the linear dump one), a reduction of DFI was observed (approximately 0.03 ± 0.01 kg). A higher DFI (approximately 0.02 ± 0.01 kg) was found in batches of barrows from SPU than in batches of females from SPU and batches of animals of mixed sex from both SPU and farrow-to-

Table 2 Description of independent categorical variables and their percentage of occurrence in the company

Variable	Percentage of batches in each category
Semester of placement[b,e]	Summer / autumn (48.76 %); winter / spring (51.24 %)
Number of animals placed[b,f]	< 500 (20.78 %); 500–1000 (55.04 %); > 1000 (24.18 %)
Number of barns[b,f]	One (42.14 %); two or more (57.86 %)
Stall age[b,f]	< 5 years (20.78 %); 5 to 10 years (53.26 %); > 10 years (25.96 %)
Reform of facilities[b,f]	Yes (21.07 %); no (78.93 %)
Number of pigs per pen [b,c,f]	< 20 (21.81 %); > 20 (78.19 %)
Building material/ barn[a,f]	Masonry (97.48 %); wood and mixed (2.52 %)
Type of feeder[b,c,f]	Conical semiautomatic (81.75 %); others (18.25 %)[d]
Type of drinker[a,f]	Nipple (98.66 %); water cup (1.34 %)
Water source[b,f]	Well / headwater (55.19 %); treated water (44.81 %)
Water pipes material[a,f]	Hose (1.48 %); PVC pipe (97.18 %); mixed (1.34 %)
Roof material[b,f]	Clay (87.39 %); asbestos / zinc (12.61 %)
Material used to separate the pens[b,f]	Wood or masonry (18.69 %); mixed (81.31 %)
Floor material[a,f]	Concrete (100 %)
Pens with shallow pools[a,f]	Yes (99.85 %); no (0.15 %)
Slurry tank[a,f]	Yes (100 %)
Electricity supply[a,f]	Yes (100 %)
Waste lagoons[a,f]	Yes (100 %)
Ventilation fans[a,f]	Yes (2.52 %); no (97.48 %)
Exhaust fans[a,f]	No (100 %)
Humidifiers / nebulizers[b,g]	Yes (25.71 %); no (74.29 %)
Composters[a,f]	Yes (98.37 %); no (1.63 %)
Trees around the facilities[b,f]	Yes (43.62 %); no (56.38 %)
Barn's position relative to the sun[b,f]	Diagonal / contrary (44.07 %); parallel (55.93 %)
Number of feed used[a,f]	Five (100 %)
Different feeds according to the sex[a,f]	No (100 %)
Feed form[a,f]	Pelleted (100 %)
Shock with antibiotics[a,f]	Yes (100 %)
Routes used to administer antibiotics[a,f]	Water (1.19 %); water and feed (98.81 %)
Programs used[a,f]	Ractopamine / immunocastration (100 %)
Labour force[b,f]	Unfamiliar (24.48 %); familiar (75.52 %)
Number of employed genetic[a,f]	Three (100 %)
Breeds used[a,e]	Large White / Landrace / Pietrain (100 %)
Sexed batches[a,f]	No (100 %)
Sex segregation in pens[a,f]	Yes (100 %)

Table 2 Description of independent categorical variables and their percentage of occurrence in the company *(Continued)*

Ileitis, enzootic pneumonia, meningitis[a,e]	Yes (100 %)
Glasser's disease, erysipela[a,e]	No (100 %)
Origin[b,c,e,i]	SPU (42.9 %); farrow-to-finish units (57.1 %)
Sex[b,c,h]	Barrows (11.85 %); females (12.92 %); mixed (75.23 %)

[a]Variables initially rejected to the statistical analysis due to the absence of variability among its categories
[b]Variables initially considered to the statistical analysis
[c]Variables included in the final models
[d]Others: composed mostly by linear dump type (17.2 %) and a few farms with a linear semiautomatic one (1.1 %)
[e]Considering 683 batches as experimental units (n)
[f]$n = 674$
[g]$n = 669$
[h]$n = 650$
[i]Percentage of batches composed by animals coming either from a specialized piglet production unit (SPU) or from different farrow-to-finish units

finish farms. The regression analysis indicated that for each kilogram of IW, there was an increase of approximately 0.008 ± 0.002 kg in DFI, and for each kilogram of FW, DFI increased by approximately 0.01 ± 0.0005 kg, as presented in Table 3.

Feed conversion ratio

The average FCR was 2.45 ± 0.12 (range 2.15 to 2.86) (Table 1). Multivariate regression analysis showed that FCR was influenced by the number of pigs per pen ($P < 0.001$), type of feeder ($P = 0.04$), ORIGSEX ($P < 0.001$), IW ($P < 0.001$), FW ($P < 0.001$) and DGF ($P < 0.001$) (Table 5). The model without predictors (the null model) for FCR had a total variance of 0.015261, where 0.002331 (15.3 %) was observed between farms whereas 0.01293 (84.7 %) was between batches from the same farm. The multivariate model reduced the residual variance of FCR to 0.005516, which indicated that approximately 64 % of its total variance was explained by the predictors in the final model (Table 6). The residual distribution of FCR is shown in Fig. 2. The percentages of variability explained between farms and between batches from the same farm were 33.5 and 69.3 %, respectively (Table 6).

Feed conversion ratio improved by 6.0 ± 1.2 points when animals were kept at less than 20 per pen compared to batches with more than 20 animals per pen. The type of feeder had also an effect, with non-automatic feeders (mainly linear dump type) improving FCR by 3.0 ± 1.4 points. Regarding ORIGSEX, there was an improvement in FCR of approximately 5.0 ± 1.0 points for batches of females from SPU and 3.0 ± 1.0 points for mixed-sex batches from SPU compared to mixed-sex batches from farrow-to-finish farms. Multivariate regression analysis showed that FCR improved by approximately 3.5 ± 0.2 points for each additional

Table 3 Estimates of the effects of the factors studied on daily feed intake (in kilograms per pig) in 683 batches from 93 grow-finishing pig farms

Variable	Category	Mean (kg)	Estimate (s.e.)	95 % CL		
				Low	Upper	P-value
Intercept		–	0.73 (0.07)	0.58	0.88	< 0.001
N° pigs per pen	< 20	2.11	−0.04 (0.01)	−0.06	−0.02	< 0.001
	> 20	2.16	0	–	–	–
Type of feeder	Others (linear dump)	2.12	−0.03 (0.01)	−0.05	−0.003	0.03
	Conical semiautomatic	2.15	0	–	–	–
ORIGSEX	SPU / barrows	2.15	0.02 (0.01)	0.005	0.04	0.009
	SPU / females	2.12	−0.01 (0.01)	−0.03	0.003	0.12
	SPU / mixed	2.13	0.0004 (0.0071)	−0.013	0.014	0.95
	Farrow-to-finish / mixed	2.13	0	–	–	–
IW		–	0.008 (0.002)	0.004	0.013	< 0.001
FW		–	0.01 (0.00)	0.01	0.01	< 0.001

s.e. standard error, *CL* confidence level, *ORIGSEX* variables "origin" and "sex" combined, *SPU* specialized piglet production unit, *IW* initial weight, *FW* final weight

kilogram of IW and by approximately 1.0 ± 0.0 points for each additional kilogram of FW. The DGF also influenced FCR, with each day in the GF phase being approximately 1.5 ± 0.0 points worse, as demonstrated in Table 5.

Discussion

In this study, all the factors included in the final models had an influence on the dependent variables, and the total variance of DFI and FCR accounted by the models was 50 and 64 %, respectively. The final models developed by Agostini et al. [14] explained 62 % of the total variance of total feed intake and 24.8 % of FCR whereas the one developed by Oliveira et al. [8] explained 81 % of the total variance of DFI. The difference between the percentages of variance explained in these studies may be due to the difference between the variability of the factors studied.

One aspect observed in this study concerns the variability explained between farms and between batches within a farm with the multivariate models of DFI and FCR. Approximately 43.3 and 69.3 % of the variability of

DFI and FCR, respectively, was explained between batches from the same farm. This greater proportion of the variability between batches explained in a farm for FCR is due to the inclusion of the variable DGF (a variable taken per batch, and not per farm) in the model; this variable is not included in the model for DFI.

With respect to the number of pigs per pen, there was a decrease of DFI and improve of FCR in pens that had less than 20 animals throughout the GF phase. The analysis of the social changes due to an increased number of animals in the pen has a great importance for animal welfare and for productivity [16]. According to Schmolke et al. [17], one concern about large group size is the reduced growth rate. Street and Gonyou [18] found that pigs housed in small groups (18 animals) during the GF phase reached 3 % more weight than those housed in large ones (108 animals). FCR was also better (6 %) in small groups, and this was more evident at the end of the study (14 % more efficient than those housed in large groups). These results were similar to

Table 4 Variance observed between farms and between batches within a farm for model without predictors (null model) and multivariate model (full model) and percentage of variance explained by the variables included in the final model for daily feed intake

Effect	Null model		Full model		Variance explained (%)
	Variance	%	Variance	%	
Farm	0.00346	36.3	0.00136	28.2	60.8
Batches (Farm)	0.00608	63.7	0.00345	71.8	43.3
Total	0.00954	100.0	0.00481	100.0	49.6

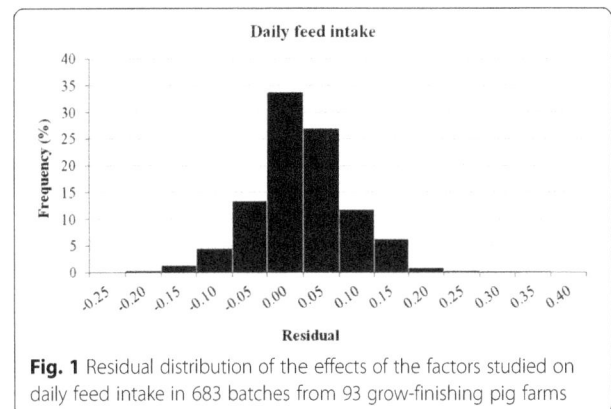

Fig. 1 Residual distribution of the effects of the factors studied on daily feed intake in 683 batches from 93 grow-finishing pig farms

Table 5 Estimates of the effects of the factors studied on feed conversion ratio in 683 batches from 93 grow-finishing pig farms

Variable	Category	Mean (kg/kg)	Estimate (s.e.)	95 % CL		
				Low	Upper	P-value
Intercept		–	1.43 (0.10)	1.23	1.62	< 0.001
N° pigs per pen	< 20	2.40	−0.05 (0.01)	−0.07	−0.03	< 0.001
	> 20	2.45	0	–	–	–
Type of feeder	Others (linear dump)	2.41	−0.03 (0.01)	−0.06	−0.00	0.04
	Conical semiautomatic	2.44	0	–	–	–
ORIGSEX	SPU/barrows	2.43	−0.02 (0.01)	−0.03	0.00	0.09
	SPU/females	2.40	−0.05 (0.01)	−0.07	−0.03	< 0.001
	SPU/mixed	2.42	−0.03 (0.01)	−0.04	−0.01	< 0.001
	Farrow-to-finish/mixed	2.44	0	–	–	–
IW		–	0.035 (0.002)	0.03	0.04	< 0.001
FW		–	−0.01 (0.00)	−0.01	−0.01	< 0.001
DGF		–	0.015 (0.001)	0.01	0.02	< 0.001

s.e. standard error, CL confidence level, ORIGSEX variables "origin" and "sex" combined, SPU specialized piglet production unit, IW initial weight, FW final weight, DGF duration of the grow-finishing phase

those found by Vermeer et al. [19], who found that pigs kept in larger groups in the GF phase grew slower. A large group size can provide greater opportunities for exploration and freedom of movement. Thus, during the grower phase, the poorer growth rate may be explained by the fact that part of dietary energy is rather directed to satisfy the demands of greater locomotor activities of animals [20], resulting in worse FCR. Some pig companies may choose to build larger pens (with more animals per pen but no change in space allowance per animal) to better use the space of the barns by reducing the area that would be used to runners and partitions. However, the increase in efficiency offered by the construction of large spaces together with the reduction of work required per pig must be counterposed to the reduction in growth rate during the phases of post-weaning and growth when animals are housed in large groups [20]. Anyway, new studies on the subject should take into account the statements made by Estevez et al. [16], in which the search for the so-called "optimum group" is somewhat guaranteed to fail. Group sizes will vary not

only according to the animal species but also according to the complexity of environmental factors involved, such as the availability and location of food.

The type of feeder significantly affected DFI and FCR. The use of "other" feeder types (most commonly, the linear dump one) resulted in reduced DFI and better FCR over the use of conical semiautomatic feeder. The cost and the need to modify the facilities make experiments with different types of feeders difficult to conduct [21]. Studies that have related the performance parameters between two type of feeders have included comparisons between those that simultaneously provide feed and water to feed animals with those that offer only dry feed [14, 22, 23], comparisons between feeders with a single space for animals versus those that offer multiple spaces [14, 22–24], and evaluations of the effects of changing the type of feeder between the growing and finishing phases [25]. Changing feeder

Table 6 Variance observed between farms and between batches within a farm for model without predictors (null model) and multivariate model (full model) and percentage of variance explained by the variables included in the final model for feed conversion ratio

Effect	Null model		Full model		Variance explained (%)
	Variance	%	Variance	%	
Farm	0.00233	15.3	0.00155	28.1	33.5
Batches (Farm)	0.01293	84.7	0.00397	71.9	69.3
Total	0.01526	100.0	0.00552	100.0	63.9

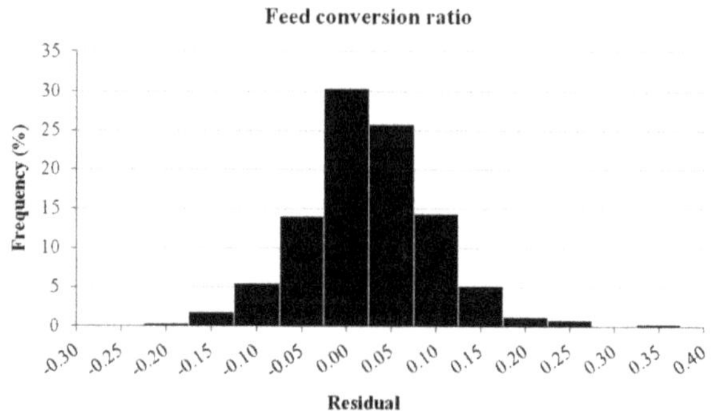

Fig. 2 Residual distribution of the effects of the factors studied on feed conversion ratio in 683 batches from 93 grow-finishing pig farms

when animals are transferred to GF housing leads to reduced feed intake and performance in the first week after the change, but no negative effect on performance over the entire finishing phase [25]. Comparisons with the results of this study are therefore limited, given the limited information on the subject and because of the wide variation in existing feeders already studied.

The type of feeder may influence feed wastage. In commercial farm conditions, as feed wastage is not subtracted from the actual consumption, the increased wastage results in higher DFI and worse FCR, since the feed is not being utilized for animal growth. Agostini et al. [14] observed a reduction in feed intake without affecting weight gain, when pigs were fed in troughs that provided a unique space associated with a drinker. This could be due to the lower feed wastage with this equipment. In the present study the lower DFI observed in pigs fed in non-conical semiautomatic feeders (mainly linear dump one) might be related to the reduced feed wastage, which leads to an enhanced FCR. In this regard, the regulation of feeders should be considered because when these equipment, such as conical semiautomatic feeders, are inappropriately regulated, feed wastage can increase significantly.

Regarding the variables ORIGSEX, barrows from SPU have a higher DFI than females and mixed-sex batches from SPU as well as mixed-sex batches from farrow-to-finish farms. As for FCR, batches of females and mixed-sex batches from SPU showed better performance than batches of barrows originating from SPU and mixed-sex batches from farrow-to-finish farms.

The company evaluated in the present study has one specialized piglet production unit (SPU), which produces about 1,600 piglets per week that are housed in GF units. SPU are very common in the Brazilian pig industry. Commonly they adopt all-in all-out management, ensuring better health for the animals sent to GF farms. However, some GF units also receive piglets from farrow-to-finish farms [26], whose investments in animal health are usually smaller. Therefore, it is not uncommon for some of these farms to also be close to other farms without proper biosecurity, which facilitates the transmission of infectious agents. The better health of piglets from SPU may explain their higher DFI and better FCR.

For sex, these results corroborate those of Morales et al. [27] who observed a higher DFI (6.1 %) for barrows than for females in the GF phase (from 62 to 174 days of age), and Bünzen et al. [28] who observed that males can consume from 10 to 19 % more feed between 60 and 105 kg than females. Sundrum et al. [29] and Brustolini and Fontes [30] showed that due to the lower feed intake, females require approximately six days extra to reach the slaughter weight of 120 kg.

Conclusions
In the evaluated conditions, the results showed that GF pigs had a higher DFI and worse FCR when: a) housed in pens with more than 20 animals, b) fed in conical semiautomatic feeder and c) batches were composed by barrows coming from specialized piglet production unit and mixed-sex coming from farrow-to-finish units.

The design of this study gives to pig company and their farms a way to predict the weight of these factors on their performance indices and it seems to be an effective tool to assist technicians and producers in taking management decisions.

Competing interests
The authors declare that they have no competing interests.

Authors' contributions
CP drafted the paper. AN, CD, RS, MJ, JN and JA participated in the design and collected the data. PA performed the statistical analysis of data and helped drafting and formatting the paper. JG and CS conceived the original idea and design and participated in the analysis of results and preparation of the manuscript. All authors read and approved the final manuscript.

Acknowledgements
Firstly, we thank the cooperative participants, who trusted us with the data from their farms so that this study could be developed. We also thank the public research project funded by the Spanish Ministry of Education (AGL 2011-29960), in which this study was developed.

Author details
[1]Departamento de Zootecnia, Universidade Estadual de Londrina, 86051-970 Londrina, Brazil. [2]Grup de Nutrició, Maneig i Benestar Animal, Department de Ciència Animal i dels Aliments, Universitat Autònoma de Barcelona, 08193 Bellaterra, Spain.

References
1. van Heugten E. Growing-finishing swine nutrient recommendations and feeding management. In: Meisinger DJ, editor. National Swine Nutrition Guide. Ames: North Carolina State University Press; 2010. p. 80–96.
2. Losinger WC. Feed-conversion ratio of finisher pigs in the USA. Prev Vet Med. 1998;36:287–305.
3. Cline TR, Richert BT. Feeding Growing finishing pigs. In: Lewis AJ, Southern LL, editors. Swine Nutrition. 2nd ed. Boca Raton: CRC Press; 2001. p. 717–24.
4. Quiles A, Hervia ML. Factores que influyen en el consumo de piensos en los cerdos. Prod Anim. 2008;248:6–19.
5. Gispert M, Font I, Furnols GM, Velarde A, Diestre A, Carrión D, et al. Relationships between carcass quality parameters and genetic types. Meat Sci. 2007;77:397–404.
6. Niemi JK, Sevón-Aimonen ML, Pietola K, Stalder KJ. The value of precision feeding technologies for grow-finish swine. Livest Prod Sci. 2010;129:13–23.
7. Martinez J, Peris B, Gómez EA, Corpa JM. The relationship between infectious and non infectious herd factors with pneumonia at slaughter and productive parameters in fattening pigs. Vet J. 2009;179:240–6.
8. Oliveira J, Yusa E, Guitián FJ. Effects of management, environmental and temporal factors on mortality and feed consumption in integrated swine fattening farms. Livest Prod Sci. 2009;123:221–9.
9. Agostini PS, Gasa J, Manzanilla EG, Silva CA, Blas C. Descriptive study of production factors affecting performance traits in growing-finishing pigs in Spain. Span J Agric Res. 2013;11:371–81.
10. Agostini PS, Manzanilla EG, Blas C, Fahey AG, Silva CA, Gasa J. Managing variability in decision making in swine growing-finishing units. Ir Vet J. 2015;68:1–13.

11. Villalba D. Construcción y utilización de un modelo estocástico para la simulación de estrategias de manejo invernal en rebaños de vacas nodrizas. Universitat de Lleida, Lleida: Tesis Doctoral; 2000.

12. Gibon A, Sibbald AR, Thomas C. Improved sustainability in livestock systems, a challenge for animal production science – Introduction. Livest Prod Sci. 1999;61:107–10.

13. Dent JB, Edwards JG, Mcgregor MJ. Simulation of ecological, social and economic factors in agricultural systems. Agric Syst. 1995;49:337–51.

14. Agostini PS, Fahey AG, Manzanilla EG, O'Doherty JV, Blas C, Gasa J. Management factors affecting mortality, feed intake and feed conversion ratio of grow-finishing pigs. Animal. 2014;8:1312–8.

15. Maes D, Duchateau L, Larriestra AJ, Deen J, Morrison RB, de Kruif A. Risk factors for mortality in grow-finishing pigs in Belgium. J Vet Med B Infect Dis Vet Public Health. 2004;51:321–6.

16. Estevez I, Andersen IL, Nævdal E. Group size, density and social dynamics in farm animals. Appl Anim Behav Sci. 2007;103:185–204.

17. Schmolke SA, Li YZ, Gonyou HW. Effect of group size on performance of growing-finishing pigs. J Anim Sci. 2003;81:874–8.

18. Street BR, Gonyou HW. Effects of housing finishing pigs in two group sizes and at two floor space allocations on production, health, behavior, and physiological variables. J Anim Sci. 2008;86:982–91.

19. Vermeer HM, de Greef KH, Houwers HWJ. Space allowance and pen size affect welfare indicators and performance of growing pigs under Comfort Class conditions. Livest Prod Sci. 2014;159:79–86.

20. Turner SP, Allcroft DJ, Edwards SA. Housing pigs in large social groups: a review of implications for performance and other economic traits. Livest Prod Sci. 2003;82:39–51.

21. Heck A. Fatores que influenciam o desenvolvimento dos leitões na recria e terminação. Acta Sci Vet. 2009;37(supl.1):211–8.

22. Gonyou HW, Lou Z. Effects of eating space and availability of water in feeders on productivity and eating behavior of grower/finisher pigs. J Anim Sci. 2000;78:865–70.

23. Patterson DC. A comparison of offering meal and pellets to finishing pigs from self-feed hoppers with and without built-in watering. Anim Feed Sci Tech. 1991;34:29–36.

24. Nielsen BL, Lawrence AB, Whittemore CT. Feeding behavior of growing pigs using single or multi-space feeders. Appl Anim Behav Sci. 1996;47:235–46.

25. Magowan E, McCan MEE, O'Connell NE. The effect of feeder type and change of feeder type on growing and finishing pig performance and behavior. Anim Feed Sci Tech. 2008;142:133–43.

26. Oliveira J, Guitián FJ, Yus E. Effect of introducing piglets from farrow-to-finish breeding farms into all-in all-out fattening batches in Spain on productive parameters and economic profit. Prev Vet Med. 2007;80:243–56.

27. Morales JI, Cámara L, Berrocoso JD, López JP, Mateos GG, Serrano MP. Influence of sex and castration on growth performance and carcass quality of crossbred pigs from 2 Large White sire lines. J Anim Sci. 2011;89:3481–9.

28. Bünzen S, Apolônio LR, Silva MA. Técnicas de manejo e alimentação para melhoria da conversão alimentar. In: Associação Brasileira dos Criadores de Suínos (ABCS), Produção de Suínos: Teoria e Prática. ABCS. Brasília. 2014; 2014:686–90.

29. Sundrum A, Aragon A, Schulze-Langenhorst C, Bütfering L, Henning M, Stalljohann G. Effects of feeding strategies, genotypes, sex, and birth weight on carcass and meat quality traits under organic pig production conditions. NJAS Wagening J Life Sci. 2011;58:163–72.

30. Brustolini APL, Fontes DO. Fatores que afetam a exigência nutricional de suínos na terminação. In: Associação Brasileira dos Criadores de Suínos (ABCS), Produção de Suínos: Teoria e Prática. Brasília: ABCS; 2014. p. 677–85.

2

Experimental inoculation of *Treponema pedis* T A4 failed to induce ear necrosis in pigs

Frida Karlsson[1], Anna Rosander[2], Claes Fellström[3] and Annette Backhans[3*] (iD)

Abstract: Ear necrosis is a syndrome affecting pigs shortly after weaning and is regarded as an animal welfare issue. The etiology is unknown but *Treponema* spp., predominantly *Treponema pedis*, are commonly detected in the lesions. Oral treponemes have been suggested as source of infection, transferred by biting and licking behavior. In this study, five pigs were intradermally inoculated with *Treponema pedis* strain T A4 with the aim of investigating if this strain would induce ear lesions. Three pigs served as controls. The inoculation was repeated after 29 days, and the study continued for 56 days. Serum samples were collected throughout the study and analyzed by ELISA for IgG antibodies towards *T. pedis* T A4 lysate. Skin biopsies were taken from the inoculation area at the end of the study. Gingival samples were collected and cultivated for treponemes, for comparison to the inoculation strain and to follow colonisation. The challenged pigs did not develop any clinical signs of infection and no spirochetes were detected in sections from skin biopsies. The number of *Treponema*-positive gingival samples increased during the study. In the challenge group, IgG towards the bacterial lysate peaked 7 days after each inoculation and decreased rapidly hereafter. In the control group a weak IgG response was observed after the second inoculation, possibly caused by the oral treponemes.

Keywords: Pig, Ear necrosis, *Treponema*, IgG, Experimental infection

Background

Ear necrosis is observed in pigs after weaning or during the early grower period, and may occur as an outbreak. The lesions involve the ventral margins or the tip of the ear and are usually bilateral [1, 2]. Severe cases are characterized by hyperemia, edema, exudation, ulceration and necrosis that may spread to involve a large part of the ear [3], and eventually the ear may be sloughed off [1]. We previously showed that *Treponema* spp., predominantly *T. pedis*, were common and abundant in both shoulder ulcers and ear necrosis [4, 5], and similar results were presented by Clegg et al. [6]. The detection of oral treponemes closely related to ulcer treponemes led us to hypothesize that treponemes are transferred to the skin by biting and licking behavior [4]. However, further studies are needed to reveal if treponemes are involved with the aetiology as the primary cause of the syndrome or if they are secondary invaders of the skin ulcers. The aim of this study was to test if inoculation with *T. pedis* T A4 could induce lesions of ear necrosis in pigs, as evaluated by clinical and histopathological examination. The immune response was analysed and gingival samples were continuously checked for treponemes to study the colonization of the gingiva and to enable comparison with the inoculation strain.

Methods

The study was performed at the department of Clinical Sciences at the Swedish University of Agricultural Sciences, Uppsala, in research animal facilities (see Declarations). The study included eight pigs (A-H) of Yorkshire/Hampshire crossbreed from two litters born by Yorkshire gilts. Two males and two females from each litter were randomly selected at four weeks, when weaned, and were allocated to the treatment group (*n* = 5, A-E) or the control group (*n* = 3, F-H). During the acclimatization period of one week a wet bandage was applied to one ear of each animal to keep the skin moist. The animals were individually housed in 3m² pens with concrete floor, infrared lamps and bedding of wooden shavings and straw. Water was given ad libitum. A commercial diet (Solo 330 P SK 25 kg, Lantmännen) and hay was fed twice daily. At day 0, the

* Correspondence: annette.backhans@slu.se
[3]Department of Clinical Sciences, Swedish University of Agricultural Sciences, SE-75007 Uppsala, Sweden
Full list of author information is available at the end of the article

pigs were 5 weeks and their weight varied between 8 and 11 kg. The bacterial strain, *T. pedis*, T A4, previously isolated from a pig with ear necrosis [7], was thawed and recultured as previously described [8] for two passages before inoculation. After 3–5 days the cultures were fully grown and in the log phase, based on visual estimation of density and phase-contrast microscopy of the spirochetes shape and motility. Broth cultures were centrifuged and the bacterial pellets were washed twice with isotonic saline, centrifuged and diluted with isotonic saline to a density of ≥5 Mc Farland Standards. The animals (A-H) were anaesthetized according to a protocol by Malavasi et al. [9]. After disinfection with ethanol, both ears were injected with 0.5 ml solution, with an estimate of 10^9 bacteria (challenge pigs, A-E) or isotonic saline (control pigs, F-H), evenly distributed at four sites, approximately ¼ in on the earlobe and 0.5 cm from the ventral margin, on both sides of the earlobes. On pigs C, E, and F a blunt trauma was made by shutting a forceps on five sites along the margin of the ear. The wet bandage was kept for one week after injection. Pig B was excluded from the study from day 7 due to fainting and vomiting. At day 29 the inoculation was repeated. Thereafter the pigs were grouped two and two in the pens (A + C, D + E, F + G), except for pig H that was individually housed. The ears and the skin of the pigs were examined daily. Serum samples were collected from *vena jugularis externa* at days 0, 7, 11, 14, 21, 29, 35, 42, 49, 56. Gingival samples were taken with cottons swabs. At day 56 biopsies were collected from each ear from all pigs under anesthesia, and the pigs were euthanized by intravenous injection with 140 mg/kg pentobarbital sodium and phenytoin sodium (Euthasol® vet. Virbac Animal Health). After fixation in formalin the biopsies were embedded in paraffin and sections of 5–7 μm were cut and stained with hematoxyline and eosin (HE) and Warthin-Starry silver staining (W-S). Gingival samples were investigated by phase contrast microscopy and inoculated and cultured as previously described [8]. Pure spirochetal isolates were analysed by PCR and subsequent sequencing of the 16S ribosomal RNA-tRNA-Ile intergenic spacer region (ISR2) and 16S ribosomal RNA genes [7, 10]. Sequences were processed in CLC Main Workbench 6.7 (CLC Bio) and the megablast algorithm BLAST was used for homology searches [11].

For the enzyme-linked immunosorbant assay (ELISA), *T. pedis* T A4 lysate was prepared by washing bacterial pellets from eight 10 ml cultures three times with isotonic saline, suspended in 8 ml of isotonic saline and subjected to ultrasonic treatment using a horn-type sonicator (Vibra-cell VC-505; Sonics & Materials Inc., Newton, NJ, USA) at a frequency of 20 kHz. The cell lysate was sterile filtered using 0.2 μm syringe filters (Sartorius, Goettingen, Germany) and quantified with Picodrop Microliter UV/Vis Spectrophotometer. Assays were performed as described by Rosander et al., 2011

[12], with the following modifications: microplates (C96 Polysorp, Nunc-immuno plate) were coated at 4 °C over night (> 16 h) with the lysate at concentrations of 5 μg/ml in 100 μl 50 mM sodium carbonate and washed three times before blocking with PBS-T (phosphate buffered saline pH 7.4 with 0.05% Tween 20) for 30–45 min at room temperature. Serum samples, diluted 1:100 in PBS-T, were added in duplicate and pig IgG was detected with anti-pig IgG (whole molecule) peroxidase conjugate antibodies developed in rabbit (Sigma), diluted 1:20,000, after which wells were washed four times with PBS-T. Optical density was measured at 450 nm after the addition of 1 mM tetramethylbenzidine and 0.006% H_2O_2 in 0.1 M potassium citrate pH 4.25, incubating the plates for 10 min at room temperature, and stopping the reaction by addition of 50 μl 10% sulfuric acid per well. The significance of difference between groups was assessed by two-sample t-test using Minitab 17 Statistical software (Minitab Inc., Harrisburg, PA, USA).

Results

No clinical signs of infection could be detected. After inoculation, a mild erythema was observed in the area of inoculation in both challenge and control pigs (Fig. 1). It decreased gradually and had disappeared within ten days. On the ears that had been exposed to a blunt trauma a brown scab could be noted up to 14 days. No differences were noted between challenged and control pigs. HE stained sections from challenged and control pigs at day 56 showed focal, mild perivascular inflammatory changes in the dermis with eosinophils and lymphocytes. No spirochetes were detected in any of the W-S sections. The results from the microscopic observations of gingival samples are shown in Table 1.

Four isolates were obtained, from challenge pigs C and E, and from control pigs F and H.

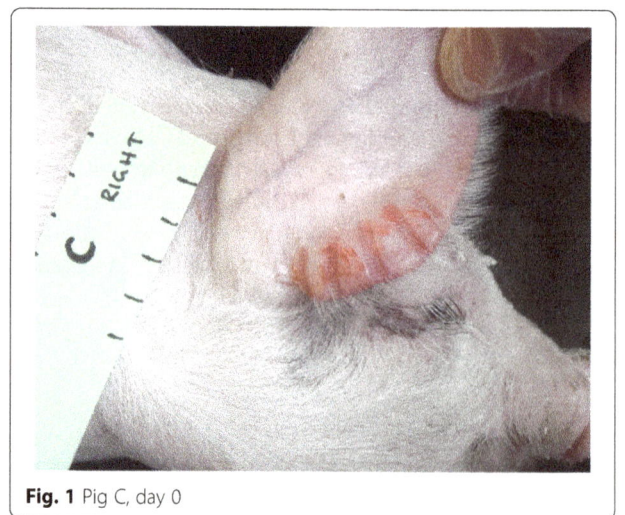

Fig. 1 Pig C, day 0

Table 1 Detection of *Treponema*-like spirochetes from gingival samples of challenge pigs (A-E) and control pigs (F-H) by phase contrast microscopy of FAB + A[a] broth cultures

Day	0	7	14	21	29	35	42	49	56
Age	5 w[b]	6 w	7 w	8 w	9 w	10 w	11 w	12 w	13 w
Pig A	−	−	−	−	+	−	−	+	−
Pig B	−	nt[c]	nt	nt	nt	nt	nt	nt	−
Pig C	−	−	+	−	+	+	+	+	+
Pig D	+	−	−	−	+	−	+	+	+
Pig E	−	−	−	−	−	+	+	+	−
Pig F	−	−	+	−	+	+	+	+	+
Pig G	−	+	−	−	+	−	+	+	−
Pig H	−	−	−	−	+	−	−	−	+

[a]FAB + A = Fastidious anaerobe broth with addition of glucose, thiamine pyrophosphate, volatile fatty acids, fetal calf serum, enrofloxacin and rifampicin [8]
[b]w = weeks[c] nt = not tested

The 316 nucleotides long ISR2 sequences of these four isolates were identical, and the homology search showed that they matched most closely (98% homology) to two strains of *T. pedis* previously isolated from pig ear necrosis; isoE1186 (accession no KC619314) and the challenge strain T A4 (CP004120), and one from pig gingiva; T M1 (KC619311). The 16S rRNA sequences of the same isolates matched most closely (99% homology) to strains T A4 (CP004120) and T M1 (FJ805835), same as above, and strain G179 (AF363634), isolated from a case of ovine foot rot. On day 7 the challenge pigs had developed an IgG response towards the *T. pedis* T A4 lysate, that thereafter decreased steadily until re-inoculation on day 29, when a similar rapid increase in antibody response was followed by a decrease (Fig. 2). In the control group, a weak response developed from day 35, and mean absorbance values were significantly higher at the end of the study on day 56 (M = 0.29, SD = 0.00958) than on day 0 (M = 0.17, SD = 0.019) (two-sample t-test, $p = 0.011$).

Discussion

To our knowledge, this is the first attempt to induce ear necrosis in pigs using a pure *Treponema* spp. culture. We used *T. pedis* as our previous studies indicated this species as the main phylotype in both ear necrosis and shoulder ulcers [4, 5]. Also, *T. pedis* is part of the treponemal consortium associated with bovine digital dermatitis (BDD) [13, 14]. The strain T A4 was selected as it originates from an outbreak of severe ear necrosis [7] and as several putative virulence related genes have been identified in its genome [15]. However, in this study T A4 did not cause any skin lesions. The reason for this negative outcome could be

that *T.pedis* is not the aetiological agent of ear necrosis. However there might be other reasons. For example, the amount of bacteria could have been insufficient, similarly to a murine model for BDD where lesion development was demonstrated to be dose dependent [16]. We applied a wet bandage to one ear of each animal to mimic the only successful reproduction of BDD-like lesions in dairy cattle using one pure treponemal strain [17]. However, to keep the bandages on the ears proved very difficult and they had to be removed after one week. For future studies we suggest a development of this approach and a longer application period. In our previous studies *T. pedis* was the main phylotype in porcine skin ulcers, but a great diversity of treponemal phylotypes was revealed [4, 5]. In older studies, ulcers were successfully reproduced in healthy animals using scraping material from ulcers containing motile spirochaetes [18, 19]. Maybe a consortium of different treponemal species is required to cause ulcers also in the pig. One approach for future challenge studies is to include a mixture of different treponemal species, possibly in combination with other putative pathogens like staphylococci or streptococci [1, 20]. The etiology of ear necrosis is suggested to involve other factors like ear biting and stress mediated by weaning, mixing of pigs and high stocking rates [20]. Thus, our experimental design with individually housed animals, chosen to avoid contamination of the inoculated area by oral treponemes through biting or licking behavior, may have prevented ear necrosis instead of inducing the disease.

There was a significant IgG response already 7 days post infection in the challenge group, but this response was short and declined rapidly. A re-inoculation boosted the response but as the study ended 26 days after the second inoculation we don't know if the levels would drop even further. In cattle the immune response to *T. phagedenis*-like spirochetes has been of short duration [21]. Our control group did show a weak IgG response at day 35, one week after re-inoculation of the challenge group. Interestingly, at that time most pigs in the study were colonized by gingival treponemes, why one could speculate that transmission of those could have occurred by biting or licking. However, also the single-housed pig showed this weak response. Presumably, colonization of gingiva is initiated already during the suckling period and, also, it cannot be ruled out that some low-dose transmission occurred between the pens and/or pigs during daily care. Our findings that treponemes 1) gradually colonized the pigs gingiva around the same age period as when ear necrosis usually occur, and 2) were identified as *T. pedis* closely related to strains isolated from

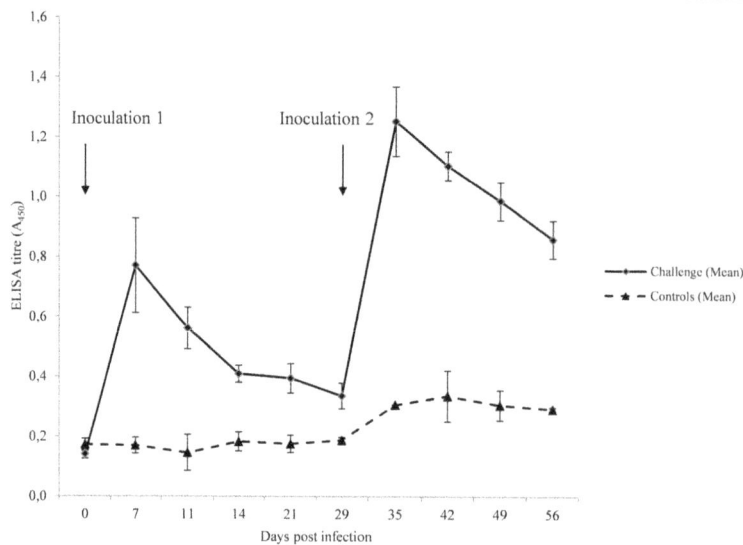

Fig. 2 Mean ELISA titres of serum IgG to *T. pedis* T A4 lysate for the pigs in challenge and control group throughout the study. Standard deviations are shown as whiskers. Inoculation time points as arrows

pig ulcers, are in line with our previous suggestion that the mouth is the reservoir for the ulcer treponemes [4].

Conclusions

In the presented model *T. pedis* T A4 failed to cause skin lesions similar to those of ear necrosis. IgG antibodies against T A4 lysate developed quickly after inoculation and then rapidly declined.

Acknowledgements
We want to thank Märit Pringle and Olov Svartström for laboratory work and valuable input on the study design.

Funding
The study was financed by the Swedish Research Council Formas (dnr 2009–1486). The funding body was not involved in the design and collection, analysis, interpretation of data or writing the manuscript.

Authors' contributions
FK: study design, draft of manuscript, main responsible for carrying out experimental study, collection of material and laboratory work. AR: main responsible for serological analysis. CF: study design, involved in experimental study. AB: study design, statistical analysis of data, final editing. All authors reviewed, edited and approved the final manuscript.

Competing interests
The authors declare that they have no competing interests.

Author details
[1]Farm and Animal Health, Klustervägen 11, SE-590 76 Vreta Kloster, Sweden. [2]Department of Biomedical Sciences and Veterinary Public Health, Swedish University of Agricultural Sciences, SE-75007 Uppsala, Sweden. [3]Department of Clinical Sciences, Swedish University of Agricultural Sciences, SE-75007 Uppsala, Sweden.

References
1. Richardson JA, Morter RL, Rebar AH, Olander HJ. Lesions of porcine necrotic ear syndrome. Vet Pathol. 1984;21(2):152–7.
2. Harcourt RA. Porcine ulcerative spirochaetosis. Vet Rec. 1973;92(24):647–8.
3. Blandford TB, Bygrave AC, Harding JD, Little TW. Suspected procine ulcerative spirochaetosis in England. Vet Rec. 1972;90(1):15.
4. Karlsson F, Svartström O, Belák K, Fellström C, Pringle M. Occurrence of *Treponema* spp. in porcine skin ulcers and gingiva. Vet Microbiol. 2013; 165(3–4):402–9.
5. Karlsson F, Klitgaard K, Jensen TK. Identification of Treponema pedis as the predominant Treponema species in porcine skin ulcers by fluorescence in situ hybridization and high-throughput sequencing. Vet Microbiol. 2014; 171(1–2):122–31.
6. Clegg SR, Sullivan LE, Bell J, Blowey RW, Carter SD, Evans NJ. Detection and isolation of digital dermatitis treponemes from skin and tail lesions in pigs. Res Vet Sci. 2016;104:64–70.
7. Pringle M, Backhans A, Otman F, Sjölund M, Fellström C. Isolation of spirochetes of genus *Treponema* from pigs with ear necrosis. Vet Microbiol. 2009;139(3–4):279–83.
8. Svartström O, Karlsson F, Fellström C, Pringle M. Characterization of *Treponema* spp. isolates from pigs with ear necrosis and shoulder ulcers. Vet Microbiol. 2013;166(3–4):617–23.
9. Malavasi LM, Jensen-Waern M, Augustsson H, Nyman G. Changes in minimal alveolar concentration of isoflurane following treatment with medetomidine and tiletamine/zolazepam, epidural morphine or systemic buprenorphine in pigs. Lab Anim. 2008;42(1):62–70.
10. Stamm LV, Bergen HL, Walker RL. Molecular typing of papillomatous digital dermatitis-associated *Treponema* isolates based on analysis of 16S-23S ribosomal DNA intergenic spacer regions. J Clin Microbiol. 2002;40:3463–9.
11. Altschul SF, Gish W, Miller W, Myers EW, Lipman DJ. Basic local alignment search tool. J Mol Biol. 1990;215(3):403–10.

12. Rosander A, Guss B, Frykberg L, Björkman C, Näslund K, Pringle M. Identification of immunogenic proteins in *Treponema phagedenis*-like strain V1 from digital dermatitis lesions by phage display. Vet Microbiol. 2011;153(3–4):315–22.

13. Klitgaard K, Bretó AF, Boye M, Jensen TK. Targeting the treponemal microbiome of digital dermatitis infections by high-resolution phylogenetic analyses and comparison with fluorescent in situ hybridization. J Clin Microbiol. 2013;51(7):2212–9.

14. Evans NJ, Brown JM, Demirkan I, Murray RD, Vink WD, Blowey RW, Hart CA, Carter SD. Three unique groups of spirochetes isolated from digital dermatitis lesions in UK cattle. Vet Microbiol. 2008;130:141.

15. Svartström O, Mushtaq M, Pringle M, Segerman B. Genome-wide relatedness of *Treponema pedis*, from gingiva and necrotic skin lesions of pigs, with the human oral pathogen *Treponema denticola*. PLoS One. 2013;8(8):e71281.

16. Elliott MK, Alt DP, Zuerner RL. Lesion formation and antibody response induced by papillomatous digital dermatitis-associated spirochetes in a murine abscess model. Infect Immun. 2007;75(9):4400–8.

17. Gomez A, Cook NB, Bernardoni ND, Rieman J, Dusick AF, Hartshorn R, Socha MT, Read DH, Döpfer D. An experimental infection model to induce digital dermatitis infection in cattle. J Dairy Sci. 2012;95(4):1821–30.

18. Osborne HG, Ensor CR. Some aspects of the pathology, aetiology, and therapeutics of foot-rot in pigs. N Z Vet J. 1955;3(3):91–9.

19. Dodd S. A disease of the pig, due to a spirochaeta. J Comp Pathol Terapeut. 1906;19:216–22.

20. Park J, Friendship RM, Poijak Z, DeLay J, Slavic D, Dewey CE. An investigation of ear necrosis in pigs. Can Vet J. 2013;54(5):491–5.

21. Trott DJ, Moeller MR, Zuerner RL, Goff JP, Waters WR, Alt DP, Walker RL, Wannemuehler MJ. Characterization of Treponema phagedenis-like spirochetes isolated from papillomatous digital dermatitis lesions in dairy cattle. J Clin Microbiol. 2003;41(6):2522–9.

3

The use of oral fluids to monitor key pathogens in porcine respiratory disease complex

Juan Hernandez-Garcia[1*] , Nardy Robben[2], Damien Magnée[2], Thomas Eley[3], Ian Dennis[4], Sara M. Kayes[5], Jill R. Thomson[5] and Alexander W. Tucker[1]

Abstract

Background: The usefulness of oral fluid (OF) sampling for surveillance of infections in pig populations is already accepted but its value as a tool to support investigations of porcine respiratory disease complex (PRDC) has been less well studied. This study set out to describe detection patterns of porcine reproductive and respiratory syndrome virus (PRRSV), porcine circovirus type 2 (PCV2), swine influenza virus type A (SIV) and *Mycoplasma hyopneumoniae* (*M. hyo*) among farms showing differing severity of PRDC.

The study included six wean-to-finish pig batches from farms with historical occurrence of respiratory disease. OF samples were collected from six pens every two weeks from the 5th to the 21st week of age and tested by real time PCR for presence of PRRSV, SIV and *M. hyo* and by quantitative real time PCR for PCV2. Data was evaluated alongside clinical and post-mortem observations, mortality rate, slaughter pathology, histopathology, and immunohistochemistry testing data for PCV2 antigen where available.

Results: PRRSV and *M. hyo* were detectable in OF but with inconsistency between pens at the same sampling time and within pens over sequential sampling times. Detection of SIV in clinical and subclinical cases showed good consistency between pens at the same sampling time point with detection possible for periods of 2–4 weeks. Quantitative testing of OF for PCV2 indicated different patterns and levels of detection between farms unaffected or affected by porcine circovirus diseases (PCVD). There was good correlation of PCR results for multiple samples collected from the same pen but no associations were found between prevalence of positive test results and pen location in the building or sex of pigs.

Conclusions: Detection patterns for PRRSV, SIV and *M. hyo* supported the effectiveness of OF testing as an additional tool for diagnostic investigation of PRDC but emphasised the importance of sampling from multiple pens and on multiple occasions. Preliminary evidence supported the measurement of PCV2 load in pooled OF as a tool for prediction of clinical or subclinical PCVD at farm level.

Keywords: Oral fluids, PCV2, *Mycoplasma hyopneumoniae*, SIV, PRRSV

Background

Respiratory disease results in major losses in the pig industry through reduced performance, increased mortality and antimicrobial use [1, 2] with negative impacts on animal welfare and public health. Multiple pathogens contribute to a polymicrobial infection known as Porcine Respiratory Disease Complex (PRDC) [3]. These pathogens can be classified as primary agents, which overcome and weaken the host defence mechanisms, or opportunistic secondary pathogens that take advantage of impaired defences resulting in aggravated disease often requiring longer periods of antimicrobial treatment. Key primary agents of PRDC include porcine reproductive and respiratory syndrome virus (PRRSV), *Mycoplasma hyopneumoniae* (*M. hyo*), swine influenza virus (SIV) and porcine circovirus type 2 (PCV2) [4].

* Correspondence: jh937@cam.ac.uk
[1]Department of Veterinary Medicine, University of Cambridge, Madingley Road, CB30ES Cambridge, England, UK
Full list of author information is available at the end of the article

Combined infection with PRDC-associated pathogens can produce synergistic effects via mechanisms that include producing immune depression, alteration of macrophage function and cytokine response, and hampering of the mucociliary clearance in the respiratory tract which enables bacterial colonization [3]. Such interactions have been described in the literature between PCV2 and other agents [4, 5], also for PRRSV [6–9], SIV [10], *M. hyo* [11, 12], and further respiratory pathogens [3].

Diagnostic investigation of PRDC at population and individual level is complicated by this polymicrobial nature of the problem but also by the dynamic progression over time, with different pathogens being dominant or detectable at different stages of the disease process [3]. Laboratory techniques have become a core element of the diagnostic process for PRDC, supplementing clinical examination, and pathological findings; A wide range of different diagnostic samples and techniques may be employed in a single case investigation, including for example antibody detection in serum, antigen detection or culture from respiratory tract fluids and tissue samples [13]. Recently, oral fluid (OF) has been used as an additional sample platform for antibody and nucleic acid detection of key PRDC pathogens [14].

The commercial use of OF-based diagnostics has grown considerably in recent years because of practical, economic and welfare advantages of collecting OF rather than serum. It is important to note that OF may also contain material from the respiratory system, environmental and faecal contamination, material from the nasal cavity, antibodies and crevicular fluid, further widening the scope for detection of infectious agents through this sample platform but also resulting in some laboratory challenges. Problems related to polymerase chain reaction (PCR) inhibitors in OF and sample degradation have been major limitations for this technique [15, 16]. However, knowledge surrounding laboratory diagnostic techniques based on OF has increased markedly since 2010 [17] including refined collection methods [18, 19] and processing [20] or preservation methods [15, 21] to optimise sample quality. In addition, optimised PCR conditions have been developed for specific respiratory pathogens including PRRSV [22, 23], SIV [24, 25] and PCV2 [26, 27]. Most focus has been on viral rather than bacterial pathogen detection in OF but the knowledge base is increasing for *Actinobacillus pleuropneumoniae, Haemophilus parasuis* [28] and *M. hyo* [29–31]. In addition, the OF platform relies on a pooled sample at pen-level from animals that may or may not interact individually with the sampling rope and may themselves be shedding pathogen, or have antibody titres, at differing levels thereby raising potential constraints related to sensitivity

of the test. The availability of data on the wide scale use of OF testing to investigate PRDC, and the implications for these concerns, remains scarce and there are only a few studies investigating multiple PRDC pathogens on the same samples [14, 32, 33].

This study set out to describe the detection of key respiratory pathogens in OF samples collected over time from commercial pig populations undergoing respiratory disease. This was achieved by a longitudinal study of PRRSV, PCV2, SIV and *M. hyo* detection in OF alongside clinical and pathological information. Although the usefulness of OF sampling for surveillance of pig populations has already been described [14], the present study set out to describe differences in detection patterns between farms more or less severely affected by PRDC, thereby providing initial insights into the usefulness of OF sampling in diagnostic investigations, in addition to its proven value as a surveillance tool.

Methods

Study design

A longitudinal survey was carried out over an eight-month period (January to August 2015) using six batches of pigs. Study batches were selected from three different breeding sources of commercial crossbred pigs from a single production pyramid. These sources were classified as low (A), medium (B) and high risk for suffering respiratory problems (C) based on the severity and incidence of historical respiratory problems, clinical observations, post mortem examinations, laboratory results and slaughter pathology evaluations during the wean-to-finish phase.

Two batches per source were selected for study making a total of six batches. Each batch was assigned at weaning (24–30 days of age) to a wean-to-finish farm: Pigs from source A (low severity of respiratory problems) were allocated in farm A1 and A2, pigs from source B (medium severity of respiratory problems) went to farm B1 and B2, and finally, pigs from source C (high severity or respiratory problems) were sent to farms C1 and C2 (Table 1). At arrival, pigs were segregated by gender and randomly allocated in pens (30 to 120 pigs/pen). Farms were composed by several barns, but just one barn per farm was considered for testing purposes. Each barn had pens arranged in a row with solid floors comprising a straw bedded area and a dunging area allowing for removal of faeces using a tractor-based scrape-through passage system. Consequently, each barn was divided into three sections: clean (pen 1 and 2 in the furthest point form the passage exit), central (pen 3 and 4 at the mid-way point along the passage) and dirty (pen 5 and 6 near the passage exit). One male pig pen and one female pig pen were selected in each section making a total of six pens per

Table 1 Pig batches included in the study with reported respiratory problems in previous batches

Source (expected severity of respiratory problems)	A (low)	B (medium)	C (high)
Expected problems based on historical records.	Source negative for PRRSV and *M. hyo*. Occasional problems with SIV.	Source positive for PRRSV but negative for *M. hyo*. Previous batches presented SIV and *Streptococcus suis* disease.	Source positive for PRRSV and *M. hyo*. Previous batches presented respiratory and *Streptococcus suis* disease.

batch that were repeatedly sampled in OF at 2-week intervals across nine time points (in weeks 5, 7, 9, 11, 13, 15, 17, 19 and 21 of age) starting in the week after arrival and finishing in the 21st week of age a few weeks prior to slaughter. Every batch was vaccinated one to seven days after weaning against PCV2 and *M. hyo*. Pigs in C1 and B2 were also vaccinated against PRRSV at the 5th week of age.

Samples and data collection
Batch clinical observations and casualties
Clinical observation data was collected during each sampling visit with categorisation of clinical signs and external lesions (respiratory, enteric, neurological, tail bitten, wasting, musculoskeletal, found dead/unknown) considering severity and incidence. Where possible, veterinary post-mortem examination was done to support the categorisation and to permit sample collection for extended investigations. Where justified by clinical or post mortem findings, PCVD diagnosis was done based on published criteria [34] on lung and inguinal lymph node tissue fixed in 10% formalin and processed for histopathological evaluation and immunohistochemistry by Cap protein specific PCV2 monoclonal antibody (INGENASA, Madrid, Spain) [35]. Wean to finish mortality data was collected for each batch.

Batch slaughter pathology data
A minimum of 10% of the pigs of each batch were examined at slaughter (without consideration of whether pigs originated from pens previously surveyed, or not, by OF); lungs were evaluated following the British Pig Executive Pig Health Scheme (BPHS) scoring system for average severity of enzootic pneumonia (EP)-like lesions and prevalence of pleurisy lesions based in the Goodwin score system [36, 37].

OF and serum samples
OF samples were collected with unbleached cotton ropes using a ratio of one rope for each 25 pigs with a 30 min exposure. Ropes were 1.5 cm thick, and 20 cm long for young pigs and 40 cm long for pigs older than 17 weekold. Ropes were hung in central parts of the pen when possible so pigs had 360° access, distributed in different points to maximize interactions. The height of the bottom part of the rope was adjusted to fit match with the average height of the pigs' shoulder joint.

Ropes were collected into individual containers and shipped under chilled conditions for next day delivery to the diagnostic laboratory. Blood samples were collected from 12 pigs in each of the six batches at 15 weeks of age as part of the farms' routine health monitoring program; these pigs were randomly selected among the six OF tested pens.

Laboratory analysis of OF and serum
Serum samples and OF samples collected from each rope were individually analysed and no pools were done. OF samples were stored at 4 °C after arrival and nucleic acids were extracted on the day of receipt. Residual OF was stored at −80 °C. Total nucleic acids were extracted using the MagMAX™ Express-96 Particle Processor (MME-96; Thermo Fisher Scientific) and the MagMAX™ -96 Viral RNA Isolation Kit (cat. no. AM1836; Thermo Fisher Scientific) following the manufacturer's OF Sample Extraction Protocol in the MagMAX™ Pathogen RNA/DNA Kit manual. Extracted nucleic acids were stored at −80 °C prior to testing by PCR.

Nucleic acid samples were tested for four porcine pathogens. PCV2, SIV and PRRSV were tested using commercial real time PCR kits (LSI VetMAX™ Porcine Circovirus Type 2 – Quantification kit, VetMAX™ Gold SIV Detection Kit, and LSI VetMAX™ PRRSV EU/NA, Thermo Fisher Scientific). The presence of *M. hyo* was determined using VetMAX™ *M. hyopneumoniae* reagents paired with VetMAX™ -plus quantitative PCR (qPCR) Master Mix (Thermo Fisher Scientific). The SIV, PRRSV and *M. hyo* assays were presence/absence tests only while the PCV2 PCR was supplied with a quantified control that allowed the quantification of viral genome copies in positive samples (genome copies/mL OF). SIV positive samples were subtyped using H1H3 Duplex and N1N2 Duplex primer/probe mixes (still in development in 2015; Thermo Fisher Scientific) in conjunction with Path-ID™ Multiplex One-Step RT-PCR Kit (Thermo Fisher Scientific). All PCRs were prepared as per the kit inserts and were run on a 7500 Real Time PCR System (Applied Biosystems). Data was analysed using the 7500 Software.

Extracted serum was tested for antibodies against PRRSV strains of genotype 1 and 2 (IDEXX PRRS X3 5/ STRIP, IDEXX), real-time PCR for PRRSV (LSI VetMAX™ PRRSV EU/NA, Thermo Fisher Scientific) and by qPCR for PCV2 LSI VetMAX™ Porcine Circovirus Type 2 – Quantification kit, Thermo Fisher Scientific).

Values of cycle threshold (Ct) below 37 were considered as positives in the case of PRRSV, Ct results between 37 and 40 were re-analysed according to the manufacturer recommendations, and considered as positive if Ct values in the second analysis were lower than 40. For SIV and *M. hyo*, Ct values below 37 were considered positive and values between 37 and 40 were reported as weak positives, according to the manufacturer recommendations, though only positives with Ct < 37 are considered in most of the downstream analysis as detailed above. In the case of PCV2, values for log10 genome copies/mL were calculated from the raw Ct values using the internal standard curve, which enables accurate quantification in a range between 1×10^4 and 1×10^8 genome copies/mL. Limits of detection for samples extracted with MagMAX™ Pathogen RNA/DNA and analysed with LSI VetMAX™ PCV2 were set in $1 \times 10^{3.48}$ genome copies/mL for OF, and $1 \times 10^{3.6}$ genome copies/mL for blood or serum. Results under the limit of detection were considered inconclusive, and viral load results out of the quantification range were expected to be inaccurate.

Data analysis

Ct values and viral load results of each rope collected were individually analysed and interpreted considering clinical signs, post-mortem lesions, histopathological findings and slaughterhouse evaluations. Agreement among results from different ropes in a pen, and different pens in a barn were assessed to estimate the robustness of this sampling method in this scenario. Pens and barns were considered positive for a pathogen where at least one of the OF samples resulted positive for PRRS, with a Ct value <37 for SIV and *M. hyo*, or presented a PCV2 viral load over the limit of detection ($1 \times 10^{3.48}$ genome copies/mL).

Correlations between Ct values for multiple OF samples collected from the same pen were evaluated using Pearson's correlation coefficient. In the case more than two ropes in a pen presented a Ct value <40, highest and lowest Ct values were selected for the analysis. Statistics were performed by using R version 3.3.1 [38].

Results

Clinical signs, causes of death and post-mortem investigations

Observations for clinical signs among the batches were grouped into three stages of production: nursery (aged 5–8 weeks), grower (age 9–15 weeks) and finisher (age 16 weeks to slaughter at around 23 weeks) (Table 2). Three out the six batches presented signs of respiratory disease commencing after weaning in A1, B2 and C1, and these continued for all or most of the growing and finishing period. In the case of B1 and C2, respiratory problems started later at the grower stage. Signs of enteric disease were observed soon after weaning in 3 of the batches namely B1, B2 and C1 but only in B2 did these signs continue into the grower phase. Neurological signs associated with suspected meningitis were observed in four of the batches with A1 and C1 experiencing problems during the nursery period but B1 and B2 experiencing problems commencing in the grower stage. Wasting was noted only in B2, throughout the grower and finisher stages, while more general uneven growth was found in B2 but also in the finisher stage of C1. No clinical signs were observed in A2.

Casualty pigs, comprised of pigs that died or were euthanized, were categorised into broad suspected causal groups (Table 3). Data were dependent on stockperson categorisation and as such should be interpreted with caution, in particular the category of 'found dead', but a total

Table 2 Clinical observations recorded during 2-weekly sampling visits and slaughter lung evaluation

	Weeks 5 to 8	Weeks 9 to 15	Week 16 to finish	Pigs evaluated at slaughter/ Number of pigs in the batch at weaning	Average EP-like lesion score at slaughter	Prevalence (%) of pleurisy lesions at slaughter
A1	Respiratory (+) Neurological (+)	Respiratory (++)	Respiratory (++)	250/786	1.2	12
A2	No signs observed	No signs observed	No signs observed	248/1005	1.4	1
B1	Enteric (+)	Respiratory (+) Neurological (++)	Respiratory (+) Tail biting. (+)	202/1204	1.4	6
B2	Enteric (+++) Respiratory (++)	Neurological (+), Enteric (+) Respiratory (+++), Wasting (++) Uneven growth (+++)	Respiratory (++) Wasting (+) Uneven growth (+++)	126/1063	7.8	1
C1	Respiratory (+) Neurological (+) Enteric (+)	Respiratory (++) Musculoskeletal (+)	Uneven growth (++) Musculoskeletal (+) Respiratory (+)	163/709	4.7	1
C2	No signs observed	Respiratory (+)	Respiratory (+++)	157/1105	1.9	2

"+" indicates an estimation of a low proportion (<15%) of affected pigs, "++" a moderate proportion (15–35%), and "+++" a high proportion (>35%) of affected pigs. EP-Like lesions based on the BPHS system based on the Goodwin scale [36]

Table 3 Categorisation of the suspected cause of death for dead and euthanized pigs

Cause recorded	Number of pigs per batch (and percentage of the total in the batch)					
	A1 $N = 786$	A2 $N = 1005$	B1 $N = 1204$	B2 $N = 1063$	C1 $N = 709$	C2 $N = 1105$
Respiratory	22 (2.7%)	0	16 (1.3%)	27 (2.5%)	6 (0.8%)	7 (0.6%)
Enteric	0	0	0	1 (0.1%)	0	0
Neurological	0	1 (0.1%)	7 (0.6%)	21 (2%)	3 (0.4%)	1 (0.1%)
Tail bitten	0	5 (0.5%)	0	0	0	0
Wasting	0	1 (0.1%)	0	16 (1.5%)	0	4 (0.3%)
Musculoskeletal	0	1 (0.1%)	2 (0.2%)	5 (0.5%)	1 (0.1%)	7 (0.6%)
Found dead/unknown	4 (0.5%)	10 (1%)	13 (1.1%)	13 (1.2%)	15 (2.1%)	9 (0.8%)
Total of casualties	26 (3.3%)	18 (1.8%)	38 (3.2%)	83 (7.8%)	25 (3.5%)	28 (2.5%)

Cause of the death was obtained from pig caretakers' records in addition to veterinary post-mortem examinations when possible. N: initial number of pigs at weaning. In brackets, percentages are based on the total number of pigs in the herd at weaning

of 48 of 220 casualties underwent post mortem examination by a veterinarian and these categorisations were confirmed. Respiratory causes were the most frequent, or jointly most frequent, recorded reason for casualty in all batches except A2, and wean to finish mortality, defined as casualty pigs that died or were euthanized, ranged from 1.8% (A2) to 7.7% (B2) (Table 3, Fig. 1).

Lung lesions were evaluated at slaughter in 126 to 250 pigs per batch (Table 2). Batch level average EP-like lesion scores ranged from 1.2 (A1) to 7.8 (B2) (Table 2); frequency distribution of EP-like lesion scores is shown in Fig. 2. The prevalence of pleurisy lesions detectable at slaughter ranged from 1% (C1, A2, B2) to 12% (A1) (Table 2, Fig. 2).

OF sample collection
Samples were successfully collected on a total of 310/320 scheduled pen sample time points. The principal reasons for failure to collect a sample were low levels of pig interaction or damage to the sampling material

caused by destructive interaction. Lack of interaction with the ropes was a major problem for recently weaned piglets and young pigs in cold weather.

Laboratory analysis of OF and serum samples
PRRSV
PRRSV nucleic acid was detected only in C1 (7/9 time points) and B2 (3/9 time points) (Fig. 3) with positive results obtained from weaning age onwards in both batches. Maximum pen-level prevalence was 6/6 for C1 but only 2/6 for B2. There was an apparent decline in pen level prevalence at later time-points. Detection patterns were irregular over time in that a pen testing positive on multiple occasions might also report interspersed negative results. All Ct values were higher than 31 indicating low levels of detectable viral RNA in the samples. Serum samples collected at 15 weeks of age were negative for PRRSV PCR for every batch, and positive for PRRSV antibodies in 12/12 pigs tested in each of C1 and B2 but all other batches gave negative results (Table 4).

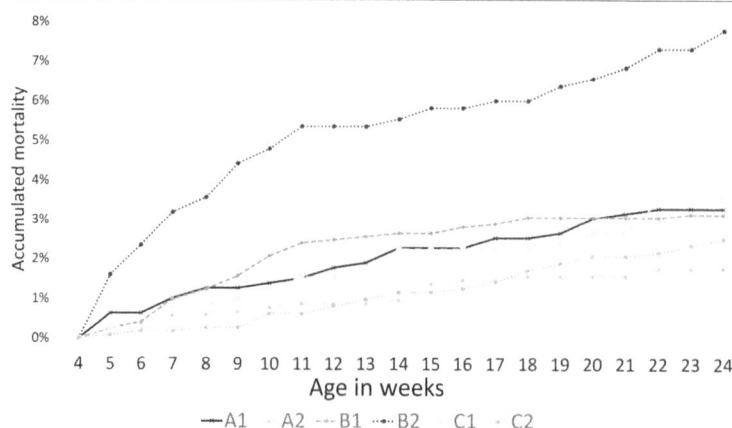

Fig. 1 Cumulative mortality per batch. Cumulative mortality, according to pig age, comprising pigs that died or were euthanized among the study batches from weaning until slaughter

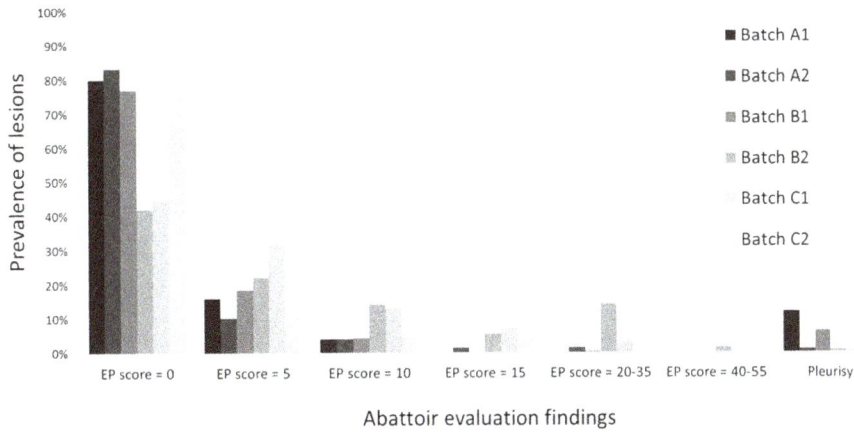

Fig. 2 Respiratory system lesions in abattoir evaluations. Frequency distribution of Enzootic Pneumonia (EP)-like lesion scores based on the Goodwin scale [36], and prevalence of pleurisy lesions were assessed for a subset (*n* = 126 – 250 pigs) of each study batch

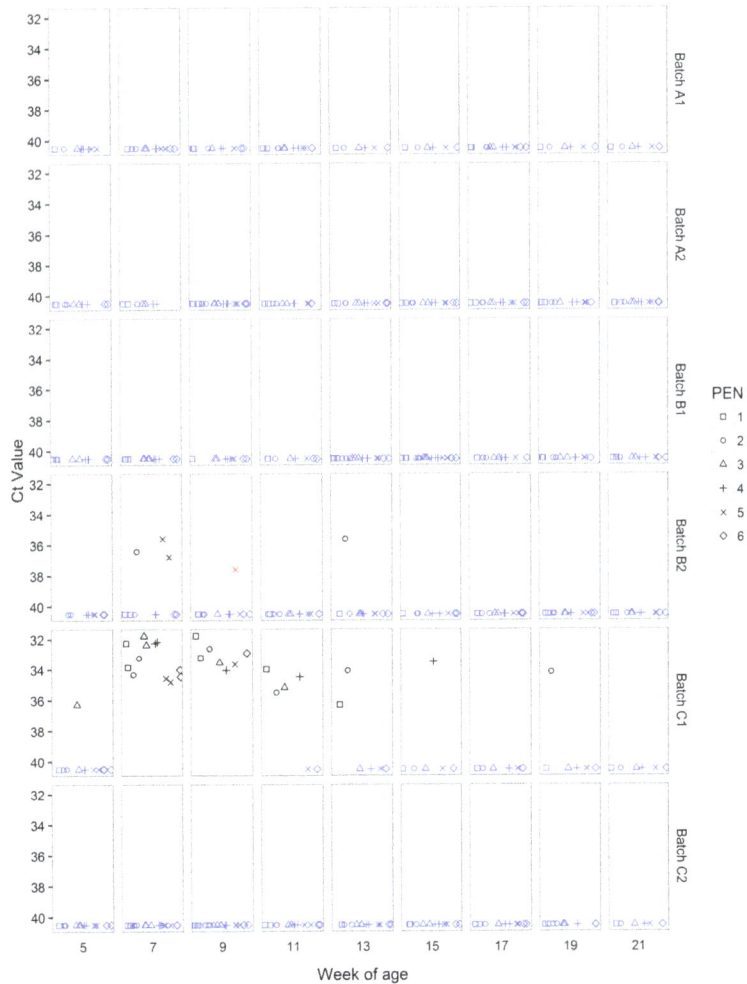

Fig. 3 PRRSV Ct values in OF samples. Real-time PCR Ct values for PRRSV in OF samples collected from pens at between 5 and 21 weeks of age. Each sample from each rope is represented regarding batch, time point and pen from which it was collected. Samples with positive detection are represented in *BLACK* (Ct values <37); inconclusive results in *RED* (Ct values ≥37 and <40); Negative results (no detection in CT ≥ 40) in *BLUE*

Table 4 Results of PRRSV antibody ELISA analysis and PCV2 qPCR in serum at 15th week

Farm/Batch	PRRSV antibody ELISA ($n = 12$ pigs per batch)	PCV2 qPCR ($n = 12$ pigs per batch)
A1	Negative (0/12)	Negative (0/12)
A2	Negative (0/12)	Negative (0/12)
B1	Negative (0/12)	Negative (0/12)
B2	Positive (12/12)	Inconclusive (4/12; $10^{2.5}$ to $10^{3.5}$ PCV2 genome copies/mL, values under the limit of detection)
C1	Positive (12/12)	Negative (0/12)
C2	Negative (0/12)	Negative (0/12)

PCV2

PCV2 DNA amplification was apparently detected by qPCR in OF at most sampling occasions across the study, ranging from 5/9 occasions for C1, through to 9/9 sampling occasions for A1, A2 and B2 (Fig. 4).

Three different patterns of detection were found. First, batches A1, B1, C1 and C2 recorded viral loads under the limit of detection of the method. There was a trend among these four batches for reduced apparent detection prevalence notably after the 13th week of age (Fig. 4).

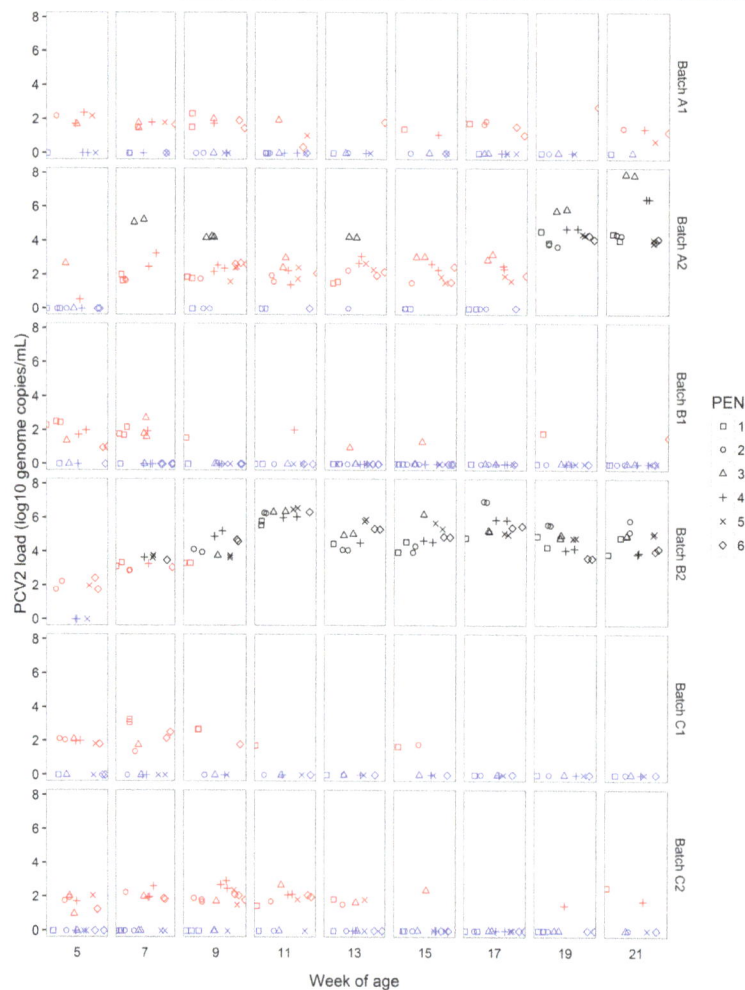

Fig. 4 PCV2 viral load in OF samples. PCV2 viral load (log10 genome copies/mL) for OF samples collected from pens at between 5 and 21 weeks of age. Each sample from each rope is represented regarding batch, time point and pen from which it was collected. In *BLACK* viral load values over the limit of detection ($1 \times 10^{3.48}$ genome copies per mL). In *BLUE*, negative samples where PCV2 DNA was not detected. In *RED*, inconclusive results with viral load values under the limit of detection. Note that viral load values under the limit of quantification (1×10^{4} genome copies per mL) could be not accurately quantified

Batches A2 and B2 each showed different patterns of PCV2 detection in OF. Both these batches recorded higher virus loads over the limit of detection on 5/9 and 8/9 sampling occasions respectively, with the positive pen prevalence being lowest at the 5th week of age. However, A2 differed from B2 in that only one pen in A2 was responsible for yielding OF samples over the limit of detection until the 19th week after which time all pens exceeded this value at the 19th and 21st week, with a peak value of $1 \times 10^{7.9}$ genome copies/mL in the 21st week. Conversely, for B2, OF samples from all pens exceeded the limit of detection at all sampling points from the 9th week onwards, peaking at 1×10^7 genome copies/mL in the 17th week of age and this batch also recorded the highest number of casualties (see Fig. 1 and Table 3).

Serum samples collected in the 15th week of age and every sample had PCV2 viral load values under limit of detection for serum (Table 4).

Post-mortem examinations reported combinations of gross lesions compatible with PCV2 including wasting, emaciation, pallor, rough coat, ascites, jaundice, discoloured liver, interstitial pneumonia, lymph node enlargement and interstitial nephritis [34, 39] in pigs from B2 while examinations on casualties from A1, B1, C1, A2 and C2 did not present suspicious combinations of lesions. Histopathological analysis and immunohistochemistry (IHC) were done on any casualty pigs with individual signs that might be suspicious of PCVD. Clinical PCVD diagnosis was confirmed by histopathology and IHC in batch B2 (4/14 pigs tested; all positive cases were from the 9–15 weeks-old grower stage). In addition 1/2 pigs tested in A2 showed patchy IHC staining for PCV2 antigen. No positive cases were reported in A1, B1 and C1 where IHC testing was done in 2, 1 and 3 pigs respectively. No pigs in C2 were tested for IHC.

SIV
SIV nucleic acid was detected in OF at two consecutive sample points in A2 (5th and 7th week of age) and B2 (9th and 11th week of age) and 3 consecutive sample points in C2 (5th to 9th week of age) (Fig. 5). The prevalence of positive pens ranged between one and five out of six. Of the three positive batches, clinical signs including respiratory problems, cough, sneezes, fever, and prostration, and lesions including interstitial pneumonia, multifocal catarrhal pneumonia; all compatible with influenza were observed only in B2. Sub-typing of all positive samples resulted in classification as H1N2.

M. hyo
M. hyo nucleic acid was detected in OF in A1, B2, C1 and C2 (Fig. 6). All batches yielded consistently negative results just after weaning (5th week of age). Detection patterns were irregular over time in that a pen testing positive on multiple occasions might also report interspersed negative results. Positive pen prevalence increased from the 17th week of age onwards with, notably, all six pens in B2 giving a positive result at all three of the final sample points before slaughter (17th, 19th and 21st week of age). Ct values were variable with a minimum Ct value (between 27 and 28) recorded in batches B2 (at the 17th week of age), C1 (at the 19th week of age), and in A1 (at the 21st week of age). These batches with the greatest number of pens positive for M. hyo across the 19th and 21st week of age sample points to presented the most severe EP-like lesion scores at slaughter (Table 2).

Correlation between multiple OF samples collected from the same pen
Two or more OF samples were collected in 219 pens (generating 484 OF samples) while single OF samples were obtained from the remaining 91 pens resulting in a total of 310 tested pens and 575 OF samples analysed.

Ropes collected at the same time in the same pen showed similar Ct values on most occasions; agreement (same results) for multiple OF samples collected from different ropes in a pen, with at least one positive rope-sample, was 67% for PRRSV (8/12 positive pens), 96% for PCV2, (51/53), 78% for SIV (21/27), and 53% for M. hyo (18/34).

In those pens where multiple samples tested positive or weak positive (in the case of SIV or M. hyo), correlations between different samples Ct values were significant ($P < 0.01$) and strong ($R^2 \geq 0.60$) for every pathogen tested PCV2 ($R^2 = 0.97$) (Fig. 7), PRRSV ($R^2 = 0.85$), SIV ($R^2 = 0.79$) and M. hyo ($R^2 = 0.60$).

Agreement among pens in a barn
A total of 54 "barns" -six barns in nine time points- were tested; 10 (19%) were positive for PRRSV, 13 (24%) were positive for PCV2, seven (13%) were positive for SIV and 18 (33%) were positive for M. hyo.

Agreement among the tested pens in a barn was low; PRRSV was detected in just a single pen in 50% of the cases (five out of 10 positive barns), 23% for PCV2 (three out of 13 positive barns), 14% (one out of seven positive barns) for SIV and 28% (five out of 18 positive barns) for M. hyo. Three or more pens out of six in a barn were positive at the same sample time point in 30% (three out of 10) of the positive barns for PRRSV, 77% (10 out of 13 positive barns) for PCV2, 71% (five out of seven positive barns) for SIV and 50% (nine out of 18 positive barns) for M. hyo.

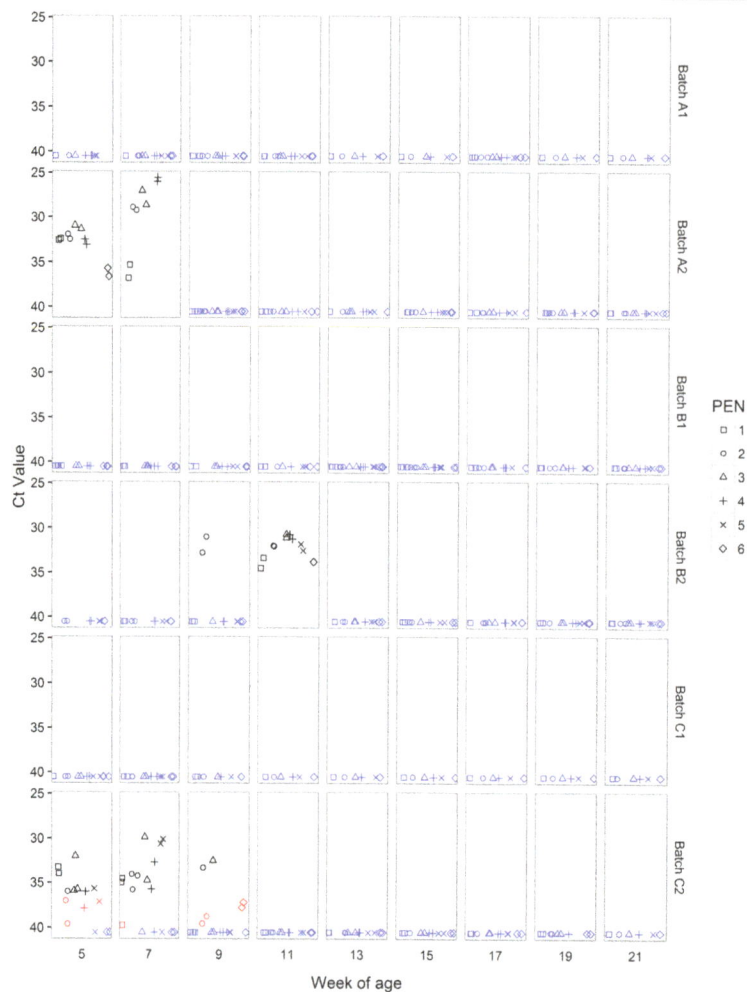

Fig. 5 Swine influenza virus Ct values in OF samples. Real-time PCR Ct values for SIV in OF samples collected from pens at between 5 and 21 weeks of age. Each sample from each rope is represented regarding batch, time point and pen from which it was collected. Samples with positive detection are represented in *BLACK* (Ct values <37); weak positive results in *RED* (Ct values ≥37 and <40); Negative results (no detection in CT ≥ 40) in *BLUE*

Consistency of pen results across time, and spatial patterns or sex effects

Detection patterns for the same pen across time were irregular especially in the case of *M. hyo*; a pen that was positive in a given time could be negative in the next sampling and positive again later on (Fig. 6). However in the case of PCV2, detection patterns were more stable and those pens with higher viral load tended to present similar results at subsequent sample points (Fig. 4).

No differences in detection patterns were seen between pens in terms of spatial distribution within the building or in terms of sex distribution.

Discussion

OF sample collection was found to be straightforward under most on-farm conditions. Sampling was difficult in younger pigs in the three days after weaning, especially when pigs were not previously exposed to ropes; this problem was more pronounced when environment conditions were cold and piglets tended to huddle. In older ages, the main cause of sample collection failure was destruction of the sampling ropes by aggressive chewing or a lack of interaction. Therefore planning of OF-based sampling strategies should take account of timing and environmental conditions in order to allow sampling to be done when pigs are most likely to interact with the collection ropes.

Five out of six batches presented respiratory problems. Severity of clinical disease was not directly related to the initial classifications; multiple post-weaning management factors at the growing farm could have had an important impact on pigs' health. It was notable that clinical signs of diseases suspected to be caused by PCV2, *M. hyo* and/or PRRSV were observed despite vaccination. All vaccinations were made on the 4th or 5th week according to the practices at each farm; however, results of OF analyses for PRRSV (in C1) and PCV2 (in A2 and B2)

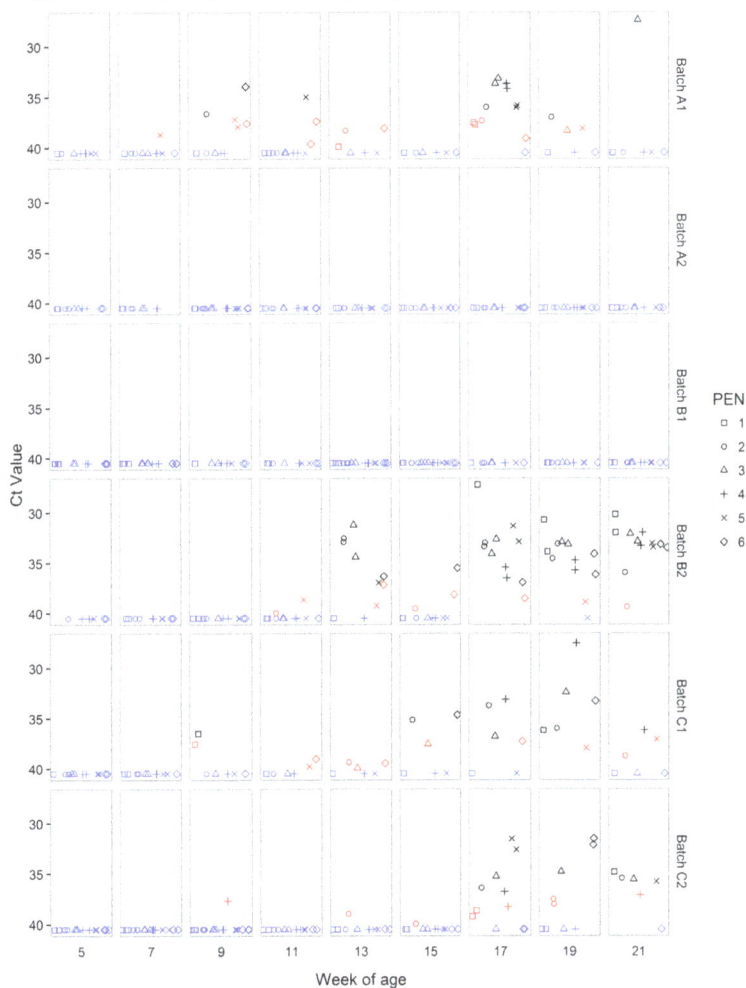

Fig. 6 *Mycoplasma hyopneumoniae* Ct values in OF samples. Real-time PCR Ct values for *M. hyo* in OF samples collected from pens at between 5 and 21 weeks of age. Each sample from each rope is represented regarding batch, time point and pen from which it was collected. Samples with positive detection are represented in *BLACK* (Ct values <37); weak positive results in *RED* (Ct values ≥37 and <40); Negative results (no detection in CT ≥ 40) in *BLUE*

suggest that viral circulation started soon after weaning indicating that vaccination timing was possibly non optimal and a contributor to clinical disease.

The observed patterns of detection of PRRSV, SIV and *M. hyo* highlighted opportunities and limitations for the use of OF testing as part of a diagnostic approach for PRDC. In terms of PRRSV detection, previous studies already reported the successful use of OF to detect PRRSV in young pigs [40] but our findings emphasised the benefit of sampling from multiple pens on a repeated basis in order to overcome recognised limitations in sensitivity of detecting PRRSV in pooled OF samples [41]. On the other hand, our findings showed the usefulness of pooled OF samples for detection of both clinical and non-clinical SIV infection with a window of two to four weeks for detection, confirming the previously reported prolonged shedding of SIV in OF [42]. Although this

study showed the usefulness of OF testing for confirmation of *M. hyo* in clinical PRDC, including in two batches (A1, B2) derived from sources believed to be *M. hyo* negative based on clinical history, it emphasised the limited sensitivity of this testing method. Results presented negative detection by PCR in pig groups that previously, and subsequently had positive detection which suggests this testing method has a poor sensitivity. Therefore the absence of detection of *M. hyo* nucleic acid in pooled OF should not be interpreted as absence of infection from the population. In addition, we found a tendency for those batches with the greatest number of pens positive for *M. hyo* across the 19th and 21st week sample points to present the most severe EP-like lesion scores at slaughter which suggests that higher prevalence and lower Ct values could be related to respiratory problems with *M. hyo* active involvement. The results in this

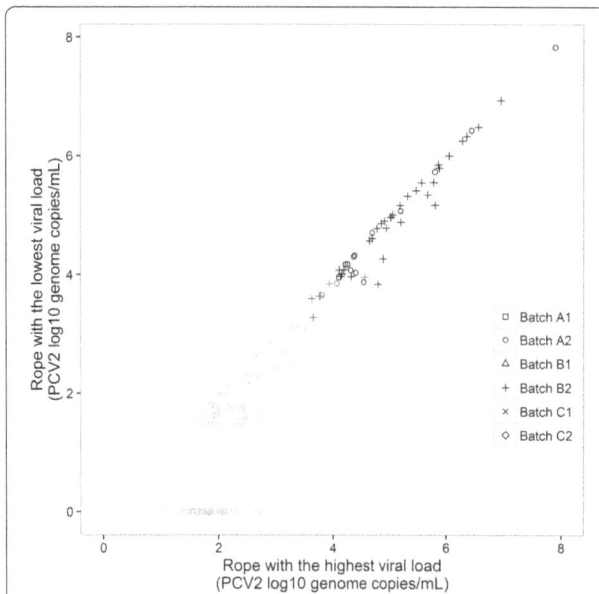

Fig. 7 PCV2 viral load for OF samples collected in the same pen. PCV2 viral load logarithmic values for pairs of OF samples collected from the same pens in the same time point. For each pen the rope with the highest and the lowest viral load were included. In *BLACK*, viral load over the limit of quantification for both ropes; as it has been not defined for OF, the authors considered the reference value for serum (1×10^4 genome copies/mL). In *BLUE*, PCV2 positive samples with at least one rope over the limit of detection ($1 \times 10^{3.48}$ genome copies/mL) but under limit of quantification (1×10^4 genome copies/mL). In *GREY*, PCV2 viral load values under the limit of detection for at least one rope; note that viral load values under the limit of quantification could be not accurately quantified. There was a strong correlation ($R^2 = 0.97$, p < 0.01) between viral load for pairs of ropes with PCV2 viral load over the limit of detection

study emphasized the potential value of OF as a sampling platform to study pen-level prevalence and PCV2 viral load in pooled pen-level samples, as previously described [14, 26]. Even though no relationships between PCV2 detection in OF and prevalence or severity of respiratory disease were apparent, the data indicated the possible use of pooled OF samples to support the diagnosis of PCVD at population level (see Fig. 4 and Table 2). The current study was limited by the small number of participating farms so observed relationships between timing and load of PCV2 detection in pen-level OF samples and results of confirmatory diagnostic tests for PCVD in those farms must be interpreted with caution. In addition, interpretations of quantitative data on PCV2 load in pooled OF samples must be made with caution due to uncertainties including the number of animals contributing to the pool and their individual level of shedding. Nevertheless, previous studies of individual pigs found relationships between the quantities of PCV2 in various samples with generally increased viral load detectable for pigs with clinical PCVD, including in OF [43–46]. Most of these studies associate serum viral load and PCVD; correlations between PCV2

viral loads in serum and individual oral fluids were reported as strong ($R^2 = 0.6$) [26], and oral fluids were described as more sensitive than serum to detect PCV2 when blood samples only represent fraction of the group [47].

Differences in viral loads and patterns of detection at pen level were observed between farms with and without PCVD problems. Farms without detectable clinical or subclinical PCVD in this study presented consistently low viral load in pooled OF samples, generally below the limit of detection, and the number of samples without any PCV2 detection increased with age (Fig. 4). In contrast, higher levels of PCV2 were detected in OF, already exceeding the limit of detection consistently across sampled pens by the 5th week of age, where clinical PCVD was confirmed from the 9th week onwards by clinical signs, gross pathology and IHC for PCV2 antigen (Batch B2). In contrast, a different detection profile was found in one batch (A2) where some evidence for subclinical infection by PCVD was found by IHC staining of viral antigen in lymph node but evidence of clinical PCVD was not found. Here, there was much less consistency in detected viral load between pens sampled at the same time point, with consistently high PCV2 viral load being detected only from the 19th week onward. These findings emphasise the potential value of further more extensive studies using qPCR on pen-level OF samples to explore further any associations between shedding load of PCV2, clinical and subclinical PCVD, and productivity parameters.

Our findings supported sampling designs that target as many pens as possible, rather than focusing resources into collecting multiple rope based OF samples from a smaller number of pens. Close correlation of Ct values between two positive OF samples from the same pen supported this, as did the finding that the proportion of detectably positive pens on a given sampling occasion could be as low as one out six pens. Further studies could support objective determination of the sensitivity of pen level OF testing for respiratory pathogens, compared to other individual sample platforms such as serum or nasal swabs. Direct comparisons are complicated by uncertainties including the relative contribution of individual animals to a pooled sampled, differences in individual shedding load between individuals, as well as differences in shedding of the target pathogen by different routes.

Conclusions

This study provided practical information on the design of OF sampling strategies to support on-farm investigations of respiratory disease in pigs involving PRRSV, SIV, *M. hyo* and PCV2. Importantly, sampling design needs to account for limitations in sensitivity of the test and for differences in herd level infection dynamics. Finally, we found preliminary evidence that measurement of PCV2 load in pooled OF might serve as a tool for prediction of clinical or subclinical PCVD at farm level.

Abbreviations
BALF: Bronchoalveolar lavage fluid; BPHS: British Pig Executive Pig Health Scheme; Ct: Cycle threshold; DNA: Deoxyribonucleic acid; EP: Enzootic pneumonia; IHC: Immunohistochemistry; *M. hyo: Mycoplasma hyopneumoniae*; OF: Oral fluid; PCR: Polymerase chain reaction; PCV2: Porcine circovirus type 2; PCVD: Porcine circovirus diseases; PRDC: Porcine respiratory disease complex; PRRSV: Porcine reproductive and respiratory syndrome virus; qPCR: Quantitative polymerase chain reaction; RNA: Ribonucleic acid; SIV: Swine influenza virus

Acknowledgements
The authors acknowledge Thermo Fisher Scientific for donation of diagnostic testing kits and SAC (Consulting) Veterinary Services for laboratory testing; Dr. Fernando Constantino-Casas and Mr. Thomas Wileman of the Department of Veterinary Medicine at Cambridge; Dr. Henny Martineau and Professor Dirk Werling of the Royal Veterinary College, London; Ms. Elise Martin of Thermo Fisher Scientific; Dr. Susanna Williamson of the UK Animal and Plant Health Agency, Christina Pettit of BQP Ltd, Stradbroke, Suffolk; Zoetis for funding of the ECPHM residency programme at Cambridge and finally the famers who collaborated in this study. SAC Consulting Veterinary Services acknowledges the funding received from the Scottish Government as part of its Public Good Veterinary and Advisory Services.

Funding
Reagents and laboratory testing were financed by Thermo Fisher Scientific. The Department of Veterinary Medicine in the University of Cambridge funded the sample collection, clinical inspections, interpretation of data, and the manuscript writing. JHG was funded by the Zoetis / Cambridge Senior Training Scholarship in Pig Health Management. The SAC, BQP, RVC and the Department of Veterinary Medicine in the University of Cambridge also contributed to fund some diagnostic work.

Authors' contributions
JHG participated in the study design, sample collection, data analysis, laboratory work, results interpretation and manuscript redaction. NR and DM collaborated in the study design and result interpretation. SMK and JRT contributed with laboratory work and participated in the result interpretation and manuscript redaction. ID collaborated in the study design and animal supervision. TE contributed with laboratory work and result interpretation. AWT participated in the study design, data analysis, result interpretation and manuscript redaction. All authors read and approved the final manuscript.

Competing interests
Authors N. Robben and D. Magnée are employees of Thermo Fisher Scientific. There are no further declared conflicts of interest affecting the authors.

Author details
[1]Department of Veterinary Medicine, University of Cambridge, Madingley Road, CB30ES Cambridge, England, UK. [2]Thermo Fisher Scientific, Waltham, MA, USA. [3]Royal Veterinary College, University of London, London, England, UK. [4]BQP Ltd., Stradbroke, England, UK. [5]SAC Consulting Veterinary, Scotland's Rural College (SRUC), Penicuik, Midlothian, Scotland, UK.

References
1. Maes D, Deluyker H, Verdonck M, Castryck F, Miry C, Vrijens B, de Kruif A. Herd factors associated with the seroprevalences of four major respiratory pathogens in slaughter pigs from farrow-to-finish pig herds. Vet Res. 2000;31(3):313–27.
2. Van Alstine WG. Respiratory system. In: Zimmerman JJ, Karriker LA, Ramirez A, Schwartz KJ, Stevenson GW, editors. Diseases of swine, vol. 10. 10th ed. Chichester: Wiley-Blackwell; 2012.
3. Opriessnig T, Gimenez-Lirola LG, Halbur PG. Polymicrobial respiratory disease in pigs. Anim Health Res Rev. 2011;12(2):133–48.
4. Opriessnig T, Halbur PG. Concurrent infections are important for expression of porcine circovirus associated disease. Virus Res. 2012;164(1–2):20–32.
5. Dorr PM, Baker RB, Almond GW, Wayne SR, Gebreyes WA. Epidemiologic assessment of porcine circovirus type 2 coinfection with other pathogens in swine. J Am Vet Med Assoc. 2007;230(2):244–50.
6. Pogranichniy RM, Yoon KJ, Harms PA, Sorden SD, Daniels M. Case-control study on the association of porcine circovirus type 2 and other swine viral pathogens with postweaning multisystemic wasting syndrome. J Vet Diagn Invest. 2002;14(6):449–56.
7. Rovira A, Balasch M, Segales J, Garcia L, Plana-Duran J, Rosell C, Ellerbrok H, Mankertz A, Domingo M. Experimental inoculation of conventional pigs with porcine reproductive and respiratory syndrome virus and porcine circovirus 2. J Virol. 2002;76(7):3232–9.
8. Fan P, Wei Y, Guo L, Wu H, Huang L, Liu J, Liu C. Synergistic effects of sequential infection with highly pathogenic porcine reproductive and respiratory syndrome virus and porcine circovirus type 2. Virol J. 2013;10:265.
9. Sinha A, Shen HG, Schalk S, Beach NM, Huang YW, Meng XJ, Halbur PG, Opriessnig T. Porcine reproductive and respiratory syndrome virus (PRRSV) influences infection dynamics of porcine circovirus type 2 (PCV2) subtypes PCV2a and PCV2b by prolonging PCV2 viremia and shedding. Vet Microbiol. 2011;152(3–4):235–46.
10. Wei H, Lenz SD, Van Alstine WG, Stevenson GW, Langohr IM, Pogranichniy RM. Infection of cesarean-derived colostrum-deprived pigs with porcine circovirus type 2 and Swine influenza virus. Comp Med. 2010;60(1):45–50.
11. Alarcon P, Velasova M, Werling D, Stärk KDC, Chang Y-M, Nevel A, Pfeiffer DU, Wieland B. Assessment and quantification of post-weaning multi-systemic wasting syndrome severity at farm level. Prev Vet Med. 2011;98(1):19–28.
12. Seo HW, Park S-J, Park C, Chae C. Interaction of porcine circovirus type 2 and Mycoplasma hyopneumoniae vaccines on dually infected pigs. Vaccine. 2014;32(21):2480–6.
13. Brockmeier S, Halbur PG, Thacker EL. Porcine respiratroy complex. In: Brogden KA, Guthmiller JM, editors. Polymicrobial diseases. Washington: ASM Press; 2002.
14. Ramirez A, Wang C, Prickett JR, Pogranichniy R, Yoon K-J, Main R, Johnson JK, Rademacher C, Hoogland M, Hoffmann P, et al. Efficient surveillance of pig populations using oral fluids. Prev Vet Med. 2012;104(3–4):292–300.
15. Decorte I, Van der Stede Y, Nauwynck H, De Regge N, Cay AB. Effect of saliva stabilisers on detection of porcine reproductive and respiratory syndrome virus in oral fluid by quantitative reverse transcriptase real-time PCR. Vet J. 2013;197(2):224–8.
16. Ochert AS, Boulter AW, Birnbaum W, Johnson NW, Teo CG. Inhibitory effect of salivary fluids on PCR: potency and removal. PCR Methods Appl. 1994;3(6):365–8.
17. Prickett JR, Zimmerman JJ. The development of oral fluid-based diagnostics and applications in veterinary medicine. Anim Health Res Rev. 2010;11(2):207–16.
18. Seddon YM, Guy JH, Edwards SA. Optimising oral fluid collection from groups of pigs: Effect of housing system and provision of ropes. Vet J. 2012;193(1):180–4.
19. Dawson LL, Edwards SA. The effects of flavored rope additives on commercial pen-based oral fluid yield in pigs. J Vet Behav Clin Appl Res. 2015;10(3):267–71.
20. Olsen C, Karriker L, Wang C, Binjawadagi B, Renukaradhya G, Kittawornrat A, Lizano S, Coetzee J, Main R, Meiszberg A, et al. Effect of collection material and sample processing on pig oral fluid testing results. Vet J. 2013;198(1):158–63.
21. Jones TH, Muehlhauser V. Effect of handling and storage conditions and stabilizing agent on the recovery of viral RNA from oral fluid of pigs. J Virol Methods. 2014;198:26–31.

22. Prickett J, Simer R, Christopher-Hennings J, Yoon KJ, Evans RB, Zimmerman JJ. Detection of porcine reproductive and respiratory syndrome virus infection in porcine oral fluid samples: a longitudinal study under experimental conditions. J Vet Diagn Investig. 2008;20(2):156–63.

23. Chittick WA, Stensland WR, Prickett JR, Strait EL, Harmon K, Yoon KJ, Wang C, Zimmerman JJ. Comparison of RNA extraction and real-time reverse transcription polymerase chain reaction methods for the detection of porcine reproductive and respiratory syndrome virus in porcine oral fluid specimens. J Vet Diagn Investig. 2011;23(2):248–53.

24. Romagosa A, Gramer M, Joo HS, Torremorell M. Sensitivity of oral fluids for detecting influenza A virus in populations of vaccinated and non-vaccinated pigs. Influenza Other Respir Viruses. 2012;6(2):110–8.

25. Detmer SE, Patnayak DP, Jiang Y, Gramer MR, Goyal SM. Detection of influenza a virus in porcine oral fluid samples. J Vet Diagn Investig. 2011;23(2):241–7.

26. Kim WI. Application of oral fluid sample to monitor porcine circovirus-2 infection in pig farms. J Vet Clin. 2010;27(6):704–12.

27. Prickett JR, Johnson J, Murtaugh MP, Puvanendiran S, Wang C, Zimmerman JJ, Opriessnig T. Prolonged detection of PCV2 and anti-PCV2 antibody in oral fluids following experimental inoculation. Transbound Emerg Dis. 2011;58(2):121–7.

28. Costa G, Oliveira S, Torrison J. Detection of Actinobacillus pleuropneumoniae in oral-fluid samples obtained from experimentally infected pigs. J Swine Health Prod. 2012;20(2):78–81.

29. Roos LR, Fano E, Homwong N, Payne B, Pieters M. A model to investigate the optimal seeder-to-naive ratio for successful natural Mycoplasma hyopneumoniae gilt exposure prior to entering the breeding herd. Vet Microbiol. 2016;184:51–8.

30. Strait E, Roe C, Levy N, Dorazio C, Kuhn M. Diagnosis of *Mycoplasma hyopneumoniae* in growing pigs. 21st IPVS 2010 proceedings. 2010(O.103):1.

31. Cheong Y, Oh C, Lee K, Cho KH. A survey of porcine respiratory disease complex (PRDC) associated pathogens among commercial pig farms of Korea via oral fluid method. J Vet Sci. 2016. http://www.vetsci.org/journal/view.html?uid=1191&vmd=Full&.

32. Biernacka K, Karbowiak P, Wróbel P, Chareza T, Czopowicz M, Balka G, Goodell C, Rauh R, Stadejek T. Detection of porcine reproductive and respiratory syndrome virus (PRRSV) and influenza A virus (IAV) in oral fluid of pigs. Res Vet Sci. 2016;109:74–80.

33. Prickett JR, Kim W, Simer R, Yoon KJ, Zimmerman J. Oral-fluid samples for surveillance of commercial growing pigs for porcine reproductive and respiratory syndrome virus and porcine circovirus type 2 infections. J Swine Health Prod. 2008;16(2):86–91.

34. Segalés J. Porcine circovirus type 2 (PCV2) infections: clinical signs, pathology and laboratory diagnosis. Virus Res. 2012;164(1–2):10–9.

35. Patterson R, Eley T, Browne C, Martineau HM, Werling D. Oral application of freeze-dried yeast particles expressing the PCV2b Cap protein on their surface induce protection to subsequent PCV2b challenge in vivo. Vaccine. 2015;33(46):6199–205.

36. Goodwin RFW, Hodgson RG, Whittlestone P, Woodhams RL. Some experiments relating to artificial immunity in enzootic pneumonia of pigs. Epidemiol Infect. 1969;67(03):465–76.

37. Holt H, Alarcon P, Velasova M, Pfeiffer D, Wieland B. BPEX Pig Health Scheme: a useful monitoring system for respiratory disease control in pig farms? BMC Vet Res. 2011;7(1):82.

38. R Core Team. R: a language and environment for statistical computing. Vienna: R Foundation for Statistical Computing; 2016.

39. Segales J, Allan G, Domingo M. Porcine circovirus. In: Zimmerman JJ, Karriker LA, Ramirez A, Schwartz KJ, Stevenson GW, editors. Diseases of swine. 10th ed. Ames: Iowa State Press; 2012. p. 405–17.

40. Kittawornrat A, Panyasing Y, Goodell C, Wang C, Gauger P, Harmon K, Rauh R, Desfresne L, Levis I, Zimmerman J. Porcine reproductive and respiratory syndrome virus (PRRSV) surveillance using pre-weaning oral fluid samples detects circulation of wild-type PRRSV. Vet Microbiol. 2014;168(2–4):331–9.

41. Olsen C, Wang C, Christopher-Hennings J, Doolittle K, Harmon KM, Abate S, Kittawornrat A, Lizano S, Main R, Nelson EA, et al. Probability of detecting porcine reproductive and respiratory syndrome virus infection using pen-based swine oral fluid specimens as a function of within-pen prevalence. J Vet Diagn Investig. 2013;25(3):328–35.

42. Decorte I, Steensels M, Lambrecht B, Cay AB, De Regge N. Detection and isolation of swine influenza A virus in spiked oral fluid and samples from individually housed, experimentally infected pigs: potential role of porcine oral fluid in active influenza A virus surveillance in swine. PLoS One. 2015;10(10):e0139586.

43. Grau-Roma L, Hjulsager CK, Sibila M, Kristensen CS, Lopez-Soria S, Enoe C, Casal J, Botner A, Nofrarias M, Bille-Hansen V, et al. Infection, excretion and seroconversion dynamics of porcine circovirus type 2 (PCV2) in pigs from post-weaning multisystemic wasting syndrome (PMWS) affected farms in Spain and Denmark. Vet Microbiol. 2009;135(3–4):272–82.

44. Brunborg IM, Fossum C, Lium B, Blomqvist G, Merlot E, Jorgensen A, Eliasson-Selling L, Rimstad E, Jonassen CM, Wallgren P. Dynamics of serum antibodies to and load of porcine circovirus type 2 (PCV2) in pigs in three finishing herds, affected or not by postweaning multisystemic wasting syndrome. Acta Vet Scand. 2010;52:22.

45. Olvera A, Sibila M, Calsamiglia M, Segales J, Domingo M. Comparison of porcine circovirus type 2 load in serum quantified by a real time PCR in postweaning multisystemic wasting syndrome and porcine dermatitis and nephropathy syndrome naturally affected pigs. J Virol Methods. 2004;117(1):75–80.

46. Segales J, Calsamiglia M, Olvera A, Sibila M, Badiella L, Domingo M. Quantification of porcine circovirus type 2 (PCV2) DNA in serum and tonsillar, nasal, tracheo-bronchial, urinary and faecal swabs of pigs with and without postweaning multisystemic wasting syndrome (PMWS). Vet Microbiol. 2005;111(3–4):223–9.

47. Finlaison D, Collins AM. Evaluation of oral fluid samples for herd health monitoring of pathogens and the immune response in pigs. 2A-108 1213. Australia: Elizabeth Macarthur Agricultural Institute; 2014.

4

Survival of porcine epidemic diarrhea virus (PEDV) in thermally treated feed ingredients and on surfaces

Michaela P. Trudeau[1], Harsha Verma[2], Pedro E. Urriola[1], Fernando Sampedro[2], Gerald C. Shurson[1] and Sagar M. Goyal[2*]

Abstract

Background: Infection with Porcine Epidemic Diarrhea Virus (PEDV) causes vomiting, diarrhea, and dehydration in young pigs. The virus made its first appearance in the U.S. in 2013, where it caused substantial neonatal mortality and economic losses in the U.S. pork industry. Based on outbreak investigations, it is hypothesized that the virus could be transmitted through contaminated feed or contaminated feed surfaces. This potential risk created a demand for research on the inactivation kinetics of PEDV in different environments. Therefore, the objective of this study was to evaluate the survival of PEDV in 9 different feed ingredients when exposed to 60, 70, 80, and 90 °C, as well as the survival on four different surfaces (galvanized steel, stainless steel, aluminum, and plastic).

Results: Overall, there were no differences ($P > 0.05$) in virus survival among the different feed matrices studied when thermally processed at 60 to 90 °C for 5, 10, 15, or 30 min. However, the time necessary to achieve a one log reduction in virus concentration was less ($P < 0.05$) when ingredients were exposed to temperatures from 70 °C (3.7 min), 80 °C (2.4 min), and 90 °C (2.3 min) compared with 60 °C (4.4 min). The maximum inactivation level (3.9 log) was achieved when heating all ingredients at 90 °C for 30 min. There were no differences in the amount of time necessary to cause a one log reduction in PEDV concentration among the different surfaces.

Conclusions: The results of this study showed that PEDV survival among the 9 feed ingredients evaluated was not different when exposed to thermal treatments for up to 30 min. However, different combinations of temperature and time resulted in achieving a 3 to 4 log reduction of PEDV in all feed ingredients evaluated. Finally, PEDV survival was similar on galvanized steel, stainless steel, aluminum and plastic.

Keywords: Thermal processing, Feed ingredients, Porcine epidemic diarrhea virus, Inactivation, Survival, Surfaces

Background

Upon infection with Porcine Epidemic Diarrhea Virus (PEDV), pigs experience vomiting, diarrhea, and dehydration leading to high mortality in suckling pigs [1]. The virus is excreted in large amounts in the feces of infected pigs, making it highly contagious and difficult to control [2]. After the virus was identified in Belgium in 1978, it slowly spread to multiple countries including Canada, Korea, and China [3]. In the United States, the virus was first detected in May of 2013, and while the mode of introduction has not yet been confirmed, contaminated feed has been suspected as the cause of transmission [4].

Recent research on PEDV survival in feed ingredients has shown that it appears to survive longer in soybean meal (greater than 180 days) compared with other commonly used feed ingredients [5]. The authors also showed that PEDV can survive for up to 30 days in blood meal, corn dried distiller's grains with solubles, meat and bone meal, red blood cells, L-lysine HCl, D, L-methionine, choice white grease, choline chloride, and complete feed. However, the research determined virus survival when samples were stored at low, uncontrolled temperatures (varying between –15 to 20 °C) and did

* Correspondence: goyal001@umn.edu
[2]Veterinary Population Medicine, University of Minnesota, 1365 Gortner Avenue, St. Paul, MN 55108, USA
Full list of author information is available at the end of the article

not investigate the impact of any thermal processing treatment. Results from other studies suggest that specific thermal processing treatments, such as spray drying (a process using dry hot air to reduce the moisture of a particle) can reduce the survival of PEDV in porcine and bovine plasma by 5 log [6, 7]. Other research has shown that conditioning and pelleting with temperatures above 54.4 °C could be effective in reducing infectivity of PEDV in swine feed [8]. However, the sole impact of thermal processing on the inactivation kinetics of PEDV in feed is still unknown.

If a feed ingredient is contaminated when it enters the feed mill, it has been shown to contaminate the feed mill surfaces [9]. Previous research has shown differences in the effectiveness of decontamination treatments between various equipment and facility surface materials including metal, plastic, rubber, and concrete [10]. This surface contamination with PEDV can then contaminate subsequent batches of feed [11]. If this type of contamination occurs, it is necessary to understand virus inactivation kinetics on different surface materials before a treatment is applied. However, the survival of PEDV on various surfaces is not well known.

The objectives of this study were to measure the effect of thermal treatment on inactivation kinetics of PEDV in nine commonly used feed ingredients, and to determine the PEDV inactivation kinetics on various equipment and facility surfaces (i.e. galvanized steel, stainless steel, aluminum, and plastic). We hypothesized that different chemical characteristics of the feed ingredients would affect PEDV survivability when subjected to different thermal treatments and PED virus inactivation would differ among material surfaces.

Methods

Virus propagation

The NVSL strain of PEDV was grown in Vero-81 cells, which were grown in Dulbecco's Modified Eagle Medium (Mediatech, Herndon, VA), 8% fetal bovine serum (FBS; HyClone, South Logan, UT), 50 μg/mL gentamicin (Mediatech, Herndon, VA), 150 μg/mL neomycin sulfate (Sigma, St. Louis, MO), 1.5 μg/mL fungizone (Sigma, St. Louis, MO), and 455 μg/mL streptomycin (Sigma, St. Louis, MO). Before inoculation, the cells were washed 3 times with phosphate buffered Saline solution (pH 7.2). After inoculation, the cells were incubated at 37 °C allowing virus absorption using maintenance medium (DMEM, antibiotics, and 10.0 μg/mL trypsin; Gibco, Life Technologies, Grand Island, NY). After 1 h, new media were added to the flask and the cells were placed in an incubator at 37 °C under 5% CO_2. The cells were examined daily for the appearance of cytopathic effects (CPE), usually appearing 4 to 5 days post-infection. After CPE was observed, the cells underwent 3 freeze-thaw cycles (−80 °C to 25 °C)

and were then centrifuged at 2500×g for 15 min at 4 °C. After centrifugation, the supernatant was collected, aliquoted in 25 mL tubes, and stored at −80 °C until used.

Feed ingredients composition

Feed ingredients (i.e. soybean meal, swine growing-finishing vitamin and trace mineral premix, spray dried porcine plasma, meat meal, meat and bone meal, blood meal, corn, and corn distillers dried grains with solubles) were obtained from the feed mill at the Southern Research and Outreach Center of the University of Minnesota (Waseca, MN). The sample of complete feed evaluated was a phase II starter diet that did not contain any animal by-products (Vita-Plus CGI, enhanced NP-NT, batch no. 831458). All feed and feed ingredients were tested and confirmed negative for PEDV by real time RT-PCR. Samples were sent to Minnesota Valley Testing Laboratory (New Ulm, MN) to analyze the nutrient composition of each ingredient (Table 1). Standard procedures established by AOAC International were used to measure moisture (method 930.15), ash (method 942.05), ether extract (method 2003.05), crude fiber (method 930.39), and crude protein (method 990.03) content [12]. The proximate analysis values were obtained from a single sample. The pH was measured by mixing 50 mL of distilled water with 5 g of each feed ingredient, premix, and complete feed. The mixture was then stirred with a magnetic stirrer for 20 min. The pH of the suspended feed was measured using a pH probe (Fisher Scientific, Waltham, MA) and recorded. All chemical composition values for each ingredient were determined from one replicate. The pH of each sample was measured in triplicate.

Virus survival in feed ingredients after thermal processing

Five gram aliquots of each ingredient were weighed into plastic scintillation vials (Fisher Scientific, Pittsburgh, PA) and placed into sealed, airtight, and water proof containers. Preliminary experiments measured the temperature of the feed and feed ingredients after being placed in the water bath and determined that 1 h was required for feed to achieve the maximum temperature of the water bath. During the experiment, the containers were placed in a water bath at 60, 70, 80 and 90 °C for 1 h to reach water bath temperature. Once the samples reached the desired temperature, they were removed and 1 mL of PEDV (passage 19, titer 3.2×10^4 TCID$_{50}$/mL) was added to the samples. During this time, the samples were removed from the water bath for about 5 min to complete the inoculation procedure. The inoculated samples were then immediately placed back into the water bath for 0, 5, 10, 15, or 30 min.

To elute the surviving virus from the samples of feed and feed ingredients, an eluent solution, 3% beef extract (Lab Scientific, Highlands, NJ) 0.05 M glycine (Sigma), pH 7.2 was used. After various time points, this solution

Table 1 Chemical composition of common feed ingredients used in diets for pigs

Ingredient[a]	Moisture (%)	Ash (%)	Ether extract (%)	Crude fiber (%)	Crude Protein[b] (%)	pH[c]
CF	8.57	9.45	4.47	2.02	24.20	5.82
SBM	12.12	6.42	0.71	3.26	45.40	6.73
C	14.90	1.55	3.86	1.55	7.03	6.21
DDGS	10.31	4.56	5.86	6.50	30.10	4.39
PM	2.41	73.77	1.42	1.62	1.91	3.49
SDPP	11.60	7.44	0.15	< 0.01	77.79	7.15
BM	11.58	1.79	0.16	0.05	92.60	8.40
MM	4.80	24.26	13.54	1.83	54.90	6.64
MBM	5.74	24.77	10.77	1.16	55.70	6.50

[a]*CF* complete feed, *SDPP* spray dried porcine plasma, *MM* meat meal, *MBM* meat and bone meal, *BM* blood meal, *SBM* soybean meal, *C* corn, *PM* vitamin-trace mineral premix, *DDGS* Corn distillers dried grains with solubles
[b]Crude protein is calculated from nitrogen content × 6.25
[c]Average of 3 replicates

was added to the sample aliquot and mixed well. After light centrifugation to remove organic debris, the supernatant was collected. To determine the concentration of surviving virus, a titration was performed by preparing serial 10-fold dilutions of the supernatant in maintenance medium. These dilutions were inoculated into monolayers of Vero-81 cells grown in 96 microtiter well plates (Nunc, Rochester, NY) at 100 μL/well using three wells per dilution. The inoculated cells were incubated at 37 °C under 5% CO_2 for 4 to 5 days and observed for CPE. The virus titer was then calculated as 50% tissue culture infective dose ($TCID_{50}$/mL) [13]. The virus titers of the supernatants were compared to those of the initial virus titer to determine the amount of virus inactivation.

Virus survival in equipment surfaces

A total of 4 surface materials were evaluated including stainless steel, aluminum, plastic, and galvanized steel. Stainless steel and aluminum sheets were purchased from Hardware Hank (St. Paul, MN). For the plastic surface, 6-well plastic plates (Nunc, New York, NY) were used, and galvanized steel (28 gal. Silver Galvanized Steel Hobby Sheet Sleeved; Model # 57321) was obtained from Home Depot (Roseville, MN).

The PEDV inoculation solution (40 μL) was applied to the center of a sample of stainless steel, aluminum, plastic, or galvanized steel. The virus was allowed to dry for 10 min, and the sheets and plates were then stored at room temperature (~25 °C) for up to 10 days. At 0, 1, 2, 5, and 10 days, surviving virus was eluted from the center of a surface using 400 μL of an elution buffer (3% beef extract in 0.05 M glycine, pH 7.2). To elute the virus, the elution buffer was applied to the surface and then removed off the surface with a pipette. At the time 0 elution point, 78% of the virus was recovered using this method. After elution, the sample was titrated in Vero-81 cells to determine virus concentration. This

experiment was then repeated once more to provide a total of two experiments.

Calculations and statistical analyses

Inactivation kinetics data on virus survival were analyzed using the Weibull model [14]. The fitting of the model to the experimental data was performed by using the GINAFiT add-in software on Microsoft excel [15]. Assuming that the temperature resistance for PEDV follows a Weibull distribution, an equation was used to predict the log concentration of surviving virus after the thermal treatment (Eq. 1):

$$Log(N) = Log(N_0) - (^t/_\delta)^n \quad (1)$$

In eq. 1, N is the surviving virus expressed as $TCID_{50}$/mL, N_0 is the initial virus titer at the start of the experiment, t is time (min), δ is the time of the first log reduction of virus concentration (min), and n is the shape parameter. The shape parameter (n) indicates the shape of the curve with a value $n > 1$ representing the formation of a shoulder-shaped curve and being convex, and $n < 1$ represented the formation of a tail-shaped curve and concave in shape, while $n = 1$ represented a linear function. The adjusted R^2 value (Adj. R^2) was used to evaluate how well the model fit the experimental data.

The delta values obtained from the Weibull model indicated the amount of time necessary to reduce the virus concentration by 1 log. The delta values were compared across treatments. Normality was assessed using the UNIVARIATE procedure of SAS. An ANOVA statistical analysis using the PROC-MIXED procedure of SAS was performed to determine statistically significant differences between feed ingredients and between temperature treatments. When evaluating virus survival between the four temperatures, feed ingredient was considered a random effect. Least squared means with a Tukey adjustment were used to determine differences among each treatment if $P < 0.05$. The experimental unit was a single vial.

Results

There were no differences ($P > 0.05$) in survival of PEDV after the thermal treatment among the 9 feed materials evaluated (Table 2). This observation was consistent at each of the 4 temperatures applied, indicating that the virus resistance to thermal treatment was not affected by the different chemical composition of the feed matrices. Delta values at 70 to 90 °C were less ($P < 0.05$) than at 60 °C (Table 3), indicating higher virus inactivation kinetics at greater temperatures. The shape parameter of the virus inactivation curves were not different among treatments, and values ranged between 0.45 and 0.60, indicating that at each temperature, curves were concave and formed tails. This behavior corresponds to a rapid decrease of virus concentration after short treatment times followed by a plateau where the virus survived for an extended period of time.

When comparing the log reduction achieved after 10, 15, or 30 min, no differences ($P > 0.05$) were observed when the virus was exposed to 60 and 70 °C, but greater reductions ($P < 0.05$) in virus concentration were achieved at 80 and 90 °C. A reduction of 1.9 to 2.0 log was achieved at 60 °C for 15 min, or 70 °C for 10 min, and a 2.2 to 2.4 log reduction occurred after treatment at 60 °C for 30 min, 70 °C for 15 min, or 80 °C for 10 min. Greater than a 3 log reduction was observed when applying 80 °C for 30 min (3.4 log), or 90 °C for 15 min (3.3 log). The maximum log reduction (3.9 log) was achieved at 90 °C for 30 min.

During the 10-day incubation period, PEDV titer was reduced by 1.3 log on all surfaces except for stainless steel, in which only a 0.83 log reduction was observed. The PEDV remained viable (10^2 $TCID_{50}/g$) on each of the four surfaces after 10 days of incubation. When delta values were compared, there were no differences among all 4 surfaces ranging from 0.7 and 7.7 days (Table 4).

Discussion

Recent investigations have shown that feed contaminated with PEDV is capable of infecting pigs [16]. Therefore, it is important to develop mitigation strategies to reduce the risk of virus transmission to swine farms through contaminated feed. Previous research has suggested that contaminated feed ingredients can be a risk factor for PEDV transmission among swine farms, and that virus survival was different among ingredients [5]. Varying PEDV survival among feed ingredients suggests that feed ingredients may need to be handled and processed differently based on virus inactivation kinetics and relative risk of transmission for a specific feed ingredient. When thermal treatment of complete feed was evaluated at high temperatures, heating complete feed at 120 °C for 25 min resulted in a 3 log reduction in PEDV [17]. However, the previous study was performed using complete feed, and there has been limited information published regarding thermal treatment of PEDV in individual feed ingredients. If a feed ingredient is contaminated, studies have shown that it can then contaminate surfaces in a feed mill [9]. After surface contamination with PEDV, subsequent batches of feed can be contaminated with the virus [11]. Therefore, it is necessary to determine if any differences in virus survival among feed ingredients requires different thermal processing conditions to reduce the risk of subsequent contamination. Additionally, it is necessary to understand the inactivation kinetics of PEDV on various surfaces of materials used in feed mills and swine farms.

Our hypothesis was that PEDV survives differently in complete feed or feed ingredient varying in chemical

Table 2 Weibull model kinetic parameters of Porcine Epidemic Diarrhea Virus survival in ingredients after thermal treatment

Temperature	60 °C		70 °C		80 °C		90 °C	
Ingredient[a]	Delta (min)[b]	Adj. R^2	Delta (min)[b]	Adj. R^2	Delta (min)[b]	Adj. R^2	Delta (min)[b]	Adj. R^2
CF	3.8 ± 1.2	0.72	1.1 ± 1.3	0.88	1.5 ± 1.6	0.84	2.0 ± 2.2	0.84
SBM	3.3 ± 2.3	0.83	1.3 ± 5.0	0.83	1.7 ± 1.8	0.68	2.0 ± 2.1	0.85
C	3.4 ± 3.2	0.85	3.3 ± 4.5	0.75	2.2 ± 1.5	0.90	1.7 ± 1.6	0.89
DDGS	2.5 ± 1.7	0.84	2.2 ± 2.4	0.87	1.3 ± 1.4	0.87	2.1 ± 1.7	0.87
PM	4.9 ± 4.3	0.89	1.4 ± 5.0	0.76	2.0 ± 2.4	0.85	2.0 ± 1.7	0.83
SDPP	3.6 ± 3.4	0.86	2.1 ± 1.8	0.86	2.3 ± 1.6	0.85	2.1 ± 3.1	0.87
BM	2.0 ± 6.0	0.83	3.5 ± 4.4	0.81	1.5 ± 2.8	0.84	0.64 ± 0.3	0.84
MM	3.0 ± 2.6	0.85	2.0 ± 1.6	0.89	2.1 ± 1.2	0.90	2.1 ± 0.9	0.84
MBM	6.0 ± 2.5	0.88	2.4 ± 1.4	0.84	2.3 ± 1.0	0.85	0.9 ± 0.9	0.75
P-Value	0.75		0.50		0.98		0.78	

[a]CF complete feed, SDPP spray dried porcine plasma, MM meat meal, MBM meat and bone meal, BM blood meal, SBM soybean meal, C corn, PM vitamin-trace mineral premix, DDGS Corn distillers dried grains with solubles
[b]Average of 6 replicates, Delta values indicates the time to achieve 1 log reduction

Table 3 Survival of Porcine Epidemic Diarrhea virus (PEDV) in feed and feed ingredients when thermally treated

Temperature	Average δ [1,2] (min)	Shape Paremeter[3]	Adj. R^2	Log reduction at 10 min[1]	Log reduction at 15 min[1]	Log reduction at 30 min[1]
60 °C	$4.4^a \pm 3.5$	0.50	0.83	$1.7^a \pm 0.4$	$2.0^a \pm 0.4$	$2.4^a \pm 0.4$
70 °C	$3.7^b \pm 3.7$	0.45	0.84	$1.9^a \pm 0.5$	$2.3^a \pm 0.4$	$2.7^a \pm 0.7$
80 °C	$2.4^b \pm 1.8$	0.50	0.85	$2.2^b \pm 0.3$	$2.8^b \pm 0.8$	$3.4^b \pm 0.9$
90 °C	$2.3^b \pm 1.9$	0.60	0.84	$2.6^c \pm 0.9$	$3.3^c \pm 1.1$	$3.9^c \pm 0.8$
P-Value	0.0002			0.0001	0.0001	0.0001

[1]Different letters in the same column differ at $P < 0.05$
[2]δ is the time of the first log reduction of virus concentration
[3]The shape parameter (n) indicates the shape of the curve with a value $n > 1$ forming shoulders and being convex, $n < 1$ forming tails and being concave, and $n = 1$ being linear

composition, and that some ingredients may require greater processing temperatures to achieve an adequate virus inactivation. Our study evaluated feed ingredients, premix, and complete feed with different chemical composition and pH values. However, no differences were observed among the virus inactivation kinetics (delta values). These results suggest that under the conditions evaluated in this study (high temperatures and long exposure times), rapid virus inactivation may occur independently of chemical composition of ingredients, and thus, similar processing conditions can be applied to all ingredients to achieve a similar reduction in virus concentration. Our results were unexpected because of the dramatic differences in the pH values of the feed matrices evaluated (3.49 to 8.40). Quist-Rybachuk et al. (2015) found that PEDV was more heat sensitive when the pH increased from 7.2 to 10.2 [18]. The lack of differences in PEDV inactivation among ingredients despite the pH differences may also be due to the use of dry ingredients instead of liquid media. Because pH is only a characteristic of solutions, the impact of the pH on virus survival in a dry ingredient with a small amount of liquid (1 mL) is likely to be minimal. In addition to this, the maximum pH in our experiment was only 8.40, which is considerably lower than the pH of 10.2 that created variation in virus sensitivity to thermal treatments in previous experiments [18].

Although there were no differences in virus survival among the feed materials evaluated between 60 and 70 °C, greater virus inactivation was achieved at 80 and 90 °C. In order to optimize the thermal processing conditions (high temperature and short time) to inactivate PEDV, our data suggest that thermal treatment at 80 °C for 15 min was necessary for achieving a 3-log reduction. This extent of inactivation could also be achieved by thermal processing at 90 °C for 10 min or heating at 70 °C for 30 min. These findings and parameters are consistent with those reported by Hoffman and Wyler (1989), who found that PEDV was relatively stable at 50 °C, but at temperatures greater than 60 °C, the virus lost total infectivity within 30 min [19]. These results were also comparable to the survival of PEDV on the metal surface of hog transport trailers, where heating at 71 °C for 10 min was capable of reducing virus titer low enough to not cause infection in any of the 4 inoculated pigs, however, the exact reduction of PEDV was not measured [20].

If a contaminated ingredient enters the feed mill, it has been demonstrated that this ingredient will contaminate feed mill surfaces and subsequent batches of feed [9]. This research has evaluated the contamination of feed mill surfaces, but limited studies have been conducted on PEDV long-term survival after a surface is contaminated. Data from this experiment suggest that PEDV can survive for extended periods of time on all of

Table 4 Concentration of viable Porcine Epidemic Diarrhea virus (PEDV) after inoculation in various surfaces

| Time (days) | Concentration of viable PEDV (Log $TCID_{50}$/mL) on: | | | |
	Stainless steel	Aluminum	Plastic	Galvanized steel
0	3.51	3.51	3.51	3.51
1	2.51	2.51	2.51	2.51
2	2.51	2.51	2.51	2.51
5	2.45	1.70	1.51	2.51
10	2.70	2.18	2.18	2.18
Weibull model				
Delta, days	7.72 ± 7.16	0.79 ± 0.10	0.69 ± 0.00	1.74 ± 0.00
Adjusted R^2	0.88	0.67	0.56	0.94
Delta P-value	> 0.05			

the material surfaces evaluated, which are in agreement with other reports in the literature. In similar experiments, Casanova et al. (2010) found that TGEV, another swine coronavirus, can remain infectious on hard nonporous surfaces for up to 28 days [21]. In that study, there was a 3.2 log reduction in TGEV after 28 days at room temperature at 80% relative humidity. Another human coronavirus, SARS, has been actively studied for its survival on different material surfaces [21]. This virus has been reported to survive for up to 36 h on stainless steel, but the initial concentration of virus in this study was not reported [22]. In a different experiment, Rabenau et al. (2005) reported a 4-log reduction in SARS virus concentration after 9 days of incubation on a polystyrene surface [23]. Furthermore, SARS virus survived on smooth plastic more than 5 days at room temperature [24]. Results from these previous studies, along with similar examples [25, 26], indicate that coronaviruses may pose a risk for transmission via contaminated surfaces in the feed mill. Our results showed longer virus survival time (greater than 10 days), which indicates that additional mitigation measures (i.e. proper cleaning and disinfection) need to be implemented to minimize risk of virus transmission on surfaces of feed mills and swine farms.

One of the limitations for applying this combined knowledge into practice is the potential experimental methodology concern of adding 1 mL of media containing the virus to feed samples. The addition of liquid media necessarily increases the moisture content of the sample, and this may affect the virus survival. More research is necessary to compare the effect of moisture content and water activity on PEDV survival, and determine the extent that this factor plays in virus inactivation. In the surface experiment, however, the media was allowed to dry, eliminating this factor as a potential limitation. It is highly likely that the amount of virus excreted by an infected pig, and potentially transmitted via feed, would be much greater than the titer used in the present study. In a study that evaluated residual material in a suspected PEDV contaminated feed bin, CT values between 19.5 and 22.2 were determined [16]. When using a calibration curve obtained from the University of Minnesota and published by Alonso et al. (2014), this amount of virus is equivalent to 8.9 to 9.2 log copies of RNA/g [27]. In this potential scenario, the maximum log reduction (3.9 log) achieved by thermal processing alone, would not be enough to completely inactivate the virus found in the feces of infected animals, and would have the potential to be transmitted via feed during a PEDV outbreak. If this scenario represents the reality, a new approach is needed that is able to achieve a greater reduction. A hurdle approach (combining multiple processing steps) may be needed to achieve the desired

virus reduction. The use of eBeam irradiation, antimicrobials, and organic acids has been effective in reducing PEDV concentration in feed [17]. If these treatments are combined with a thermal processing as described in this study, an overall increase on virus inactivation will be expected.

Conclusions

Complete feed, vitamin-trace mineral premix, and feed ingredients are potential biosecurity risk factors in the widespread of PEDV to pork production facilities around the world if they become contaminated. The results of this study indicate that there are no differences in virus survival among complete feed, premix, and ingredients with different chemical composition when thermally treated at temperatures greater than 70 °C, suggesting that similar processing conditions will be effective to inactivate PEDV across all types of feed materials. A maximum of 4-log reduction was achieved when applying 90 °C for 30 min. PEDV inactivation kinetics (delta values) did not differ among surfaces tested, which indicated that all surfaces have the same relative risk of PEDV transmission.

Abbreviations
CPE: Cytopathic effects; DMEM: Dulbecco's Modified Eagle Medium; PEDV: Porcine Epidemic Diarrhea Virus; SDPP: Spray dried porcine plasma; $TCID_{50}$: Median Tissue Culture Infectious Dose

Acknowledgements
The authors would like to acknowledge Jonathon Erber for his assistance with data collection.

Funding
This study was funded by the National Pork Board. The funding source was not involved in the design of the study and collection, analysis, and interpretation of data or in writing the manuscript.

Authors' contributions
MPT data collection, statistical analysis, draft of manuscript. HV study design and data collection. FS statistical analysis and support drafting manuscript. PEU study design, statistical analysis and support drafting manuscript. GCS study design and support drafting manuscript. SMG study design, data collection, support drafting manuscript. All authors read and approved the final manuscript.

Competing interests
The authors declare that they have no competing interests.

Author details
[1]Department of Animal Science, University of Minnesota, 1988 Fitch Ave, Falcon Heights, MN 55108, USA. [2]Veterinary Population Medicine, University of Minnesota, 1365 Gortner Avenue, St. Paul, MN 55108, USA.

References

1. Stevenson GW, Hoang H, Schwartz KJ, Burrough EB, Sun D, Madson D, et al. Emergence of porcine epidemic diarrhea virus in the United States: clinical signs, lesions, and viral genomic sequences. J Vet Diagn Investig. 2013;25: 649–54.
2. Pensaert MB, de Bouck P. A new coronavirus-like particle associated with diarrhea in swine. Arch Virol. 1978;58:243–7. doi:10.1007/BF01317606.
3. Song D, Park B. Porcine epidemic diarrhoea virus: a comprehensive review of molecular epidemiology, diagnosis, and vaccines. Virus Genes. 2012;44: 167–75.
4. Bowman AS, Krogwold RA, Price T, Davis M, Moeller SJ. Investigating the introduction of porcine epidemic diarrhea virus into an Ohio swine operation. BMC Vet Res. 2015;11:38.
5. Dee S, Neill C, Clement T, Singrey A, Christopher-hennings J, Nelson E. An evaluation of porcine epidemic diarrhea virus survival in individual feed ingredients in the presence or absence of a liquid antimicrobial. Porc Heal Manag. 2015:1–10. doi:10.1186/s40813-015-0003-0.
6. Gerber PF, Xiao CT, Chen Q, Zhang J, Halbur PG, Opriessnig T. The spray-drying process is sufficient to inactivate infectious porcine epidemic diarrhea virus in plasma. Vet Microbiol. 2014;174:86–92.
7. Pujols J, Segales J. Survivability of porcine epidemic diarrhea virus (PEDV) in bovine plasma submitted to spray drying processing and held at different time by temperature storage conditions. Vet Microbiol. 2014;174:427–32.
8. Cochrane RA, Schumacher LL, Dritz SS, Woodworth JC. Effect of pelleting on survival of porcine epidemic diarrhea virus – contaminated feed 1. J Anim Sci. 2017;95:1170–8.
9. Schumacher LL, Cochrane RA, Evans CE, Kalivoda JR, Woodworth JC, Stark CR, et al. Evaluating the effect of manufacturing Porcine Epidemic Diarrhea Virus (PEDV) -contaminated feed on subsequent feed mill environmental surface contamination evaluating the effect of manufacturing porcine epidemic diarrhea virus. Kansas Agric Exp Stn Res Rep. 2015;1:4.
10. Huss AR, Schumacher LL, Cochrane RA, Poulsen E, Bai J, Woodworth JC, et al. Elimination of porcine epidemic diarrhea virus in an animal feed manufacturing facility. PLoS One. 2017;12:e0169612.
11. Schumacher LL, Cochrane RA, Woodworth JC, Stark CR. Utilizing feed sequencing to decrease the risk of Porcine Epidemic Diarrhea Virus (PEDV) cross- contamination during feed manufacturing utilizing feed sequencing to decrease the risk of porcine epidemic. Kansas Agric Exp Stn Res Rep. 2015;1:3.
12. Horwitz W, Latimer GW. Official methods of analysis of AOAC international. Gaithersburg: AOAC International; 2005.
13. Karber G. Fifty percent endpoint calculation. Arch Exp Path Pharmak. 1931; 162:480–7.
14. Mafart P, Couvert O, Gaillard S, Leguerinel I. On calculating sterility in thermal preservation methods : application of the Weibull frequency distribution model. Acta Hortic. 2001;72:107–14. doi:10.1016/S0168-1605(01)00624-9.
15. Geeraerd AH, Valdramidis VP, Van Impe JF. GInaFiT, a freeware tool to assess non-log-linear microbial survivor curves. Int J Food Microbiol. 2005;102:95–105.
16. Dee S, Clement T, Schelkopf A, Nerem J, Knudsen D, Christopher-Hennings J, et al. An evaluation of contaminated complete feed as a vehicle for porcine epidemic diarrhea virus infection of naive pigs following consumption via natural feeding behavior: proof of concept. BMC Vet Res. 2014;10:176.
17. Trudeau MP, Verma H, Sampedro F, Urriola PE, Shurson GC, McKelvey J, et al. Comparison of thermal and non-thermal processing of swine feed and the use of selected feed additives on inactivation of Porcine Epidemic Diarrhea Virus (PEDV). PLoS One. 2016;11:e0158128.
18. Quist-rybachuk GV, Nauwynck HJ, Kalmar ID. Sensitivity of porcine epidemic diarrhea virus (PEDV) to pH and heat treatment in the presence or absence of porcine plasma. Vet Microbiol. 2015;181:283–8. doi:10.1016/j.vetmic.2015.10.010.
19. Hofmann M, Wyler R. Quantitation, biological and physicochemical properties of cell culture-adapted porcine epidemic diarrhea coronavirus (PEDV). Vet Microbiol. 1989;20:131–42. doi:10.1016/0378-1135(89)90036-9.
20. Thomas P, Karriker LA, Ramirez A, Zhang J, Ellingson JS, Holtkamp DJ. Methods for inactivating PEDV in hog trailers. In: Twenty-second annual swine disease conference for swine Parctitioners; 2014. p. 43–50.
21. Casanova LM, Jeon S, Rutala WA, Weber DJ, Sobsey MD. Effects of air temperature and relative humidity on coronavirus survival on surfaces. Appl Environ Microbiol. 2010;76:2712–7.
22. Organization WH, Organization WH. First data on stability and resistance of SARS coronavirus compiled by members of WHO laboratory network. Geneva. http://www.who.int/csr/sars/survival_2003_05_04/en/index.html: World Heal Organ; 2003.
23. Rabenau HF, Cinatl J, Morgenstern B, Bauer G, Preiser W, Doerr HW. Stability and inactivation of SARS coronavirus. Med Microbiol Immunol. 2005;194:1–6.
24. Chan KH, Peiris JS, Lam SY, Poon LL, Yuen KY, Seto WH. The effects of temperature and relative humidity on the viability of the SARS coronavirus. Adv Virol. 2011;2011:734690.
25. Bean B, Moore BM, Sterner B, Peterson LR, Gerding DN, Balfour HH Jr. Survival of influenza viruses on environmental surfaces. J Infect Dis. 1982; 146:47–51.
26. Blachere FM, Lindsley WG, Pearce TA, Anderson SE, Fisher M, Khakoo R, et al. Measurement of airborne influenza virus in a hospital emergency department. Clin Infect Dis. 2009;48:438–40.
27. Alonso C, Goede DP, Morrison RB, Davies PR, Rovira A, Marthaler DG. Evidence of infectivity of airborne porcine epidemic diarrhea virus and detection of airborne viral RNA at long distances from infected herds. Vet Res. 2014;45:1–5.

5

Effectiveness of composting as a biosecure disposal method for porcine epidemic diarrhea virus (PEDV)-infected pig carcasses

Sarah Vitosh-Sillman[1*], John Dustin Loy[1], Bruce Brodersen[1], Clayton Kelling[1], Kent Eskridge[2] and Amy Millmier Schmidt[3]

Abstract

Background: Porcine epidemic diarrhea virus (PEDV) is an enteric disease of swine that has emerged as a worldwide threat to swine herd health and production. Substantial research has been conducted to assess viability of the virus on surfaces of vehicles and equipment, in feed and water, and on production building surfaces, but little is known about the persistence in PEDV-infected carcasses and effective disposal methods thereof. This study was conducted to quantify the persistence of PEDV RNA via quantitative real-time reverse transcription polymerase chain reaction (qRT-PCR) at various time-temperature combinations and in infected piglet carcasses subjected to composting. Although this method does not distinguish between infectious and noninfectious virus, it is a rapid and sensitive test to evaluate materials for evidence of virus genome.

Results: In the first study, PEDV was suspended in cell culture media at 1×10^5 TCID50 per sample (1 mL sample size) and subjected to various time and temperature combinations in triplicate including temperatures of 37, 45, 50, 55, 60, 65, 70 °C and exposure times of 0, 1, 2, 3, 4, 5, 7, and 14 days. At all temperatures, viral RNA copies declined over time, with the decline most marked and rapid at 65 and 70 °C. Detectable RNA did persist throughout the trial in all but the most extreme condition, where two of three samples incubated at 70 °C yielded undetectable viral RNA after 14 days. In the second study, PEDV-infected piglet carcasses were subjected to two cycles of composting lasting 36 and 37 days, respectively, for a total compost time of 73 days. Composting was performed in triplicate windrow sections housed inside biosecure, climate-controlled rooms using insulated bins designed to represent a continuous windrow compost pile. Temperatures reached 35–57 °C for 26 days of cycle 1 and 35–45 °C for 3 days of cycle 2. Samples consisting of carbon material with or without decomposed tissue as available per sample site collected at ten locations throughout the cross-section of each windrow section following the primary and secondary compost cycles yielded no detectable viral RNA.

Conclusions: Composting appears to be an effective disposal method for PEDV-infected piglet carcasses under the conditions examined. The combination of time and high temperature of the compost cycle effectively degraded viral RNA in cell culture media that should provide optimum stability. Complex compost material matrices collected from windrow sections yielded undetectable PEDV RNA by qRT-PCR after one 36-day compost cycle despite incomplete decomposition of soft tissue.

Keywords: Porcine epidemic diarrhea virus, Composting, Temperature, Mortality, Carcass disposal

---

* Correspondence: sarah.vitosh@unl.edu
[1]School of Veterinary Medicine and Biomedical Sciences, University of Nebraska-Lincoln, Fair Street and East Campus Loop, Lincoln, NE 68583, USA
Full list of author information is available at the end of the article

Background

Porcine epidemic diarrhea virus (PEDV), an RNA virus of the family *Coronaviridae*, genus *Alphacoronavirus*, causes an economically devastating enteric disease of swine [1]. The virus can infect all ages of swine and is characterized by clinical disease of watery diarrhea, vomiting, and dehydration, with high morbidity and mortality – often near 100% – in naïve suckling piglets [2]. In May 2013, PEDV was detected in outbreaks of porcine diarrhea in Iowa, United States, and quickly spread to over half of the states in the U.S. and subsequently to Canada [3, 4]. Prior to this outbreak, cases of PEDV infection had been limited to Europe and Asia [5]. Extensive investigation into how PEDV arrived in the U.S. and quickly disseminated throughout the swine industry has implicated PEDV-contaminated feed or feed ingredients as the potential origin of virus introduction [6–9]. A comprehensive root cause investigation report organized by the United States Department of Agriculture (USDA) identified flexible intermediate bulk containers, commonly used to transport feed ingredients, as the most likely source of PEDV introduction to the country [10]. These findings demonstrate the critical need to understand PEDV persistence in multiple complex matrices, including those in the environment, so that transmission of the disease can be prevented.

With nearly 100% mortality in pre-weaned piglets, the large number of carcasses and volume of infectious material generated during PEDV outbreaks was substantial. Proven, biosecure methods for carcass disposal are sought to control on-farm virus proliferation and limit site-to-site transmission. Major mortality disposal methods available to swine producers in the U.S. include rendering, incineration, burial, land-filling, and composting [11]. Although composting is widely accepted in the U.S. and Canada, it is not legally permitted for swine producers in the European Union, which are primarily limited to the methods of rendering and incineration [12]. Composting requires relatively low input costs, poses little environmental risk when properly designed and managed, and offers greater biosecurity than methods involving transport of infected carcasses beyond the farm boundary. Furthermore, in situations of disease-associated mortalities, composting is capable of inactivating the pathogen of concern when the system is managed to achieve and maintain pile temperature targets. Several studies have demonstrated this concept with carcasses and manure from virus-infected animals. Windrow-composted poultry manure from Newcastle disease virus (NDV)-infected birds was found to be free of detectable virus by virus isolation [13]. Avian influenza (AI) and NDV were inactivated following 7 days of composting at temperatures reaching 50–65 °C [14]. Compost piles containing AI-infected chicken carcasses were determined AI-negative by virus isolation after

10 days [15]. Pseudorabies virus-infected pig carcasses composted at temperatures that reached 27 to 51 °C contained undetectable virus by isolation techniques in samples collected at days 7 and 14, and compost samples collected after 35 days of composting were negative via bioassay conducted on naïve exposed sentinel pigs [16]. For pig carcasses infected with foot-and-mouth disease (FMD) virus, a more environmentally stable non-enveloped virus than those previously discussed, compost pile temperatures reaching 50 °C at 10 days of composting was successful at virus inactivation [17]. Given these demonstrated successes, the USDA published guidance to promote composting as a disposal method for birds infected by highly pathogenic AI in response to outbreaks of this disease in 2016 [18]. Overall, composting has been proven effective for managing important viral pathogens in animal production waste products by multiple testing modalities and may also be a biosecure on-farm disposal method for use by swine producers to control PEDV transmission.

PEDV is an enveloped virus that is demonstrably sensitive to a variety of disinfectants, extremes of pH, and elevated temperature [19, 20]. Therefore, exposing PEDV-infected dead animals to the elevated temperatures during routine composting may be an effective method of virus elimination. The present study was performed to evaluate the persistence of PEDV RNA with qRT-PCR in matrices and temperature conditions representative of composting in order to determine the potential effectiveness of this method for PEDV mortality disposal. The study consisted of two trials: a laboratory phase examining the rate of virus RNA degradation under a controlled application of time and temperature combinations in physiologic media; and a composting phase where PEDV-infected piglet carcasses were incorporated into compost windrow sections and monitored for temperature and virus degradation over two composting cycles.

Results

Time-temperature trial qRT-PCR

PEDV RNA was detectable at all time and temperature combinations tested, except for two of three samples on day 14 at 70 °C. Viral RNA reduction kinetics varied greatly among temperature treatments; however, the rate of reduction peaked after the initial days of temperature treatments above 37 °C and then slowed (Table 1). This is reflected by the increase in mean quantification cycle (Cq) of the qRT-PCR over time, which corresponds with a reduction in RNA targets in the sample (Fig. 1). At 37 °C, viral RNA steadily degraded at an average rate of 0.29 log per day throughout the temperature treatment. The amount of viral RNA detected from day 1 to 7 at 37 °C was significantly different from all other temperature treatments on those days. At 45 °C, viral

Table 1 Summary of time-temperature trial qRT-PCR assay results as RNA copy equivalents

Days	qRT-PCR mean log RNA copies/mL (± SD)						
	37 °C	45 °C	50 °C	55 °C	60 °C	65 °C	70 °C
0	8.57 (0.02)	8.43 (0.02)	8.40 (0.08)	8.44 (0.03)	8.41 (0.08)	8.41 (0.11)	8.57 (0.36)
1	8.45 (0.05)	7.53 (0.04)	6.58 (0.32)	5.53 (0.15)	4.69 (0.11)	4.58 (0.51)	4.67 (0.12)
2	8.26 (0.03)	6.27 (0.42)	4.67 (0.10)	4.85 (0.25)	4.83 (0.02)	4.41 (0.60)	4.35 (0.12)
3	7.85 (0.09)	5.25 (0.08)	4.91 (0.06)	4.85 (0.13)	5.03 (0.08)	4.37 (0.08)	3.81 (0.40)
4	7.64 (0.19)	4.43 (0.11)	4.56 (0.19)	4.89 (0.07)	5.16 (0.06)	4.65 (0.32)	3.79 (0.48)
5	7.48 (0.11)	4.43 (0.17)	4.69 (0.11)	4.79 (0.31)	4.60 (0.06)	4.34 (0.05)	3.58 (0.09)
7	6.02 (0.06)	5.16 (0.75)	5.27 (0.19)	4.69 (0.82)	5.09 (0.28)	3.91 (0.18)	3.13 (0.07)
14	4.55 (0.22)	4.43 (0.50)	5.21 (0.05)	4.83 (0.05)	4.41 (0.09)	3.16 (0.65)	0.78 (0.13)[a]

[a]2 of 3 samples negative (below detection limit of 8.8 RNA copies per reaction)

RNA reduction was more rapid from days 0 to 4 (average 1 log reduction per day) with no mean log change thereafter. The 50 °C treatment yielded a mean rate of RNA reduction from days 0 to 2 of 1.87 log of RNA per day, but the remainder of time treatment (2 to 14 days) did not reveal further significant decrease of viral RNA. At 55 °C, RNA decreased by 2.91 log during the first day of treatment, 0.68 log during the second day, and remained generally stable from days 2 through 14 with no further significant decrease in RNA. For 60, 65, and 70 °C treatments, viral RNA reduction was greatest – between 3.72 and 3.9 log – in the first day with no difference ($p < .05$) among the temperatures. From 1 to 14 days, viral RNA decreased a total of 0.28, 1.42, and 2.44 log at 60, 65, and 70 °C, respectively. Despite the similar rapid decrease at day 1, the quantity of viral RNA remaining at day 14 was significantly different among all of these high treatment temperatures.

Piglet infection

All piglets exhibited clinical diarrhea by day 3 post-inoculation. On day 5 post-inoculation, which coincided with infection period termination and necropsy, all piglets incorporated into the compost windrow sections displayed a diffusely dilated and thin-walled small intestine with fluidic intestinal content, which was considered consistent with PEDV infection. Microscopically, there was evident atrophic enteritis. All piglets were qRT-PCR positive for PEDV on fecal swab (mean Cq 23.07, range 19.93 to 34.75) and were strongly positive by PEDV immunohistochemistry in the small intestine and mesenteric lymph node.

Compost pile temperature performance

Despite prior testing of temperature loggers under prolonged high temperature and moisture conditions, the majority of the loggers failed early in the composting process for both compost cycles. The temperature loggers were not monitored continuously, nor were they periodically checked throughout the trial for function, to avoid disturbing their position, so the failure was not realized until the end of the trial. To ensure robust data collection, manual temperature monitoring was also performed and temperatures recorded throughout both

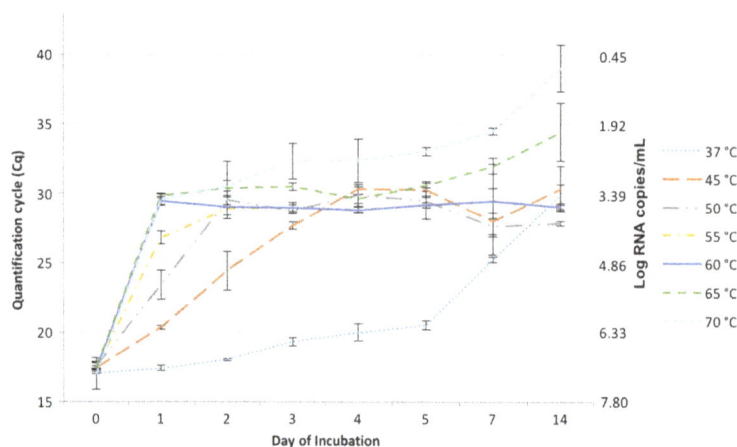

Fig. 1 Mean (*n* = 3) quantification cycle and RNA concentration over time by treatment. Error bars represent SD

compost cycles. Prior to failure during compost cycle 1, temperatures of 45 to 58 °C were recorded at the core of each compost windrow section. Mean manually recorded temperatures of windrow sections for cycles 1 and 2 are illustrated in Figs. 2 and 3, respectively. Manual temperature monitoring throughout the duration of each compost cycle revealed that mean windrow section temperatures of at least 40 °C (104 °F) were sustained for at least 14 d at all points monitored during cycle 1, while a mean temperature of at least 50 °C (122 °F) was sustained for 9 d at point 1 during cycle 1. During cycle 2, a mean temperature of 40 °C (104 °F) was achieved at points 2 and 3 for approximately 3 d, while 50 °C (122 °F) was not attained for any of the monitoring points in the windrow sections.

Using the EPA 503b rule as the criteria for determining successful composting of the carcasses for microbial reductions, benchmarks of 40 °C for 120 h (5 d) and 55 °C for 4 h must be achieved [21]. From the data presented, windrow sections achieved the benchmark of 40 °C for at least 120 h during compost cycle 1, but only the core of the windrow sections achieved 55 °C for greater than 4 h. During compost cycle 2, points 2 and 3 reached a mean temperature of 40 °C for approximately 72 h, which falls short of the EPA 503b rule criteria by 48 h, while no points achieved the benchmark of 55 °C for 4 h.

Detection of PEDV RNA in mortality composting pile

PEDV RNA was not detected by qRT-PCR in any of the compost samples collected following the first or second compost cycles.

Discussion

Elimination of PEDV RNA in composted pig carcasses achieved in this study is comparable to others demonstrating genomic RNA degradation in viruses directly subjected to composting, although experimental conditions may vary considerably. AI- and NDV-spiked chicken litter composted at temperatures reaching 50–65 °C were void of detectable viral RNA in 10 days [14]. For FMD virus associated with infected pig carcasses, composting at temperatures reaching 50–70 °C for several days was able to degrade viral RNA below RRT-PCR detection by day 21 [17]. FMD, a non-enveloped virus, is likely more environmentally persistent and resistant to organic solvents than enveloped viruses such as AI, NDV, and PEDV [22]. Therefore, the absence of detectable PEDV RNA in samples from the end of the first compost cycle at day 36 in this study is consistent with previous reports and is a reasonable result considering the variable physical properties of viruses. One problem with making a direct comparison between studies is differences in compost pile temperatures, especially when time and temperature treatment is presumed to be a vital component of pathogen destruction. The compost windrow sections in this study did not consistently achieve published compost temperature benchmarks or comparable maximum temperatures, as a mean temperature of 55 °C for 4 h was only achieved at the core of the windrow sections during cycle 1. While the temperature profile of compost piles does affect the rate of decomposition and pathogen inactivation, virus degradation in compost material has also been shown to partly rely on factors other than temperature, such as microbial activity. AI and NDV in sealed vials subjected to composting were detected by RRT-PCR at the end of testing on day 21,

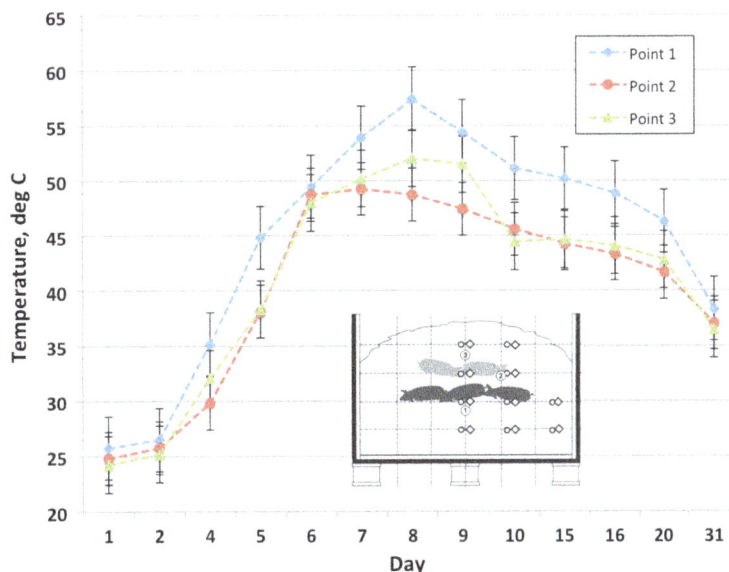

Fig. 2 Mean (n = 3) manually recorded temperatures of compost windrow sections during compost cycle 1

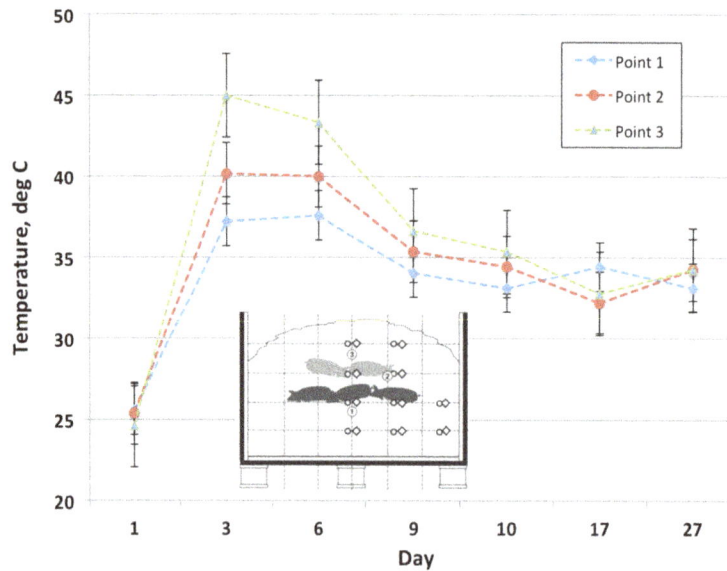

Fig. 3 Mean (n = 3) manually recorded temperatures of compost windrow sections during compost cycle 2

whereas the viruses spiked into chicken manure, used litter, feed, and a homogenate of virus-infected embryonated chicken eggs contained in mesh bags and composted were not detectable by day 10 [14]. In the same experiment, virus-inoculated embryonated chicken eggs that remained intact during composting contained detectable viral RNA, but RNA had degraded beyond detection in those that were crushed. Similarly, with virus survival, another study where NDV and avian encephalomyelitis virus (AEV) were composted in sealed vials or permeable cassettes demonstrated markedly reduced virus survival within the cassettes [23]. NDV in cassettes survived no more than 7 days, while the virus in vials survived up to 28 days. Likewise, AEV in cassettes was inactivated in about 7 days, while the vials contained infectious virus for at least 49 days. Therefore, the exposure of viruses to the complex microbial environment and decomposition by-products of compost is associated with accelerated pathogen destruction beyond the effects of temperature. Because the compost windrow sections of the current study were relatively small and constructed of wood shavings and piglet carcasses without the addition of other carbon and nitrogen sources, microbial activity or temperatures comparable to what would be expected for on-farm mortality compost piles were not able to be sustained. Even under less than ideal composting conditions, PEDV appears to be sufficiently susceptible to composting conditions and comparable to other tested viruses.

The time-temperature trial was designed to examine the effect of temperature on virus persistence in cell culture medium, an optimum environment to test virus stability. Initially, this also included re-isolation of the virus following treatments. PEDV was completely inactivated at the lowest temperature treatment, 37 °C, by 24 h;

therefore virus isolation following higher temperature treatments was not performed. Comparable experiments showed cell culture PEDV in virus media was completely inactivated when exposed to ≥60 °C for 30 min [20]. Infectivity was reduced to 0.05% of the original value when heated to 50 °C for 3 h, indicating rapid inactivation at high temperatures [20]. At 37 °C, PEDV retained infectivity after incubation for 6 h, but only at pH 6 to 8 [20]. Although pH was not monitored over the duration of the current trial, the initial pH of virus media was about 7.75, which was within the stable pH range. The upper 95% confidence level of the time required to inactivate 8 $\log_{10}$ TCID50 PEDV/mL matrix for minimal essential media, pH 7.2, and temperature 40 °C was 21.7 h [24]. The presence of plasma and alkalinization of the sample potentiated thermal inactivation. Therefore, the inactivation of PEDV under the conditions tested is comparable to other results.

Persistence of PEDV RNA has been tested in many matrices, such as feed, plasma, and manure. Consistently, low temperatures promote virus survival and long-term PCR detection of PEDV RNA, while high temperatures rapidly degrade PEDV. This may explain in part, the seasonal increase in PEDV cases that has been observed during the winter months in the United States following introduction [25]. Additionally, the persistence of PEDV RNA has been reported in open earthen manure storages for up to 9 months where environmental temperatures tend to be lower (−30 to 23 °C) [26]. In controlled laboratory studies, PEDV-spiked manure slurry stored at 25, 4, and −20 °C and PEDV-spiked feed slurry or dry feed maintained at room temperature (about 25 °C) contained RNA for at least 28 days [27]. PEDV-spiked spray-dried bovine plasma contained detectable RNA for at least 21 days at a temperature of 4 °C, although the virus survived less 7 days 22 °C [28]. PEDV-spiked fresh feces exposed to 50 and 60 °C temperatures over a range of relative humidity contained detectable virus RNA up to 7 and 3 days, respectively [27]. The time-temperature trial conducted in this study demonstrated that PEDV RNA persisted in sterile virus media for at least 14 days at temperatures of 37 to 65 °C and was degraded to an undetectable concentration at 70 °C in two of three samples. Compared to those results for PEDV-spiked fresh feces exposed to 50 and 60 °C, this indicates that the complex matrix of manure at high temperatures more effectively degrades RNA. From 37 to 60 °C, the average Cq of media at 14 days was about 30; not a significant difference despite clearly different treatment. RNA was often relatively stable in these treatments after an initial decrease in the first time points. While temperature may provide for virus inactivation and significant RNA decrease in a sterile environment, microbial or enzymatic factors are thought to promote elimination from manure and compost. This provides data to support field observations that while many environmental samples may be positive for PED RNA by qRT-PCR, this detection does not necessarily translate to the presence of infectious virus as RNA is likely detectable for an extended period of time even at elevated temperatures [26].

While this study evaluated outcomes with qRT-PCR, there are limitations of testing for viral RNA. The presence of PEDV RNA does not indicate the presence of infectious virus, which could be detected by cell culture isolation or bioassay techniques. The application of viability PCR has also shown promise in distinguishing infectious and noninfectious viruses in matrices such as water and swine manure, although PEDV has not been tested with this method and studies of virus detection in complex environmental samples, such as manure, are few [29, 30]. However, this may provide a potential method to distinguish this in future studies. In the current study, it is presumed the absence of viral RNA indicates complete destruction of the virus by composting. Extracting virus from compost and PCR techniques both have a limit of sensitivity. The lowest infectious dose of PEDV in feed has been estimated at 5.6×10^1 TCID50/g, well below the detectable limit of virus in this study [31]. While data regarding PEDV persistence in various matrices exposed to high temperature and microbial activity comparable to composting indicates it is readily inactivated, further confirmation could be provided by bioassay in piglets with composted materials.

Conclusions

Composting appears to be an effective disposal method for PEDV-infected piglet carcasses under the conditions

examined. The combination of time and high temperature representative of the compost cycle has been shown to effectively degrade viral RNA in cell culture media, a matrix that promotes stability. Windrow sections achieved a benchmark mean temperature of 55 °C for 4 h at the core during compost cycle 1, which was successful at degrading PEDV RNA. Standard benchmark temperatures for composting also include 40 °C for 120 h and 55 °C for 4 h at all points within the windrow sections during compost cycle 2, which are above the maximum temperatures achieved in this study experimentally. Because these experimental compost windrow sections were constructed of fresh wood shavings and piglet carcasses without the addition of other carbon and nitrogen sources that can improve pile conditions to promote microbial activity, and because these windrow sections were considerably smaller than field-scale compost windrows or piles, temperatures in on-farm animal carcass compost piles commonly achieve and sustain target temperatures much more readily. The complex compost material matrices from experimental compost windrow sections did not contain detectable PEDV RNA by qRT-PCR after one 36-d compost cycle, which supports the premise that greater temperatures sustained for longer periods during on-farm composting will provide effective biosecure disposal of PEDV-infected carcasses. Given our findings of both time and temperature incubations and experimental scale composting, these support the use of on farm composting for virus mitigation on farms.

Methods

Time-temperature trial

PEDV propagation and quantification

Vero cells were maintained in minimal essential media (MEM) containing 10% fetal bovine serum (FBS) and 100 μg/mL gentamicin. Two-day-old confluent monolayers of Vero cells in 150 cm² flasks were washed two times with MEM containing 2 μg/mL L-(tosylamido-2-phenyl) ethyl chloromethyl ketone (TPCK)-treated trypsin prior to inoculation. Monolayers were infected at approximately 0.01 multiplicity of infection (MOI) of PEDV (USA/Colorado/2013, GenBank accession no. KF272920) in MEM containing 2 μg/mL TPCK-treated trypsin, and incubated at 37 °C until maximum cytopathic effect (CPE) (48 to 96 h). Flasks were cycled through two brief freeze-thaw cycles and stored at –80 °C until further processing. For purification, frozen flasks were thawed and the contents centrifuged at 2000 x g for 10 min. The media supernatant was collected, pooled, mixed, and divided into aliquots that were stored at –80 °C until needed.

The PEDV virus material was assessed for the quantity of infectious virus particles. The sample was diluted in MEM TPCK-treated trypsin at 1:10 (10^{-1}) and ten-fold serially diluted to 10^{-8}. Prepared two-day-old confluent monolayers of Vero cells in 96-well plates were washed two times with MEM TPCK-treated trypsin. For each diluted sample, 50 μL was added to eight wells. The plates were incubated for 72 h at 37 °C and then fixed with 50% methanol-50% acetone for 10 min. The plates were stained with PEDV monoclonal antibody SD6 ascites (Medgene, Brookings, SD, U.S.) for 30 min at 37 °C, washed with PBS 2×, stained with anti-mouse IgG-FITC (Sigma-Aldrich Inc., St. Louis, MO, U.S.), and washed 2× to allow for visualization of infected cells. Stock virus TCID50/mL was determined by using standard Reed and Muench method [32] and was diluted to the elected TCID50/mL for each respective experiment.

Application of treatments
The trial was constructed with combinations of 37, 45, 50, 55, 60, 65, 70 °C and exposure times of 0, 1, 2, 3, 4, 5, 7, and 14 days, with three vials (replicates) of virus sample for each time-temperature treatment. Each virus sample was allocated into a sealed 1.5 mL sterile conical vial (Midsci, St. Louis, MO, U.S.) at a volume of 1 mL and was comprised of 1×10^5 TCID50 of cell-culture propagated PEDV in MEM containing 2 μg/mL TPCK-treated trypsin, 10% FBS, and 100 μg/mL gentamicin. The temperature treatment was performed in an incubator (Heratherm General Protocol Incubator, Thermo Fisher Scientific, Waltham, MA, U.S.) and monitored for temperature consistency throughout the trial. Following treatment, the vials were transferred to –80 °C for storage until qRT-PCR.

For times 0 and 1 day, virus isolation was completed using 500 μL of the treated sample. The virus sample was concentrated by centrifugation at 100,000 x g for 1 h at 4 °C (Beckman Coulter Optima L-90 K Ultracentrifuge, Brea, CA, U.S.) and the pellet re-suspended in 500 μL of MEM containing 2 μg/mL TPCK-treated trypsin. For each sample, 50 μL was added to eight wells of a 96-well plate containing 2-day-old Vero cells which had been washed two times with MEM TPCK-treated trypsin. After 3 days of incubation at 37 °C, the cells were fixed and indirect fluorescence performed with PEDV monoclonal antibody as previously described to classify as PEDV positive or negative.

Extraction of RNA
Time-temperature trial samples diluted 1:2 (to conserve sample) and rectal swabs eluted into MEM containing 100 μg/mL gentamicin were subjected to qRT-PCR analysis. For viral RNA extraction, 250 μL of each sample was aliquoted into a tube and extracted using a viral RNA isolation kit (TRIzol, Invitrogen, Carlsbad, CA, U.S.) according to the manufacturer's instructions, with the addition of 2 μL RNase-free glycogen to the aqueous phase. At least one negative extraction control consisting of all reagents

and normal horse serum was included in each extraction. RNA pellets were reconstituted in 20 μL RNase-free water and stored at –20 °C until PCR.

Quantitative real time reverse-transcription PCR
Reagents for the PEDV qRT-PCR assay were obtained from a commercially available reaction kit (QIAGEN One Step RT-PCR reagent kit; QIAGEN, Valencia, CA, U.S.), with the addition of magnesium (Sigma-Aldrich Inc., St. Louis, MO, U.S.). The PEDV primers and probes were developed according to a previously published method [33] and ordered from a commercial supplier (IDT, Iowa City, IA, U.S.). The RT-PCR reaction mix consisted of 5 μL 5× Reaction Buffer, 1 μL nucleotide triphosphates, 2 μL of 25 μM/mL $MgCl_2$, 5 μL nuclease-free water, 2 μL PEDV forward and reverse primers (10 μM each), 1 μL PEDV HEX-labeled probe (5 μM), 1 μL One Step RT-PCR Enzyme mix, and 8 μL extracted RNA. Each RT-PCR sample was analyzed on a Cepheid Smart Cycler Detection System (Cepheid, Sunnyvale, CA, U.S.) under the following conditions: 50 °C for 30 min; 95 °C for 15 min; and 45 cycles of 94 °C for 30 s, 60 °C for 60 s with optics on, and 72 °C for 30 s. Validated PCR positive controls consisting of PEDV RNA and negative extraction controls were included in each run. Samples were considered positive if the mean fluorescence exceeded 30 fluorescent units prior to 40 cycles and negative and positive PCR controls were properly classified.

PCR quantification
The amplified PEDV RT-PCR cDNA product was cloned using a commercial kit according to the manufacturer's directions using 4 μL of PCR product and the provided vector (TA Cloning Kit with One Shot TOP10 Chemically Competent *E. coli*, pCR™4-TOPO® Vector; Invitrogen, Carlsbad, CA, U.S.). Transformed colonies were selected on lysogeny broth agar plates containing 100 μg/mL ampicillin. The plasmid DNA was purified using a commercial kit (PureLink Quick Plasmid Miniprep Kit; Invitrogen, Carlsbad, CA, U.S.), and DNA was quantified with ultraviolet spectrophotometry (SmartSpec 3000 Spectrophotometer, Bio Rad Laboratories, Hercules, CA, U.S.). Copy number was calculated based on the double-stranded DNA plasmid size of 4154 bp. The nucleic acid concentration equivalent to 8.82×10^{12} copies was utilized for serial dilutions and subsequent qRT-PCR analysis (Fig. 4). Serial dilution of PEDV virus was performed to compare quantification cycle (Cq) values to TCID50/mL equivalents (Fig. 5).

Compost trial
Windrow composting bin construction
Insulated platforms were constructed on wood pallets measuring 121.92 cm (W) × 101.6 cm (L). Internal dimensions of platforms were 121.92 cm (W) × 93.46 (L) cm × 97.53 cm

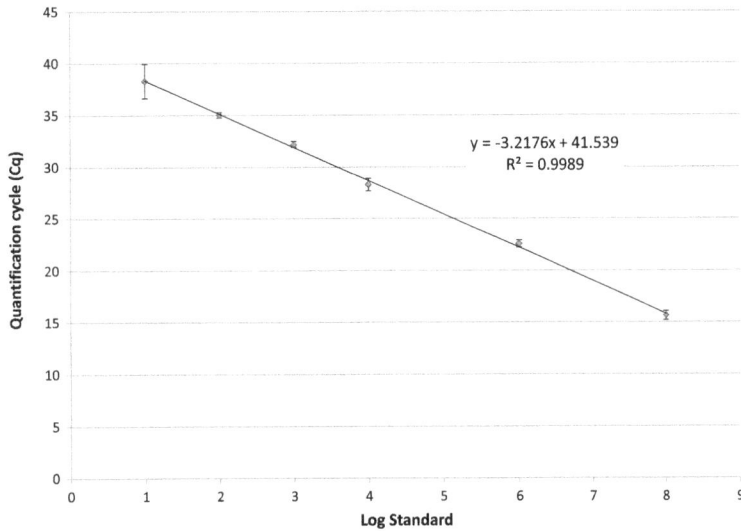

Fig. 4 Log of PEDV standard nucleic acid target (8.82 to 8.82E + 8 copies/reaction). Error bars represent standard deviation

(H) to contain a windrow section (Fig. 6). Platform walls were constructed of an outer layer of plywood (12.7 mm) and an inner layer of non-porous PolyBoard sheeting (4 mm). Foam board insulation (24 mm) was placed between these layers to achieve a composite R-value of 17.3 m^2KW^{-1}. This effort was taken to simulate the linear continuation of the windrow and the insulative properties of a compacted soil base.

Animal infection

This experiment was conducted in a biosecure (ABSL-2) room at the University of Nebraska – Lincoln Life Science Annex. All procedures involving animals were in accordance with the UNL Institutional Animal Care and Use Committee and Institutional Biosafety Committee. Twenty-seven, 21-day-old piglets were acquired from a PEDV-naïve herd and tested negative for PEDV by qRT-PCR via rectal swab on arrival to the facility. The sows from the herd of origin were serologically negative by PEDV indirect immunofluorescence assay (IFA). The piglets were allowed 3 days of acclimation prior to the start of the study and maintained on a commercial diet free of porcine-origin ingredients.

Virus stock and MEM were mixed so that each piglet inoculum was a 5-mL volume containing 1 X 10^6 TCID50 of PEDV. This inoculum was administered to piglets via syringe and gavage needle immediately following dilution.

Piglet testing and necropsy

Fecal swabs were collected at 3 and 5 days post-infection to confirm infection via viral shedding. Rectal swabs eluted

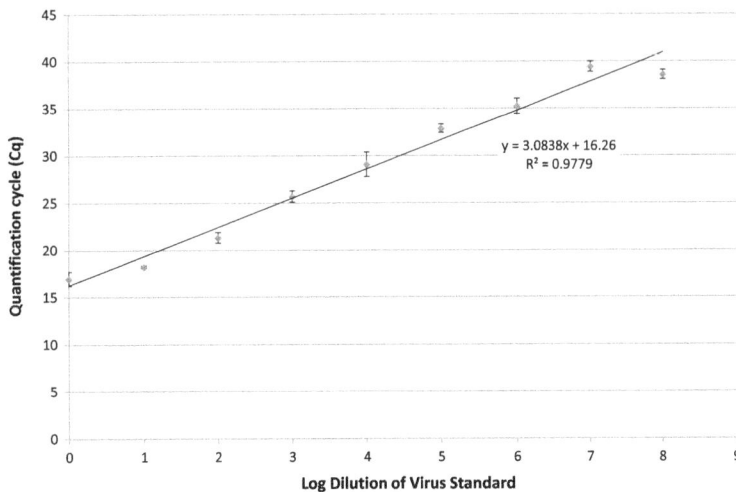

Fig. 5 Log dilution of cell culture propagated PEDV (1.00E + 6 to 1.00E-3 TCID50/mL). Error bars represent standard deviation

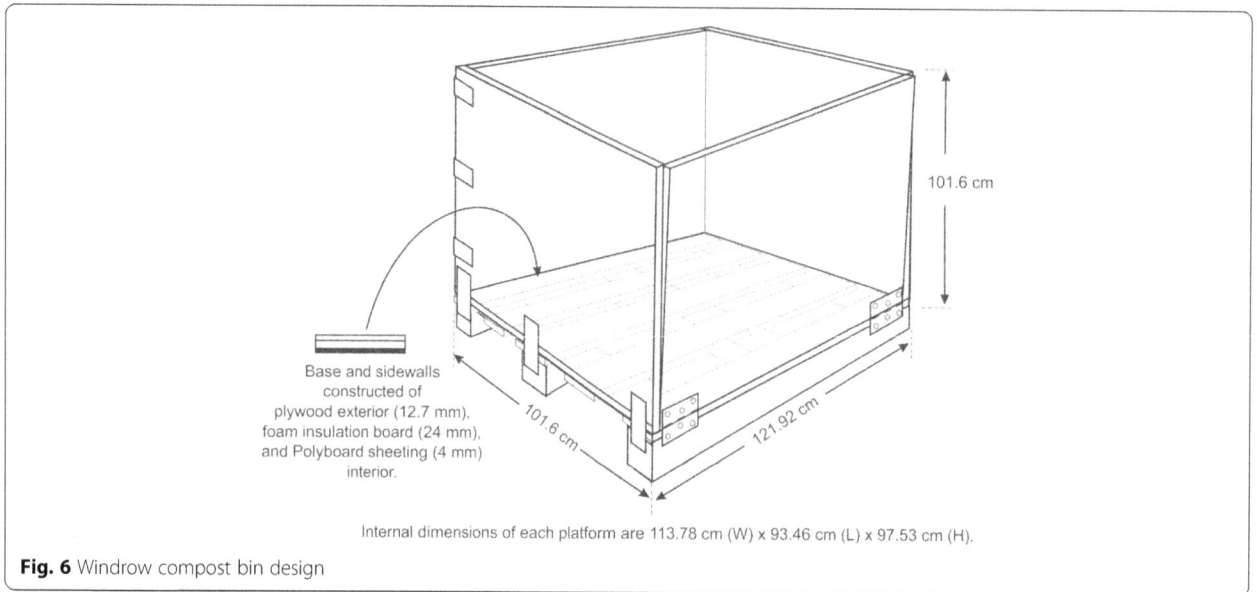

Fig. 6 Windrow compost bin design

into minimal essential media (MEM) containing 100 µg/mL gentamicin were subjected to qRT-PCR analysis.

Humane euthanasia and necropsy were performed on day 5 post-infection. Fresh and formalin fixed tissues were collected, including two segments of jejunum, one segment of ileum, and mesenteric lymph node. The remaining carcass was incorporated into the compost bin housed within the biosecure room.

Compost windrow section construction

Windrow test sections were constructed in an environmentally controlled, biosecurity level 2 room (4.27 m × 3.66 m) at the University of Nebraska-Lincoln Life Sciences Annex,

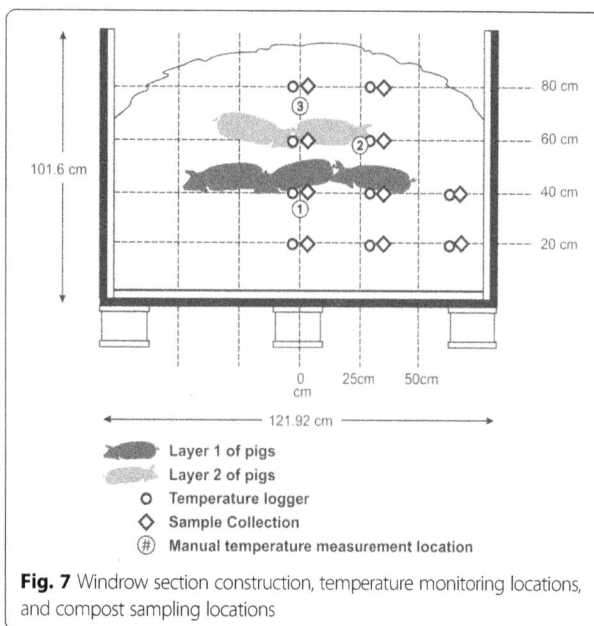

Fig. 7 Windrow section construction, temperature monitoring locations, and compost sampling locations

Lincoln, NE. A single trial was conducted with three windrow test sections. Room conditions were maintained at 16–27 °C and 50–80% relative humidity for the duration of the trial.

Pine wood shavings (Tractor Supply Co., Lincoln, NE, U.S.) were placed in the bottom of each compost bin to a depth of 20 cm and water from a municipal source was added to wet the material to a target moisture content of 55–60% w.b. Construction of each windrow section was accomplished in 20-cm layers to accommodate placement of temperature loggers. Water addition was performed following each layer of construction. Grab samples of carbon material were collected throughout windrow section construction for analysis of actual moisture content. Once a windrow section depth of 40-cm was achieved, 10 cm of shavings were placed in the pile and three animals were placed along the centerline of the windrow section with minimal space between animals (Fig. 7). A 10-cm layer of wood shavings was placed across the entire windrow section and temperature loggers were placed on the surface of this layer. Two additional animals were then placed along the centerline of the windrow section directly over the temperature loggers. At least 30 cm of clearance was maintained between the animals and platform walls for both layers of animals. The second layer of animals was covered with 20 cm of wetted wood shavings followed by an additional 20 cm of dry shavings to cap the sections with a slight mounding shape along the centerline of the windrow.

Compost pile temperature monitoring

Temperature in the windrow sections was measured on a 25-cm × 20-cm spatial grid (Fig. 7) with Apresys Temp Trak Temperature Recorders (Apresys Inc., Duluth, GA, U.S.). Symmetry was assumed along the vertical centerline of the windrow section to minimize the number of spatial sampling locations. Temperatures were recorded on a temporal sampling interval of 20 min throughout each compost cycle. Manual temperature measurements were also collected throughout each compost cycle at three locations in each windrow section (Fig. 7) using a long-handled compost thermometer (REOTEMP Instrument Corp., San Diego, CA, U.S.). The thermometer was inserted and allowed to stabilize for at least 1 min prior to temperatures being recorded.

Windrow management

Two consecutive compost cycles, lasting 36 and 37 d, respectively, were performed. Manual temperature monitoring was conducted regularly (daily during the first week of each compost cycle and at least every 3 days beyond the first week of each cycle) to monitor progression of the compost process. When temperatures failed to increase, or declined, water was added to windrow sections from a municipal source to achieve a damp sponge feel of the carbon material. In response to a slow temperature rise in all windrow sections, 5.5 kg of Roebic compost accelerator (Roebic Laboratories Inc., New Haven, CT, U.S.) was added to each windrow section on day 2 of the first compost cycle. On day 5, 0.4 kg of granular fertilizer (Lesco 18–0-18 fertilizer, Home Depot, Lincoln, NE, U.S.) was added to all windrows to further accelerate microbial activity. To add both the compost accelerator and granular fertilizer, carcasses were carefully uncovered and the products were evenly distributed across the exposed surface. Carbon material was then returned to the original configuration following fertilizer addition. Once manual temperature measurements reflected a sustained temperature of less than 100 °C in all windrows, windrows were disassembled, temperature recorders were retrieved, compost material samples were collected, and windrows were reconstructed following the same protocol described previously to initiate a second compost cycle. During the second compost cycle, temperatures were monitored as previously described and moisture added as needed. As with the first compost cycle, once temperature measurements reflected a sustained temperature of less than 100 °C in all windrows, windrows were disassembled for retrieval of temperature recorders and collection of compost material samples and remaining materials were incinerated.

Compost sample collection and processing

Compost samples were collected at ten locations in each windrow section corresponding to temperature recorder locations (Fig. 7) at the completion of the first and second compost cycles. To collect samples, windrow sections were carefully deconstructed in layers until temperature recorders were exposed. Grab samples of approximately 50 g of compost material consisting of wood and carbon material with or without decomposed tissue as available per sample site were then collected near the location of each temperature recorder and placed into sterile Whirl-pak bags (Nasco, Fort Atkinson, WI, U.S.). A new pair of nitrile exam gloves was worn during each individual sample collection. Samples were stored at −80 °C until testing.

For processing, 20 g of sample was placed into a sterile Whirl-pak bag along with 50 mL of MEM containing 100 µg/mL gentamicin. The bag was closed and subjected to stomacher blending (Stomacher® 400 Circulator; Seward Limited, Worthing, West Sussex, UK) for 2 min at 230 rpm, assuring that all compost material and organic matter had been thoroughly washed with media solution. The supernatant media was separated into a 50-mL conical vial and stored at −80 °C until qRT-PCR. This procedure was demonstrated to reliably detect 3×10^4 TCID50/ g of compost using the same compost material spiked with a known amount of the previously generated cell culture PEDV.

Necropsy tissue analysis

The formalin fixed tissues were routinely processed and embedded in paraffin blocks. The tissues were sectioned at 4 µm, stained with hematoxylin and eosin, and examined with light microscopy. Immunohistochemistry was performed on the same formalin-fixed paraffin-embedded tissues examined histologically. One section was evaluated for each tissue. The sections were cut at 4 µm and applied to slides, which were deparaffinized and stained using an automated immunohistochemical stainer (BenchMark ULTRA; Ventana Medical Systems, Inc., Tucson, AZ, U.S.). The primary antibody consisted of anti-PEDV monoclonal mouse ascites (Medgene, Brookings, SD, U.S.). Positive and negative controls consisted of a slide containing known positive tissue, which was used previously for validating this IHC procedure, along with slides of test samples using an irrelevant antibody: negative mouse serum. After deparaffinization on the immunohistochemistry stainer, the slides were incubated with a cell conditioning solution for 64 min. Primary incubation was for 1 hr at 40 °C. Secondary antibody incubation and staining were conducted with commercial reagents using manufacturer recommended protocols. Tissues were counterstained with hematoxylin for 4 min and coverslipped with glass coverslips. The slides were examined with light microscopy for positive immunoreactivity.

Data analysis

Data analysis was performed using version 9.4 of SAS software package (SAS Institute Inc., Cary, NC, U.S.).

Abbreviations
AEV: avian encephalomyelitis virus; AI: avian influenza; Cq: quantification cycle; FMD: foot-and-mouth disease; NDV: Newcastle disease virus; PEDV: porcine epidemic diarrhea virus; qRT-PCR: quantitative real-time reverse transcription polymerase chain reaction; RRT-PCR: real-time reverse transcriptase polymerase chain reaction; TCID50: 50% tissue culture infective dose; USDA: United States Department of Agriculture

Acknowledgements
The project team wishes to acknowledge Ashley Schmit, undergraduate student researcher, for assistance with piglet necropsies, compost pile management and sample collection, and time-temperature trial sample collections, and Jared Korth, undergraduate student researcher, for construction and assembly of compost bins.

Funding
Funding for this research was provided via Nebraska Pork Producers Association grant #14–239. JDL is supported by USDA Multistate Project NC229.

Authors' contributions
SJV drafted the manuscript and made substantial contributions to project conception and design, acquisition of data, and analysis and interpretation of data; AMS and JDL made substantial contributions to project conception and design, acquisition of grant funds, acquisition of data, analysis and interpretation of data, and were involved in drafting the manuscript and revising it critically for important intellectual content; BWB contributed substantially to acquisition and interpretation of data; CK contributed substantially to project conception and design, and acquisition of data; and KE made substantial contributions to analysis and interpretation of data. All authors read and approved the final manuscript.

Competing interests
JDL, co-author, has served as a consultant for, and thus has disclosed a significant financial interest in, Harrisvaccines, Inc. In accordance with its Conflict of Interest policy, the University of Nebraska-Lincoln's Conflict of Interest in Research Committee has determined that this must be disclosed.

Author details
[1]School of Veterinary Medicine and Biomedical Sciences, University of Nebraska-Lincoln, Fair Street and East Campus Loop, Lincoln, NE 68583, USA. [2]Department of Statistics, University of Nebraska-Lincoln, Lincoln, NE 68583, USA. [3]Department of Biological Systems Engineering and Department of Animal Science, University of Nebraska-Lincoln, Lincoln, NE 68583, USA.

References
1. Alvarez J, Sarradell J, Morrison R, Perez A. Impact of porcine epidemic diarrhea on performance of growing pigs. PLoS One. 2015;10(3):e0120532. doi:10.1371/journal.pone.0120532.
2. Zimmerman JJ. Diseases of swine. 10th ed. Wiley-Blackwell: Chichester, West Sussex; 2012.
3. Stevenson GW, Hoang H, Schwartz KJ, Burrough ER, Sun D, Madson D, et al. Emergence of porcine epidemic diarrhea virus in the United States: clinical signs, lesions, and viral genomic sequences. J Vet Diagn Invest. 2013;25(5): 649–54. doi:10.1177/1040638713501675.
4. Ojkic D, Hazlett M, Fairles J, Marom A, Slavic D, Maxie G, et al. The first case of porcine epidemic diarrhea in Canada. Can Vet J. 2015;56(2):149–52.
5. Song D, Park B. Porcine epidemic diarrhoea virus: a comprehensive review of molecular epidemiology, diagnosis, and vaccines. Virus Genes. 2012;44(2): 167–75. doi:10.1007/s11262-012-0713-1.
6. Bowman AS, Krogwold RA, Price T, Davis M, Moeller SJ. Investigating the introduction of porcine epidemic diarrhea virus into an Ohio swine operation. BMC Vet Res. 2015;11:38. doi:10.1186/s12917-015-0348-2.
7. Dee S, Clement T, Schelkopf A, Nerem J, Knudsen D, Christopher-Hennings J et al. An evaluation of contaminated complete feed as a vehicle for porcine epidemic diarrhea virus infection of naive pigs following consumption via natural feeding behavior: proof of concept. BMC veterinary research. 2014; 10. doi:Artn 176 10.1186/S12917-014-0176-9.
8. Dee S, Neill C, Clement T, Singrey A, Christopher-Hennings J, Nelson E. An evaluation of porcine epidemic diarrhea virus survival in individual feed ingredients in the presence or absence of a liquid antimicrobial. Porcine Health Manag. 2015;1:9. doi:10.1186/s40813-015-0003-0.
9. Dee S, Neill C, Singrey A, Clement T, Cochrane R, Jones C et al. Modeling the transboundary risk of feed ingredients contaminated with porcine epidemic diarrhea virus. BMC veterinary research. 2016;12. doi:ARTN 5110. 1186/s12917-016-0674-z.
10. Scott A, McCluskey B, Brown-Reid M, Grear D, Pitcher P, Ramos G, et al. Porcine epidemic diarrhea virus introduction into the United States: root cause investigation. Prev Vet Med. 2016;123:192–201. doi:10.1016/j. prevetmed.2015.11.013.
11. Schwager M, Baas TJ, Glanville TD, Lorimor J, Lawrence J. Mortality Disposal Analysis. Swine Research Report, 2001. Paper 24. Iowa State University, Ames, IA. 2002. Available at: http://lib.dr.iastate.edu/ swinereports_2001/24.
12. Gwyther CL, Williams AP, Golyshin PN, Edwards-Jones G, Jones DL. The environmental and biosecurity characteristics of livestock carcass disposal methods: a review. Waste Manag. 2011;31(4):767–78. doi:10.1016/j.wasman. 2010.12.005.
13. Kinde H, Utterback W, Takeshita K, McFarland M. Survival of exotic Newcastle disease virus in commercial poultry environment following removal of infected chickens. Avian Dis. 2004;48(3):669–74. doi:10.1637/ 7161-020104R.
14. Guan J, Chan M, Grenier C, Wilkie DC, Brooks BW, Spencer JL. Survival of avian influenza and Newcastle disease viruses in compost and at ambient temperatures based on virus isolation and real-time reverse transcriptase PCR. Avian Dis. 2009;53(1):26–33. doi:10.1637/8381-062008-Reg.1.
15. Senne DA, Panigrahy B, Morgan RL. Effect of composting poultry carcasses on survival of exotic avian viruses: highly pathogenic avian influenza (HPAI) virus and adenovirus of egg drop syndrome-76. Avian Dis. 1994;38(4):733–7.
16. Garcia-Siera JRD, Straw BE, Thacker BJ, Granger LM, Fedorka-Cray PJ, Gray JT. Studies on survival of pseudorabies virus, Actinobacillus pleuropneumoniae, and Salmonella serovar Choleraesuis in composted swine carcasses. J Swine Health Prod. 2001;9(5):225–31.
17. Guan J, Chan M, Grenier C, Brooks BW, Spencer JL, Kranendonk C, et al. Degradation of foot-and-mouth disease virus during composting of infected pig carcasses. Can J Vet Res. 2010;74(1):40–4.
18. Agriculture TUSDo. FY2016 HPAI response: mortality composting protocol for avian influenza infected flocks. 2016.
19. Bowman AS, Nolting JM, Nelson SW, Bliss N, Stull JW, Wang Q, et al. Effects of disinfection on the molecular detection of porcine epidemic diarrhea virus. Vet Microbiol. 2015;179(3–4):213–8. doi:10.1016/j.vetmic.2015.05.027.
20. Hofmann M, Wyler R. Quantitation, biological and physicochemical properties of cell culture-adapted porcine epidemic diarrhea coronavirus (PEDV). Vet Microbiol. 1989;20(2):131–42.
21. USEPA Standards for the Use or Disposal of Sewage Sludge, 40 C.F.R. § 503B. 1993.
22. Maclachlan NJ, Dubovi EJ, ed. Fenner's veterinary virology. 5th ed. Academic Press. Cambridge: United States; 2017.
23. Glanville TD, Ahn HK, Richard TL, Harmon JD, Reynolds DL, Akinc S. Effect of envelope material on biosecurity during emergency bovine mortality composting. Bioresour Technol. 2013;130:543–51. doi:10.1016/j.biortech. 2012.12.035.
24. Quist-Rybachuk GV, Nauwynck HJ, Kalmar ID. Sensitivity of porcine epidemic diarrhea virus (PEDV) to pH and heat treatment in the presence or absence

of porcine plasma. Vet Microbiol. 2015;181(3–4):283–8. doi:10.1016/j.vetmic.2015.10.010.

25. USDA. Swine Enteric Coronavirus Disease (SECD) Situation Report - Mar 30, 2017. Available at: https://www.aphis.usda.gov/aphis/ourfocus/animalhealth/animal-disease-information/swine-disease-information/ct_ped_weekly_sit_report_archive. Accessed 5 Apr 2017.

26. Tun HM, Cai Z, Khafipour E. Monitoring survivability and infectivity of porcine epidemic diarrhea virus (PEDv) in the infected on-farm earthen manure storages (EMS). Front Microbiol. 2016;7:265. doi:10.3389/fmicb.2016.00265.

27. Goyal S. PEDV research updates: Environmental stability of PED (porcine epidemic diarrhea virus). University of Minnesota, US National Pork Board. 2014. Available at: http://www.pork.org/pedv-2013-research/. Accessed 5 May 2017.

28. Pujols J, Segales J. Survivability of porcine epidemic diarrhea virus (PEDV) in bovine plasma submitted to spray drying processing and held at different time by temperature storage conditions. Vet Microbiol. 2014;174(3–4):427–32. doi:10.1016/j.vetmic.2014.10.021.

29. Fongaro G, Hernandez M, Garcia-Gonzalez MC, Barardi CR, Rodriguez-Lazaro D. Propidium Monoazide coupled with PCR predicts infectivity of enteric viruses in swine manure and biofertilized soil. Food Environ Virol. 2016;8(1):79–85. doi:10.1007/s12560-015-9225-1.

30. Parshionikar S, Laseke I, Fout GS. Use of propidium monoazide in reverse transcriptase PCR to distinguish between infectious and noninfectious enteric viruses in water samples. Appl Environ Microbiol. 2010;76(13):4318–26. doi:10.1128/AEM.02800-09.

31. Schumacher LL, Woodworth JC, Jones CK, Chen Q, Zhang J, Gauger PC, et al. Evaluation of the minimum infectious dose of porcine epidemic diarrhea virus in virus-inoculated feed. Am J Vet Res. 2016;77(10):1108–13. doi:10.2460/ajvr.77.10.1108.

32. Reed L, Muench H. A simple method of estimating fifty per cent endpoints. Am J Hyg. 1938;27(3):493–7.

33. Kim SH, Kim IJ, Pyo HM, Tark DS, Song JY, Hyun BH. Multiplex real-time RT-PCR for the simultaneous detection and quantification of transmissible gastroenteritis virus and porcine epidemic diarrhea virus. J Virol Methods. 2007;146(1–2):172–7. doi:10.1016/j.jviromet.2007.06.021.

6

Impact of two mycotoxins deoxynivalenol and fumonisin on pig intestinal health

Alix Pierron[1,2], Imourana Alassane-Kpembi[1] and Isabelle P. Oswald[1*]

Abstract

Mycotoxins are secondary metabolites of fungi that grow on a variety of substrates. Due to their high consumption of cereals and their sensitivity, pigs are highly impacted by the presence of mycotoxins. At the European level, regulations and recommendations exist for several mycotoxins in pig feed. Among these toxins, fumonisin B_1 (FB_1), and deoxynivalenol (DON) have a great impact on the intestine and the immune system. Indeed, the intestine is the first barrier to food contaminants and can be exposed to high concentrations of mycotoxins upon ingestion of contaminated feed. FB_1 and DON alter the intestinal barrier, impair the immune response, reduce feed intake and weight gain. Their presence in feed increases the translocation of bacteria; mycotoxins can also impair the immune response and enhance the susceptibility to infectious diseases. In conclusion, because of their effect on the intestine, FB_1 and DON are a major threat to pig health, welfare and performance.

Keywords: Pig, Fumonisin B_1, Deoxynivalenol, Feed contamination, Intestine, Barrier function, Immune response

Background

Food safety is a major issue throughout the world. In this respect, much attention needs to be paid to the possible contamination of food and feed by fungi and the risk of mycotoxin production. Mycotoxins are secondary metabolites produced by filamentous fungi, mainly by species from the genus *Aspergillus*, *Fusarium* and *Penicillium*. They are produced on a wide variety of substrates before, during and after harvest. Mycotoxins are very resistant to technological treatments and difficult to eliminate; therefore they can be present in human food and animal feed [1]. The ingestion of mycotoxin-contaminated feed can induce acute diseases, and the ingestion of low doses of fungal toxins also causes damage in case of repeated exposure [2, 3].

Monogastric livestock, pig and poultry, are particularly vulnerable to mycotoxins because of the high percentage of cereals in their diet and because they lack a rumen with a microbiota able to degrade mycotoxins before their intestinal absorption. From an intestinal pig health perspective, the most notorious mycotoxins (Fig. 1) are fumonisins, especially fumonisin FB_1 (FB_1) and trichothecenes, especially

deoxynivalenol (DON) [4]. In the European Union, some recommendations exist for both toxins in pig feed (Table 1).

This review will summarize the effect of FB_1 and DON on the intestine and analyze the consequences in terms of pig health.

Toxicity of DON and FB1

Toxicity of DON

DON is a 12,13-epoxy-3α,7α,15-trihydroxytrichothec-9-en-8-on (Fig. 1). Numerous studies bring information on the toxic effects of DON in mamals, especially rodents [5–7]. At the molecular level, DON targets the ribosome. It binds to the A-site of the peptidyl transferase center (PTC) of this organelle [8]. This binding is linked to the epoxy- and C3- group of the DON molecule [9]. Interaction with the ribosome leads to an inhibition of the elongation of chain elongation step of protein synthesis leading to an inhibition of RNA, DNA and protein synthesis [6]. This ribosome binding activates several ribosome-associated mitogen activated protein kinases (MAPKs), including p38, c-Jun N-terminal Kinase (JNK), and extracellular signal-regulated kinase 1 and 2 (ERK1/2), an effect called "ribotoxic stress" response [10].

* Correspondence: isabelle.oswald@toulouse.inra.fr
[1]ToxAlim Research Centre in Food Toxicology, INRA, UMR 1331, ENVT, INP Purpan, 180 chemin de Tournefeuille, BP93173, 31027 Toulouse, Cedex 03, France
Full list of author information is available at the end of the article

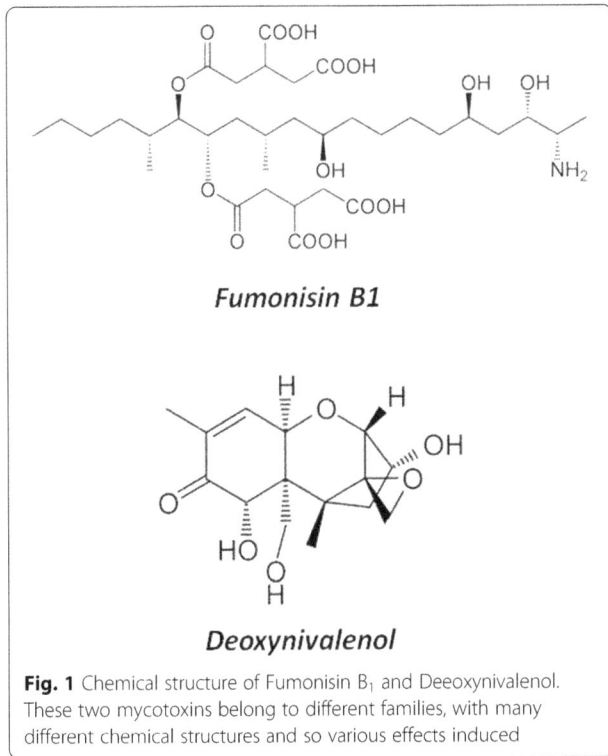

Fig. 1 Chemical structure of Fumonisin B$_1$ and Deeoxynivalenol. These two mycotoxins belong to different families, with many different chemical structures and so various effects induced

A high concentration DON causes effects and symptoms similar to those observed during an exposure to ionizing radiation, such as abdominal distress, salivation, discomfort, diarrhea, vomiting, leukocytosis and gastrointestinal bleeding. This mycotoxin also has high emetic and anorexic effects resulting in growth suppression [11, 12]. The colloquial name of DON is "vomitoxin" due to its strong emetic effects observed in pigs [13]. The underlying mechanisms for anorexia are not yet fully understood. Two major mediators of DON-induced anorexia, *i.e.* pro-inflammatory cytokines and satiety hormones, have emerged from studies carried out mainly in mice [10, 14]. It is worth to point out that, contrary to humans or pigs, emesis cannot occur in rodents, but the abnormal food intake behaviour observed

Table 1 Recommendations for DON and FB$_1$ in pigs feed and feedstuffs. Depending of the mycotoxin and the type of feed intended to pigs, different directive and recommendation exist about the concentration authorized. (EC Recommendations 2006/576/EC and 2013/165/EU)

Mycotoxins	Pig feeds	Max. content mg/Kg (ppm)
DON	Cereals (without maize by-products)	8 (12)
	Complete and complementary feeding stuffs for pigs	0.9
FB$_1$ + FB$_2$	Cereals	60
	Complete and complementary feeding stuffs for pigs, horse and rabbit	5

in mice (or other rodents) is considered indicative of nausea-induced anorexia [6].

The immune system is sensitive to DON and can be either stimulated or suppressed depending on dose, exposure frequency, timing and the functional immune assay being employed [10]. Leukocytes, most notably mononuclear phagocytes, play a likely central role in the acute and chronic toxicity evoked by DON. Low concentrations of DON induce expression of early response and pro-inflammatory genes at the mRNA and protein levels, while high concentrations promote rapid onset of leukocyte apoptosis. This immune dysregualtion is a consequence of the ribotoxic stress. Indeed, activation of p38 and ERK1/2 triggers two competing signaling pathways, one downstream of p38 favoring apoptosis and one downstream of ERK1/2 favoring survival and cytokine expression [6]. DON also impairs humoral and cell-mediated responses, alters serum IgA levels, IgA-associated nephropathy [15].

Others studies show, that DON can also have reproductive and teratological effects, with increase of skeletal abnormalities, neural arch defects or fusion, and genotoxic effects with the induction of oxydative stress mediated DNA damage on cells [16]. By contrast, there is inadequate evidence in experimental animals for the carcinogenicity of DON and the International Agency for Research on Cancer (IARC), placed DON in Group 3, "not classifiable as to its carcinogenicity to humans".

Toxicity of FB1

Fumonisin B$_1$ (FB$_1$) is the diester of propane-1,2,3-tricarboxylic acid and 2-amino-12,16-dimethyl- 3,5,10,14,15-pentahydroxyeicosane (Fig. 1). Its toxicity have been broadly reviewed [17, 18]. The primary amine function and the tricarballylic acid side chains appears necessary for the biological activity of FB$_1$, as N-substituted fumonisin and hydrolized fumonisin fail to elicit effects both *in vitro* and *in vivo* [19, 20]. FB$_1$ has an unsubstituted primary amino group at C2 and competitively inhibits ceramide synthase, which results in disruption of the *de novo* biosynthesis of ceramide and alteration of the sphingolipid metabolism. An immediate consequence of the ceramide synthase inhibition is accumulation of the enzyme's substrates sphinganine (Sa) and, to a lesser degree, sphingosine (So) in tissues, serum, and urine. In facts, increase in the Sa:So ratio in tissues and bio-fluids are explored as biomarker to fumonisin exposure in several species though these modifications of sphingoid base profiles are transient [21, 22].

A correlation between the fumonisin-induced Sa accumulation and the onset of apoptosis and mitosis has been shown in the liver and kidney of several species including pig [23, 24]. Moreover, the depletion of specific sphingolipids associated to the membrane lipid rafts involved in folate transport was suggested as the mechanism by which

FB$_1$ disrupts the 5-methyltetrahydrofolate uptake in cells [25]. The primary consequence of the disrupted folate uptake may be the teratogenic effect reported with FB$_1$ given intraperitoneally to pregnant dams leading to neural tube defects in embryo [26]. Folate deficiency as a risk factor for neural tube defects is well established [27]. Besides the neural tube defects in newborns, the symptoms induced by FBs are unusually broad and include, brain lesions in horses, lung edema in swine as well as cancer in experimental animals. The International Agency for Research on Cancer (IARC) classified FB$_1$ in Group 2B as 'possibly carcinogenic to humans'.

Especially in pigs, fumonisins are poorly absorbed from the gastrointestinal tract. The calculated bioavailability for FB$_1$ was approximately 0.041 of the dose [28]. The absorbed fraction remains in the tissues (preferentially in liver and kidneys) for an extended period of time, and enterohepatic recirculation contributes to the long biological half-life of the mycotoxin [28, 29].

The fumonisin toxicosis in pig is well documented. Historically, outbreaks of a fatal disease in pigs fed *Fusarium verticillioides*-contaminated maize crop in mid-western and south-eastern USA in 1989 led to the identification of FB$_1$ as the causative agent of porcine pulmonary edema (PPE) [30]. Within 4–7 days of initial feeding of highly contaminated feed, pigs show respiratory distress and cyanosis that is rapidly followed by death due to acute pulmonary edema and hydrothorax [31]. Non-lethal pulmonary edema has also been reported following longer term, lower dose exposures [32]. The fumonisin-induced pulmonary edema appears to result from acute left-sided heart failure, as FB$_1$ has been shown to decrease cardiac contractility, mean systemic arterial pressure, heart rate and cardiac output, and increases mean pulmonary artery pressure and pulmonary artery wedge pressure [33, 34]. This cardiotoxicity was also documented in horse following intraveinous administration of purified FB$_1$ [35].

Additional findings reported in pig from chronic exposure studies include right ventricular hypertrophy due to pulmonary hypertension, hepatic injury characterized by icterus with severe hepatic fibrosis and nodular hyperplasia and effects on both specific and non-specific immunity [36, 37]. FB$_1$ decreased phagocytosis and inhibited sphingolipid biosynthesis in pig pulmonary macrophages, and decreased clearance of particles and bacteria from the pulmonary circulation [38, 39].

Regarding the immunity, dietary exposure to FB$_1$, even at low doses is associated to sex-specific decrease of antibody titers following vaccination and increased swine susceptibility to opportunistic pathogens [40, 41]. Of note, gender-dependent immunosuppression following subacute exposure to FB$_1$ has also been described in mice, and the authors hypothetized that the selective alterations in lymphocyte functions and dramatic reduction in specific thymocytes in females may be related to FB$_1$-induced alterations in estrogen metabolism and signaling [42].

Effects of DON and FB1 on the pig intestine

The toxicity of DON and FB$_1$ varies according to several parameters such as the dose, the duration of exposure, the age and the sex of the animal, as well as nutritional factors [43–45]. Their effects on performance are greater in males and young pigs [41, 45].

The intestinal tract is the first target for mycotoxins following ingestion of contaminated feed. The intestinal epithelium is a single layer of cells lining the gut lumen that acts as a selective filter, allowing the absorption of dietary nutrients, essential electrolytes, and water from the intestinal lumen into the blood circulation [46]. It also constitutes the largest and most important barrier to prevent the passage of harmful intraluminal substances from the external environment into the organism, including foreign antigens, microorganisms, and their toxins [47, 48]. Following the ingestion of mycotoxin-contaminated feed, intestinal epithelial cells may be exposed to high concentrations of toxins, potentially affecting intestinal functions [49–51].

Effect on Feed intake

DON and to a letter extend FB$_1$ have an effect on feed intake and subsequent animal growth.

The colloquial name of DON, vomitoxin, refers to its emetic effect observed both in field reports and in experimental intoxications where high doses of the toxin were given orally or intravenously to pigs. Complete feed refusal was observed at levels of 12 and vomiting at 20 mg DON/kg feed. Pig feeding trials with naturally or artificially contaminated diets have shown decreased feed consumption and weight gain at doses from 0.6 to 3 mg DON/kg feed [52]. A meta-analysis showed that deoxynivalenol reduced feed intake and weight gain by 26 %; the same analysis also demonstrated a 16 % reduction of feed intake in response to aflatoxin B$_1$ (AFB$_1$) [45].

Consumption of pure FB$_1$ or FB$_1$-contaminated feed also induces a slight reduction of feed intake and body weight in piglets. Although FB$_1$ is poorly absorbed and metabolized in the intestine, it induces intestinal disturbances (abdominal pain or diarrhea) and cause extra-intestinal organ pathologies [53].

Effect on intestinal digestion and nutrient absorption

At the molecular level DON and FB$_1$ have been shown to alter the absorptive functionality of the intestine.

The sodium-glucose dependent transporter (SGLT-1) activity is particularly sensitive to DON. SGLT-1 is the main apical transporter for active glucose uptake in the small intestine [54]. Inhibition of SGLT-1 by DON has nutritional consequences and could explain diarrhea associated with DON ingestion, since this transporter is responsible for daily absorption of water in the gut [5]. DON not only impairs the intestinal absorption of sugars (glucose and fructose), but also alters the uptake of palmitate and monocarboxilates in the jejunum [55].

In contrast to DON, sodium-dependent glucose absorption is up-regulated in pig after acute or long term exposure to FB_1 [56, 57]. Pigs consuming corn culture extracts containing FB also showed a markedly lowered activity of aminopeptidase N [56]. Likewise, exposure to 1.5 mg/kg b.w. FB_1 has been shown to induce sphingo-lipid depletion in pig intestinal epithelium, which can result in a deficiency of folate uptake [50, 58].

Effect on intestinal histomorphology

Consumption of mycotoxin-contaminated feed induces histological damage on intestinal tissue. Epithelial lesions (multifocal atrophy, villi fusion, apical necrosis of villi, vacuolation of enterocytes and edema of lamina propria) in the intestine of pigs fed with a diet naturally contaminated with DON have been observed [52, 59]. No effect was observed on crypt depth. Jejunal lesions, including shortened and coalesced villi, lysis of enterocytes, and edema, were also observed in an *ex-vivo* model of intestinal tissues after exposure to DON [60–62]. Exposure to FB also induces changes in intestinal villi morphology such as reduced villi height and villi fusion and atrophy [52]. As described in poultry, the morphological changes may lead to a decrease of nutrients absorption by enterocytes, a reduced energy and nutrient uptake and impaired growth [63].

Effect on barrier function

Both DON and FB_1 alter intestinal barrier functions. Several studies have investigated the effect of DON on the transepithelial electrical resistance (TEER), a good indicator of the integrity of the barrier function. DON decreases TEER in pig intestinal epithelial cells in a time and dose dependant manner [9, 51, 60, 64]. In piglets jejunal explants the paracellular passage, assessed in Ussing chambers, was significantly increased in presence of 20 to 50 µM of DON [65]. Similarly to DON, FB_1 impaired the integrity of porcine intestinal epithelial cell line derived from the jejunum (IPEC-J2) monolayer via altered viability and reduced TEER [66]. It has also been observed that a prolonged exposure to FB_1 prevents the establishment of the TEER and alters the resistance of an already established monolayer of porcine intestinal epithelial cells [67].

At the molecular level, these toxins affect the intestinal epithelium permeability through modulation of the tight junction complexes [50, 51]. A defective expression of occludin and E-cadherin has been observed in the ileum of piglets fed low doses of FB_1 [61]. The FB-induced alteration of the sphingolipid biosynthesis pathway and the associated lipid rafts could also contribute to impairing the establishment and maintenance of tight junctions [53]. Likewise, the activation of MAPKs by DON affects the expression and cellular localization of proteins forming or being associated with tight junctions such as claudins and ZO-1, which results in increased intestinal paracellular permeability [60].

The loss of tight junction integrity and resulting increased paracellular permeability may lead to increased bacterial translocation across the intestine and increased susceptibility to enteric infections. Such an increase in bacterial passage through intestinal epithelial cells has major implications for pig health in terms of sepsis, inflammation and enteric infection.

Differentiated IPEC-J2 cells treated 24 h with 0.1-10 µM DON in a co-exposure with *Salmonella* Typhimurium bacteria show a significant increase of the translocation of the bacteria across intestinal epithelial cells [68]. On differentiated IPEC-1 cells treated 48 h with DON an increase translocation of *Escherichia coli* was observed in 17, 50 and 63 % with 5, 10 and 20 µM DON respectively [65]. So, DON is able to increase the passage of macromolecule and bacteria in intestinal epithelial cells.

Two separate studies analyzed the effect of low to moderate doses of FB_1 on intestinal colonization and mucosal response to pathogenic strains of *E. coli* [69, 70]. They both demonstrated a higher susceptibility of intestinal *E. coli* infection of piglets exposed to the toxin. Translocation of bacteria to the mesenteric lymph nodes and dissemination to the lungs, and to a lesser extent to liver and spleen, were observed in FB_1-treated pigs in comparison to untreated animals [70].

Modulation of intestinal immune response

DON and FB_1 impact the systemic and/or the local immune response (review [5, 10, 53]). As far as pig is concerned, several studies have investigated the effect of theses mycotoxins on the intestinal immune system.

The effect of ingestion of FB_1 was measured on the intestinal production of 5 inflammatory cytokines (IL-1β, IL-6, IL-12, TNF-β and IL-8). Both *in vitro* and *in vivo* data indicate that FB_1 specifically decreases expression of IL-8 mRNA [71]. IL-8 being involved in the recruitment of inflammatory cells in the intestine during infection [72–74], this specific decrease of intestinal IL-8 may contribute to the observed increased susceptibility of FB_1-treated piglets to *E. coli* infection [70]. The increased susceptibility to intestinal infection is also correlated with a reduced intestinal expression of IL-12p40, an impaired function of intestinal antigen presenting cells (APC), a decreased upregulation of Major Histocompatibility Complex Class II molecule (MHC-II) and reduced T cell stimulatory capacity [69].

DON modulates intestinal immunity both directly (through activation of signalling pathways) and indirectly (through crossing of luminal bacterial antigens, which was observed together with bacterial translocation following mucus layer alteration and tight junction opening) [75]. In a pig jejunal explant model, DON has been shown to trigger the innate as well as adaptative immunity [76]. Intestinal exposure to DON induced a pro-inflammatory response with a significant increase of expression of TNF-α, IL-1α, IL-1β, and IL-8. Moreover, DON up-regulated the expression of genes involved in the differentiation of Th17 cells (STAT3, IL–17A, IL-6, IL-1b) at the expenses of the pathway of regulatory T cells (FoxP3, RALDH1). DON also induced genes related to the pathogenic Th17 cells subset such as IL–23A, IL-22 and IL-21 and not genes related to the regulatory Th17 cells such as TGF-b and IL-10 [76]. Likewise, DON potentiated the up-regulation of IL-1β, IL-8, MCP1 and IL-6 induced by *S.* Typhimurium in pig intestinal loops [68].

Intestinal microbiota

As other fungi secondary metabolites especially antibiotics, several mycotoxins have demonstrated antimicrobial properties [77, 78]. As a consequence, mycotoxins may modify the intestinal microflora. Surprisingly, this impact of mycotoxins has been poorly investigated. Two studies have investigated the impact of DON and FB_1 on the intestinal microflora [79, 80].

The first study investigated the impact of DON on the intestinal microflora by Capillary Electrophoresis Single-Stranded Conformation Polymorphism (CE-SSCP). Consumption of feed naturally contaminated with DON (2.8 mg/kg feed) for four weeks had a moderate effect on total faecal Aerobic Mesophilic Bacteria and Anaerobic Sulfite-Reducing. By constrast, DON changed the faecal microflora balance; it did not impact the diversity index but modulate the richness index [79].

In the second study, pigs received feed contaminated with 12 mg FB/kg feed for 63 days. This diet transiently

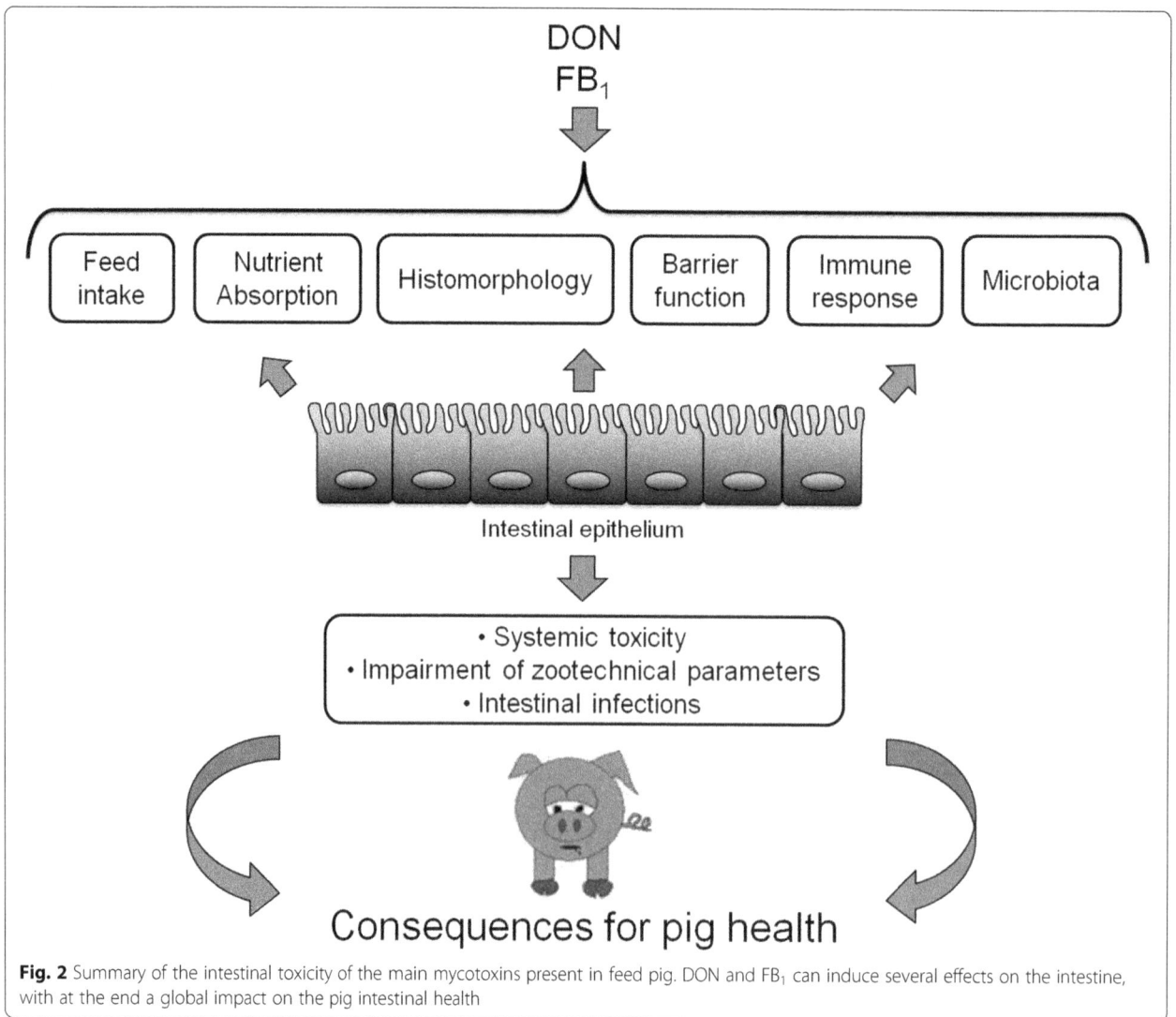

Fig. 2 Summary of the intestinal toxicity of the main mycotoxins present in feed pig. DON and FB_1 can induce several effects on the intestine, with at the end a global impact on the pig intestinal health

affected the balance of the digestive microbiota during the first four weeks of exposure as measured by SSCP feacal microbiota profiles; a co-infection with *S.* typhimurium amplified this phenomenon and change the microbiota profile. As already observed with DON, aerobic mesophylic bacteria count was not change by FB_1 treatment [80].

Conclusion

Regulations and recommendations exist for six mycotoxins (AF, FB, Ochratoxin A (OTA), zearalenone (ZEN), T2/HT2 toxins (T2/HT2) and DON) present in pig feed. Among them, DON and FB have been studied for their toxicity in the intestine of pig. The intestine is a target for mycotoxins and as illustrated in this paper, the fact that the intestine is a target for DON and FB_1 have some consequences in terms of pig health (Fig. 2). Theses mycooxins are not only locally toxic for the intestine, but also dysregulate many intestinal functions and impair the local immune response. This results in systemic toxicity leading to many symptoms, alteration of zootechnical parameters. Feed contamination with mycotoxins also increases impair the barrier function of the intestine, leading to translocation of bacteria across the intestine and thus intestinal and systemic infections.

Global surveys indicate that animals are generally exposed to more than one mycotoxin [81]. Indeed fungi are able to produce several mycotoxins simultaneously; and it is common practice to use multiple grains in animal diets. Unfortunately, the toxicity of mycotoxin mixtures cannot be predicted based on their individual toxicities. Interactions between concomitantly occurring mycotoxins can be antagonistic, additive, or synergistic [82]. The data on combined toxicity of mycotoxins are limited and therefore, the health risk from exposure to a combination of mycotoxins is incompletely understood [83, 84] and deserves further investigation.

Abbreviations
AFB_1, Aflatoxin B_1; AFB_2, Aflatoxin B_2; CE-SSCP, Capillary Electrophoresis Single-Stranded Conformation Polymorphism; DNA, Deoxyribonucleic acid; DON, Deoxynivalenol; ERK 1/2, Extracellular Signal Regulated Kinase 1 and 2; FB_1, Fumonisin B_1; FoxP3, Forkhead box P3; HT2, HT2 toxin; IARC, International Agency for Research on Cancer; Ig, Imunoglobulin; IL, Interleukin; IPEC-J2, Porcine Intestinal Epithelial Cell line derived from the jejunum; JNK, C-Jun N-terminal Kinase; MAPKs, Mitogen Activated Protein Kinases; MCP1, Monocyte chemoattractant protein-1; MHC-II, Major Histocompatibility Complex - Class II; OTA, Ochratoxin A; OVA, Ovalbumin; PPE, porcine pulmonary edema ; PTC, Peptidyl Transferase Center; RALDH1, Retinaldehyde dehydrogenase 1; RNA, Ribonucleic acid; Sa, Sphinganine; SGLT-1, Sodium-glucose dependent transporter; So, Sphingosine; STAT3, Signal transducer and activator of transcription 3; T2, T2 toxin; TEER, Trans Epithelial Electrical Resistance; TGF, Transforming Growth Factor; TNF, Tumor Necrosis Factor; ZEN, Zearalenone

Acknowledgment
The authors thank Ryan Hines, Biomin, for language editing.

Funding
A. Pierron was supported by a fellowship from CIFRE (2012/0572, jointly financed by the BIOMIN Holding GmbH, Association Nationale de la Recherche Technique and INRA). This work was supported in part by the projects Liporeg (APP-ICSA 2015) and PHC STEFANIK 2016.

Authors' contributions
All authors agree fully to the content of the review. All authors read and approved the final manuscript.

Author's information
IPO, Research director at INRA Toxalim, Head of the team "Biosynthesis and Toxicity of Mycotoxins".
AP, 3rd year PhD student at INRA Toxalim, in the team "Biosynthesis and Toxicity of Mycotoxins".
IAK is a postdoctoral research fellow in the INRA Toxalim team "Biosynthesis and Toxicity of Mycotoxins".

Competing interests
The authors declare that they have no competing interests.

Author details
^{1}ToxAlim Research Centre in Food Toxicology, INRA, UMR 1331, ENVT, INP Purpan, 180 chemin de Tournefeuille, BP93173, 31027 Toulouse, Cedex 03, France. ^{2}BIOMIN Research Center, Technopark 1, 3430 Tulln, Austria.

References
1. Hazel CM, Patel S. Influence of processing on trichothecene levels. Toxicol Lett. 2004;153:51–9.
2. Bryden WL. Mycotoxin contamination of the feed supply chain : Implications for animal productivity and feed security. Anim Feed Sci Technol. 2012;173:134–58.
3. Maresca M, Fantini J. Some food-associated mycotoxins as potential risk factors in humans predisposed to chronic intestinal inflammatory diseases. Toxicon. 2010;56:282–94.
4. CAST. Potential economic costs of mycotoxins in United States. In: Task Force Report 138. Mycotoxins: Risks in plant, animal and human systems. Ames: Council for Agricultural Science and Technology; 2003. p. 136–42.
5. Maresca M. From the gut to the brain: journey and pathophysiological effects of the food-associated mycotoxin Deoxynivalenol. Toxins. 2013;5:784–820.
6. Pestka JJ. Deoxynivalenol: mechanisms of action, human exposure, and toxicological relevance. Arch Toxicol. 2010;84(6):663–79.
7. Wang Z, Wu Q, Kuca K, Dohnal V, Tian Z. Deoxynivalenol: signaling pathways and human exposure risk assessment–an update. Arch Toxicol. 2014;88(11):1915–28.
8. Garreau de Loubresse N, Prokhorova I, Holtkamp W, Rodnina MV, Yusupova G, Yusupov M. Structural basis for the inhibition of the eukaryotic ribosome. Nature. 2014;513(7519):517–22.
9. Pierron A, Mimoun S, Murate LS, Loiseau N, Lippi Y, Bracarense A-PFL, et al. Microbial biotransformation of DON: molecular basis for reduced toxicity. Sci Rep. 2016;6:29105.
10. Pestka JJ. Deoxynivalenol-induced proinflammatory gene expression: mechanisms and pathological sequelae. Toxins (Basel). 2010;2(6):1300–17.
11. Pestka JJ, Smolinski AT. Deoxynivalenol: toxicology and potential effects on humans. J Toxicol Environ Health B Crit Rev. 2005;8:39–69.
12. Haschek WM, Voss KA, Beasley V. Selected mycotoxins affecting animal and human health. In: Haschek WM, Rousseaux CG, Wallig MA, editors. Handbook of Toxicological Pathology. New York: Academic; 2002. p. 645–99.

13. Vesonder RF, Ciegler A, Jensen AH. Isolation of the emetic principle from Fusarium-infected corn. Appl Microbiol. 1973;26:1008–10.

14. Lebrun B, Tardivel C, Felix B, Abysique A, Troadec JD, Gaige S, et al. Dysregulation of energy balance by trichothecene mycotoxins: Mechanisms and prospects. Neurotoxicology. 2015;49:15–27.

15. Sobrova P, Adam V, Vasatkova A, Beklova M, Zeman L, Kizek R. Deoxynivalenol and its toxicity. Interdiscip Toxicol. 2010;3:94–9.

16. Sun XM, Zhang XH, Wang HY, Cao WJ, Yan X, Zuo LF, et al. Effects of sterigmatocystin, deoxynivalenol and aflatoxin G1 on apoptosis of human peripheral blood lymphocytes in vitro. Biomed Environ Sci. 2002;15:145–52.

17. Escriva L, Font G, Manyes L. In vivo toxicity studies of fusarium mycotoxins in the last decade: a review. Food Chem Toxicol. 2015;78:185–206.

18. Voss KA, Smith GW, Haschek WM. Fumonisins: Toxicokinetics, mechanism of action and toxicity. Anim Feed Sci Tech. 2007;137:299–325.

19. Howard PC, Couch LH, Patton RE, Eppley RM, Doerge DR, Churchwell MI, et al. Comparison of the toxicity of several fumonisin derivatives in a 28-day feeding study with female B6C3F(1) mice. Toxicol Appl Pharm. 2002;185:153–65.

20. Grenier B, Bracarense AP, Schwartz HE, Trumel C, Cossalter AM, Schatzmayr G, et al. The low intestinal and hepatic toxicity of hydrolyzed fumonisin B_1 correlates with its inability to alter the metabolism of sphingolipids. Biochem Pharmacol. 2012;83:1465–73.

21. Enongene EN, Sharma RP, Bhandari N, Miller JD, Meredith FI, Voss KA, et al. Persistence and reversibility of the elevation in free sphingoid bases induced by fumonisin inhibition of ceramide synthase. Toxicol Sci. 2002;67:173–81.

22. Voss KA, Plattner RD, Riley RT, Meredith FI, Norred WP. In vivo effects of fumonisin B(1)-producing and fumonisin B(1)-nonproducing Fusarium moniliforme isolates are similar: Fumonisins B(2) and B(3) cause hepato- and nephrotoxicity in rats. Mycopathologia. 1998;141:45–58.

23. Gumprecht LA, Beasley VR, Weigel RM, Parker HM, Tumbleson ME, Bacon CW, et al. Development of fumonisin-induced hepatotoxicity and pulmonary edema in orally dosed swine: morphological and biochemical alterations. Toxicol Pathol. 1998;26:777–88.

24. Gumprecht LA, Marcucci A, Weigel RM, Vesonder RF, Riley RT, Showker JL, et al. Effects of intravenous fumonisin B1 in rabbits: nephrotoxicity and sphingolipid alterations. Nat Toxins. 1995;3:395–403.

25. Stevens VL, Tang J. Fumonisin B1-induced sphingolipid depletion inhibits vitamin uptake via the glycosylphosphatidylinositol-anchored folate receptor. J Biol Chem. 1997;272:18020–5.

26. Gelineau-van Waes J, Starr L, Maddox J, Aleman F, Voss KA, Wilberding J, et al. Maternal fumonisin exposure and risk for neural tube defects: mechanisms in an in vivo mouse model. Birth Defects Res A Clin Mol Teratol. 2005;73:487–97.

27. Pitkin RM. Folate and neural tube defects. Am J Clin Nutr. 2007;85:285S–8.

28. Prelusky DB, Trenholm HL, Rotter BA, Miller JD, Savard ME, Yeung JM, et al. Biological fate of fumonisin B1 in food-producing animals. Adv Exp Med Biol. 1996;392:265–78.

29. Prelusky DB, Trenholm HL, Savard ME. Pharmacokinetic fate of 14C-labelled fumonisin B1 in swine. Nat Toxins. 1994;2:73–80.

30. Osweiler GD, Ross PF, Wilson TM, Nelson PE, Witte ST, Carson TL, et al. Characterization of an Epizootic of Pulmonary-Edema in Swine Associated with Fumonisin in Corn Screenings. J Vet Diagn Invest. 1992;4:53–9.

31. Haschek WM, Motelin G, Ness DK, Harlin KS, Hall WF, Vesonder RF, et al. Characterization of Fumonisin Toxicity in Orally and Intravenously Dosed Swine. Mycopathologia. 1992;117:83–96.

32. Zomborszky-Kovacs M, Vetesi FF, Kovacs F, Bata A, Toth A, Tornyos G. Preliminary communication: Examination of the harmful effect to fetuses of fumonisin B-1 in pregnant sows. Teratogen Carcin Mut. 2000;20:293–9.

33. Constable PD, Smith GW, Rottinghaus GE, Tumbleson ME, Haschek WM. Fumonisin-induced blockade of ceramide synthase in sphingolipid biosynthetic pathway alters aortic input impedance spectrum of pigs. Am J Physiol Heart Circ Physiol. 2003;284:H2034–44.

34. Smith GW, Constable PD, Tumbleson ME, Rottinghaus GE, Haschek WM. Sequence of cardiovascular changes leading to pulmonary edema in swine fed culture material containing fumonisin. Am J Vet Res. 1999;60:1292–300.

35. Smith GW, Constable PD, Foreman JH, Eppley RM, Waggoner AL, Tumbleson ME, et al. Cardiovascular changes associated with intravenous administration of fumonisin B-1 in horses. Am J Vet Res. 2002;63:538–45.

36. Casteel SW, Turk JR, Cowart RP, Rottinghaus GE. Chronic Toxicity of Fumonisin in Weanling Pigs. J Vet Diagn Invest. 1993;5:413–7.

37. Harvey RB, Edrington TS, Kubena LF, Elissalde MH, Rottinghaus GE. Influence of Aflatoxin and Fumonisin B-1-Containing Culture Material on Growing Barrows. Am J Vet Res. 1995;56:1668–72.

38. Haschek WM, Gumprecht LA, Smith G, Tumbleson ME, Constable PD. Fumonisin toxicosis in swine: an overview of porcine pulmonary edema and current perspectives. Environ Health Perspect. 2001;109 Suppl 2:251–7.

39. Smith GW, Constable PD, Haschek WM. Cardiovascular responses to short-term fumonisin exposure in swine. Fund Appl Toxicol. 1996;33:140–8.

40. Marin DE, Gouze ME, Taranu I, Oswald IP. Fumonisin B1 alters cell cycle progression and interleukin-2 synthesis in swine peripheral blood mononuclear cells. Mol Nutr Food Res. 2007;51:1406–12.

41. Marin DE, Taranu I, Pascale F, Lionide A, Burlacu R, Bailly JD, et al. Sex-related differences in the immune response of weanling piglets exposed to low doses of fumonisin extract. Br J Nutr. 2006;95:1185–92.

42. Johnson VJ, Sharma RP. Gender-dependent immunosuppression following subacute exposure to fumonisin B1. Int Immunopharmacol. 2001;1:2023–34.

43. Bryden WL. Mycotoxins in the food chain: human health implications. Asia Pac J Clin Nutr. 2007;16 Suppl 1:95–101.

44. Wild CP. Aflatoxin exposure in developing countries: the critical interface of agriculture and health. Food Nutr Bull. 2007;28(2 Suppl):S372–80.

45. Andretta I, Kipper M, Lehnen CR, Hauschild L, Vale MM, Lovatto PA. Meta-analytical study of productive and nutritional interactions of mycotoxins in growing pigs. Animal. 2012;6:1476–82.

46. Prelusky DB. A study on the effect of deoxynivalenol on serotonin receptor binding in pig brain membranes. J Environ Sci Health B. 1996;31:1103–17.

47. Bouhet S, Oswald IP. The effects of mycotoxins, fungal food contaminants, on the intestinal epithelial cell-derived innate immune response. Vet Immunol Immunopathol. 2005;108:199–209.

48. Oswald IP. Role of intestinal epithelial cells in the innate immune defence of the pig intestine. Vet Res. 2006;37:359–68.

49. Alassane-Kpembi I, Oswald IP. Effects of feed contaminants on the intestinal health of monogastric farm animals. In: Nieworld T, editor. Intestinal health: key to optimise production. Wageningen: Wageningen Academic Publishers; 2015. p. 169–90.

50. Grenier B, Applegate TJ. Modulation of intestinal functions following mycotoxin ingestion: meta-analysis of published experiments in animals. Toxins (Basel). 2013;5:396–430.

51. Ghareeb K, Awad WA, Bohm J, Zebeli Q. Impacts of the feed contaminant deoxynivalenol on the intestine of monogastric animals: poultry and swine. J Appl Toxicol. 2015;35:327–37.

52. Bracarense AP, Lucioli J, Grenier B, Drociunas Pacheco G, Moll WD, Schatzmayr G, et al. Chronic ingestion of deoxynivalenol and fumonisin, alone or in interaction, induces morphological and immunological changes in the intestine of piglets. Br J Nutr. 2012;107:1776–86.

53. Bouhet S, Oswald IP. The intestine as a possible target for fumonisin toxicity. Mol Nutr Food Res. 2007;51:925–31.

54. Awad WA, Aschenbach JR, Setyabudi FM, Razzazi-Fazeli E, Bohm J, Zentek J. In vitro effects of deoxynivalenol on small intestinal D-glucose uptake and absorption of deoxynivalenol across the isolated jejunal epithelium of laying hens. Poult Sci. 2007;86:15–20.

55. Dietrich B, Neuenschwander S, Bucher B, Wenk C. Fusarium mycotoxin-contaminated wheat containing deoxynivalenol alters the gene expression in the liver and the jejunum of broilers. Animal. 2012;6:278–91.

56. Lessard M, Boudry G, Seve B, Oswald IP, Lalles JP. Intestinal physiology and peptidase activity in male pigs are modulated by consumption of corn culture extracts containing fumonisins. J Nutr. 2009;139:1303–7.

57. Lalles JP, Lessard M, Boudry G. Intestinal barrier function is modulated by short-term exposure to fumonisin B(1) in Ussing chambers. Vet Res Commun. 2009;33:1039–43.

58. Loiseau N, Debrauwer L, Sambou T, Bouhet S, Miller JD, Martin PG, et al. Fumonisin B1 exposure and its selective effect on porcine jejunal segment: sphingolipids, glycolipids and trans-epithelial passage disturbance. Biochem Pharmacol. 2007;74:144–52.

59. Eriksen GS, Pettersson H. Toxicological evaluation of trichothecenes in animal feed. Anim Feed Sci Technol. 2004;114:205–39.

60. Pinton P, Oswald IP. Effect of deoxynivalenol and other Type B trichothecenes on the intestine: a review. Toxins (Basel). 2014;6:1615–43.

61. Lucioli J, Pinton P, Callu P, Laffitte J, Grosjean F, Kolf-Clauw M, et al. The food contaminant deoxynivalenol activates the mitogen activated protein kinases in the intestine: Interest of ex vivo models as an alternative to in vivo experiments. Toxicon. 2013;66:31–6.

62. Kolf-Clauw M, Castellote J, Joly B, Bourges-Abella N, Raymond-Letron I, Pinton P, et al. Development of a pig jejunal explant culture for studying the gastrointestinal toxicity of the mycotoxin deoxynivalenol: Histopathological analysis. Toxicol In Vitro. 2009;23:1580–4.

63. Yunus AW, Blajet-Kosicka A, Kosicki R, Khan MZ, Rehman H, Böhm J. Deoxynivalenol as a contaminant of broiler feed: intetsinal development, absorptive functionality, and metabolism of the mycotoxin. Poult Sci. 2012; 91:852-61.

64. Pierron A, Mimoun S, Murate LS, Loiseau N, Lippi Y, Bracarense AP, et al. Intestinal toxicity of the masked mycotoxin deoxynivalenol-3-beta-D-glucoside. Arch Toxicol. 2016;90:2037–46.

65. Pinton P, Nougayrede JP, Del Rio J-C, Moreno C, Marin DE, Ferrier L, et al. The food contaminant deoxynivalenol, decreases intestinal barrier permeability and reduces claudin expression. Toxicol Appl Pharmacol. 2009;237:41–8.

66. Goossens J, Pasmans F, Verbrugghe E, Vandenbroucke V, De Baere S, Meyer E, et al. Porcine intestinal epithelial barrier disruption by the Fusarium mycotoxins deoxynivalenol and T-2 toxin promotes transepithelial passage of doxycycline and paromomycin. BMC Vet Res. 2012;8:245.

67. Bouhet S, Hourcade E, Loiseau N, Fikry A, Martinez S, Roselli M, et al. The mycotoxin fumonisin B1 alters the proliferation and the barrier function of porcine intestinal epithelial cells. Toxicol Sci. 2004;77:165–71.

68. Vandenbroucke V, Croubels S, Martel A, Verbrugghe E, Goossens J, Van Deun K, et al. The mycotoxin deoxynivalenol potentiates intestinal inflammation by Salmonella typhimurium in porcine ileal loops. PLoS One. 2011;6:e23871.

69. Devriendt B, Gallois M, Verdonck F, Wache Y, Bimczok D, Oswald IP, et al. The food contaminant fumonisin B(1) reduces the maturation of porcine CD11R1(+) intestinal antigen presenting cells and antigen-specific immune responses, leading to a prolonged intestinal ETEC infection. Vet Res. 2009;40(4):40.

70. Oswald IP, Desautels C, Laffitte J, Fournout S, Peres SY, Odin M, et al. Mycotoxin fumonisin B1 increases intestinal colonization by pathogenic *Escherichia coli* in pigs. Appl Environ Microbiol. 2003;69:5870–4.

71. Bouhet S, Le Dorze E, Peres S, Fairbrother JM, Oswald IP. Mycotoxin fumonisin B1 selectively down-regulates the basal IL-8 expression in pig intestine: in vivo and in vitro studies. Food Chem Toxicol. 2006;44: 1768–73.

72. Hoch RC, Schraufstatter IU, Cochrane CG. *In vivo, in vitro,* and molecular aspects of interleukin-8 and the interleukin-8 receptors. J Lab Clin Med. 1996;128:134–45.

73. Zachrisson K, Neopikhanov V, Wretlind B, Uribe A. Mitogenic action of tumour necrosis factor-alpha and interleukin-8 on explants of human duodenal mucosa. Cytokine. 2001;15:148–55.

74. Maheshwari A, Lacson A, Lu W, Fox SE, Barleycorn AA, Christensen RD, et al. Interleukin-8/CXCL8 forms an autocrine loop in fetal intestinal mucosa. Pediatr Res. 2004;56:240–9.

75. Maresca M, Yahi N, Younes-Sakr L, Boyron M, Caporiccio B, Fantini J. Both direct and indirect effects account for the pro-inflammatory activity of enteropathogenic mycotoxins on the human intestinal epithelium: stimulation of interleukin-8 secretion, potentiation of interleukin-1beta effect and increase in the transepithelial passage of commensal bacteria. Toxicol Appl Pharmacol. 2008;228:84–92.

76. Cano PM, Seeboth J, Meurens F, Cognie J, Abrami R, Oswald IP, et al. Deoxynivalenol as a new factor in the persistence of intestinal inflammatory diseases: an emerging hypothesis through possible modulation of Th17-mediated response. PLoS One. 2013;8:e53647.

77. Ali-Vehmas T, Rizzo A, Westermarck T, Atroshi F. Measurement of antibacterial activities of T-2 toxin, deoxynivalenol, ochratoxin A, aflatoxin B1 and fumonisin B1 using microtitration tray-based turbidimetric techniques. Zentralbl Veterinarmed A. 1998;45:453–8.

78. Burmeister HR, Hesseltine CW. Survey of the sensitivity of microorganisms to aflatoxin. Appl Microbiol. 1966;14:403–4.

79. Wache YJ, Valat C, Postollec G, Bougeard S, Burel C, Oswald IP, et al. Impact of deoxynivalenol on the intestinal microflora of pigs. Int J Mol Sci. 2009;10:1–17.

80. Burel C, Tanguy M, Guerre P, Boilletot E, Cariolet R, Queguiner M, et al. Effect of low dose of fumonisins on pig health: immune status, intestinal microbiota and sensitivity to Salmonella. Toxins (Basel). 2013;5: 841–64.

81. Streit E, Schatzmayr G, Tassis P, Tzika E, Marin D, Taranu I, et al. Current situation of mycotoxin contamination and co-occurrence in animal feed-focus on Europe. Toxins (Basel). 2012;4:788–809.

82. Alassane-Kpembi I, Puel O, Oswald IP. Toxicological interactions between the mycotoxins deoxynivalenol, nivalenol and their acetylated derivatives in intestinal epithelial cells. Arch Toxicol. 2015;89:1337–46.

83. Grenier B, Oswald IP. Mycotoxin co-contamination of foods and feeds: meta-analysis of publications describing toxicological interactions. World Mycotoxin J. 2011;4:285–313.

84. Alassane-Kpembi I, Schatzmayr G, Taranu I, Marin D, Puel O, Oswald IP. Mycotoxins co-contamination: Methodological aspects and biological relevance of combined toxicity studies. Crit Rev Food Sci Nutr. 2016. In press.

7

Effect of oral KETOPROFEN treatment in acute respiratory disease outbreaks in finishing pigs

Outi Hälli[1][*] , Minna Haimi-Hakala[1], Tapio Laurila[1], Claudio Oliviero[1], Elina Viitasaari[1], Toomas Orro[2], Olli Peltoniemi[1], Mika Scheinin[4], Saija Sirén[4], Anna Valros[3] and Mari Heinonen[1]

Abstract

Background: Infection with respiratory pathogens can influence production as well as animal welfare. There is an economical and ethical need to treat pigs that suffer from respiratory diseases. Our aim was the evaluation of the possible effects of oral NSAID medication given in feed in acute outbreaks of respiratory disease in finishing pigs. The short- and long-term impact of NSAID dosing on clinical signs, daily weight gain, blood parameters and behaviour of growing pigs in herds with acute respiratory infections were evaluated. Four finishing pig farms suffering from acute outbreaks of respiratory disease were visited thrice after outbreak onset (DAY 0, DAY 3 and DAY 30). Pigs with the most severe clinical signs ($N = 160$) were selected as representative pigs for the herd condition. These pigs were blood sampled, weighed, evaluated clinically and their behaviour was observed. After the first visit, half of the pens (five pigs per pen in four pens totalling 20 representative pigs per herd, altogether 80 pigs in four herds) were treated with oral ketoprofen (target dose 3 mg/kg) mixed in feed for three days and the other half (80 pigs) with a placebo. In three of the herds, some pigs were treated also with antimicrobials, and in one herd the only pharmaceutical treatment was ketoprofen or placebo.

Results: Compared to the placebo treatment, dosing of ketoprofen reduced sickness behaviour and lowered the rectal temperature of the pigs. Clinical signs, feed intake or blood parameters were not different between the treatment groups. Ketoprofen treatment was associated with somewhat reduced weight gain over the 30-day follow-up period. Concentration analysis of the *S*- and *R*-enantiomers of ketoprofen in serum samples collected on DAY 3 indicated successful oral drug administration.

Conclusions: Ketoprofen mainly influenced the behaviour of the pigs, while it had no effect on recovery from respiratory clinical signs. However, the medication may have been started after the most severe clinical phase of the respiratory disease was over, and this delay might complicate the evaluation of treatment effects. Possible negative impact of ketoprofen on production parameters requires further evaluation.

Keywords: Behaviour, Daily weight gain, Acute phase proteins, *Actinobacillus pleuropneumoniae*, NSAID, Per os medication

* Correspondence: outihalli75@gmail.com
[1]Faculty of Veterinary Medicine, University of Helsinki, Paroninkuja 20, 04920 Saarentaus, FI, Finland
Full list of author information is available at the end of the article

Background

Respiratory disease can influence production as well as animal welfare [1, 2]. For example, acute infection by one of the most common respiratory pathogens of pigs in Finland, *Actinobacillus pleuropneumoniae* (APP) is characterised by dyspnoea, cough, fever, reduced feed and water intake [3] and changes in white blood cell counts [3, 4].

Sickness behaviour is a consequence of inflammation. Typical sickness behaviour in pigs includes lethargy, reduced appetite, decreased motor activity and changes in thermal regulation. These changes help to preserve energy and to fight infection [5]. This response has been examined in experimental challenge studies. For example, pigs suffering from respiratory infection caused by porcine reproductive and respiratory (PRRS) virus spent more time lying in contact with another pig compared with non-infected controls [2]. In addition, PRRSv-inoculated pigs spent more time lying in ventral position and in contact with a penmate and less time in feeding compared to non-inoculated pigs [6].

Animals react to infections through an inflammatory response involving elevated levels of acute phase proteins in serum. In the pig, haptoglobin (Hp) is one of the most extensively investigated acute phase proteins. The concentration of Hp increases in serum within 48 h after infection [7, 8]. Respiratory infections can induce prominent increases in Hp levels as shown under experimental [9, 10] and clinical conditions [11, 12]. Another major acute phase protein in pig serum is amyloid A (SAA), which has shown the biggest difference in measured values between non-infected vs. infected animals of all investigated acute phase proteins [9, 13]. It has been suggested that acute phase proteins could be used as indicators of changes in animal health status or as aids in clinical diagnosis during infections as they are sensitive markers of infection [9].

There is an economical [14] and ethical need to treat pigs that suffer from respiratory diseases. Often, antimicrobial treatment is used. Recent evidence, however, indicates that non-steroidal anti-inflammatory drugs (NSAIDs) can also be beneficial in the treatment of respiratory diseases in pigs. NSAIDs (especially ketoprofen) have been reported to have a good ability to reduce fever [15–21] and at least to some extent to alleviate clinical signs [15–18, 20–22]. However, significant effects on blood parameters and growth have not been reported [15, 20, 21]. Evidence of the effects of NSAIDs on sickness behaviour is scarce and more information is needed; one recent study reported favourable impact of NSAID medication on sickness behaviour after lipopolysaccharide (LPS) administration [22].

The aim of our field study was to evaluate possible effects of NSAID medication administered in feed to finishing pigs during acute respiratory outbreaks in clinical conditions. Medication mixed in feed would be a practical alternative for medicating groups of diseased pigs instead of labour-intensive individual drug administration. However, sick animals usually eat less and hence it is important to evaluate whether medication mixed in feed could be successfully employed. We followed the short- and long-time impact of NSAID dosing on clinical signs, daily weight gain, blood parameters, Hp and SAA concentrations as well as on behaviour of pigs in groups of animals suffering from an acute outbreak of respiratory infection. Our assumption was that ketoprofen given in feed would alleviate clinical signs, reduce inflammation and decrease the behavioural effects of the disease, hence, improve the welfare of pigs and their daily weight gain.

Methods

This study was a randomised, double-blinded, placebo-controlled clinical trial. It was also a substudy of a study focusing on respiratory diseases in pigs in Finland aiming to determine the main pathogens responsible for acute respiratory diseases [23]. Local practicing veterinarians and farmers were asked to inform the research group about acute outbreaks of respiratory clinical signs in Finnish finishing pig herds during 2011–2014. The herds were included in the bigger study according to the same inclusion criteria that were applied for the current substudy (see below).

In this study, clinical signs refer to signs detected during a basic clinical examination, excluding behavioural observations. Accordingly, by sickness behaviour we mean observations regarding posture or activity of pigs, as explained in the ethogram (see Table 1).

After the first notification of an acute outbreak of respiratory disease, the research group personnel contacted the farm and ensured that the farm and the disease outbreak fulfilled the inclusion criteria: 1) the herd was rearing finishing pigs; 2) the herd showed acute respiratory signs e.g. cough, lowered appetite, apathy or mortality of animals; 3) the herd had either feeding arrangements that allowed all pigs in one pen to eat at the same time or automatic feeding devices that allowed individual feeding and medication for dosing of the oral medication; 4) the location of the herd had to be close enough (within 250 km driving distance) to the university clinic located in Mäntsälä, Southern Finland, for the research team to be able to organise the sampling and behavioural observations; and 5) the farmer was willing to participate. Altogether four farms were eligible for study enrolment.

Table 1 The ethogram used in the behavioural analysis of representative pigs in herds with respiratory disease outbreaks

BEHAVIOUR	DEFINITION
Posture	
Walk	Moving all 4 legs.
Stand	Standing on 4 legs motionless.
Sit	Hindquarters touching floor.
Lie lateral	Lying on either side.
Lie sternal	Lying on the belly.
Lie alone	Lying on side or belly, without contact to other pigs.
Activity	
Active	Head up, alert while lying, sitting or standing (if cannot be identified as nosing, eating or drinking).
Eat	Head in the trough
Drink	Snout in contact with water nipple.
Nosing	Touching pen mate or pen structures with snout
Passive	Standing, sitting or lying motionless, head down, not alert.
Other	Invisible or none of the above.

Farm visits and data collection

A scheme depicting the study design containing the farm visits, the treatment intervention and the numbers of study animals is presented in Fig. 1. The research group first visited the farm for a baseline visit (DAY 0) within two days after the first notification of the acute outbreak. The farm visit started approximately 3.5 h before the midday feed was given to the pigs, allowing for behavioural observations two hours prior to feeding. Researchers first identified, after consulting the farm personnel, one compartment with the most profound clinical respiratory signs. During the first farm visit (DAY 0), three pigs per herd with acute respiratory clinical signs were selected for

euthanasia and pathological examination to discern the pathogens involved in the outbreak. The lungs of these pigs were chilled and transported to the laboratory (Finnish Food Safety Authority Evira) for pathological, virological and bacteriological investigations to be begun on the next day.

From the selected compartment, eight pens containing the pigs with the most severe clinical signs were included in the study. Four pairs of two adjacent pens sharing one feeding trough were selected on the three farms using trough feeding. On the fourth farm using automated individual feeders, eight pens in one room were selected for sampling. Despite the shared trough, pigs in adjacent pens could not restrict the pigs in the other pen from approaching the feeding trough as there was a solid fence between the adjacent pens. The study pens housed an average of 11.3 (sd 1.4) pigs. From each pen, five representative pigs for the herd condition (altogether 40 pigs per farm) with the most severe clinical signs were numbered on their backs with marking spray from one to five. Half of the pens were randomly allocated for ketoprofen administration and the other half to the placebo treatment. Because of the shared feeding troughs, the pair of adjacent pens was always allocated to the same treatment. Each farm thus had 20 representative pigs divided into four pens receiving ketoprofen and another 20 pigs in four pens serving as a control group receiving treatment with placebo.

Two persons followed the behaviour of the representative pigs by direct observation with scan sampling every five minutes for two hours before the midday feeding equalling 24 observations per pig. The ethogram used is presented in Table 1.

After behavioural follow-up, the same 40 animals were evaluated clinically. Presence of clinical signs (YES/NO;

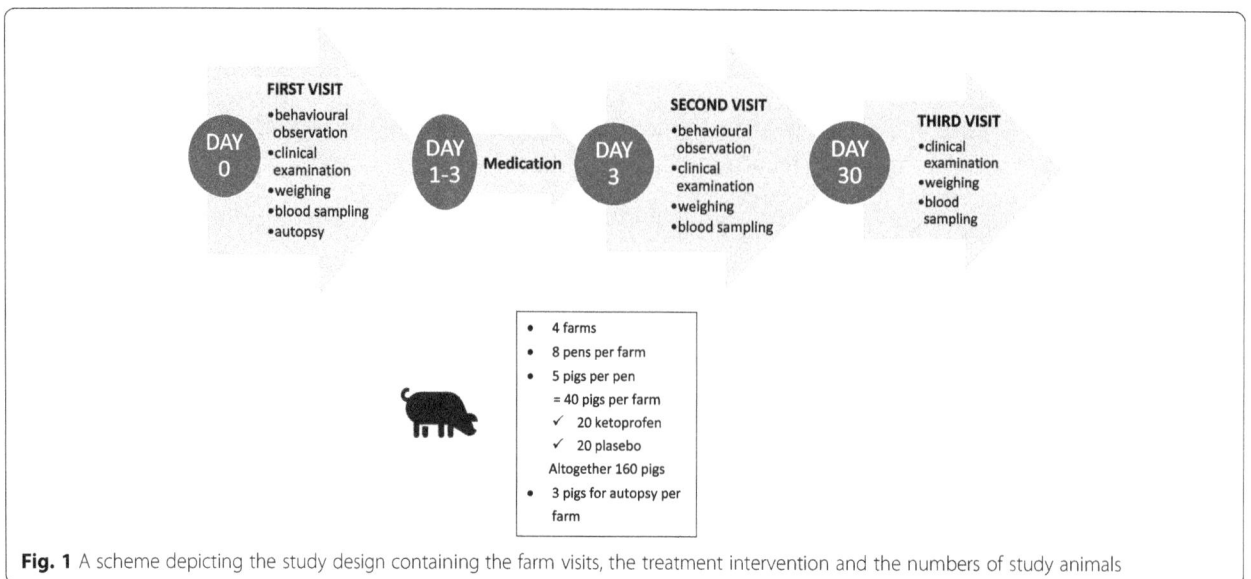

Fig. 1 A scheme depicting the study design containing the farm visits, the treatment intervention and the numbers of study animals

tear staining, tail bitten, and any other clinical sign) were recorded. The farmer had been instructed to mark all pigs with colour that were seen coughing on DAY 0 before the researchers arrived. In addition, all pigs that were seen coughing during the farm visit in the selected compartment were recorded as having a cough. Rectal body temperature was measured and one EDTA and one serum blood sample was taken from the *vena jugularis* after catching the pig with a snout snare. An ear mark with an individual number was attached to the ear of these 40 pigs. Finally, each of these 40 pigs was weighed. Unfortunately, the scale used at farm #4 turned out to be unreliable and weighing results from this farm had to be discarded. Also, approximately half of DAY 30 weighing results from farm #1 are missing because of human error.

The second farm visit was carried out three days later (DAY 3). Behavioural and clinical evaluations were repeated, and the pigs were weighed, and blood was sampled (EDTA and serum samples). About 30 days (range 21–34 days) later (DAY 30), the farm was visited for the third time. The same pigs were evaluated clinically and weighed, and blood was sampled (only serum). Unfortunately, the data recordings made during the third farm visits were incomplete regarding clinical signs, leading to many missing values in the data.

Medication

All pigs in the same pens with the representative pigs were given either ketoprofen 3 mg/kg or a placebo per os once a day for three days starting in the morning of DAY 1. The doses were calculated according to the number and weighing results of the representative pigs and the visually estimated weights of the rest of the pigs in each pen. The daily medications for each pen were dosed in small plastic bags. Herds 1–3 had long troughs, where all pigs fit to eat simultaneously. The farmers of these herds were instructed to mix the medication with small amounts (5–10 l) of regular pig feed and give the mixture by hand into the feeding trough once a day before the morning feeding. The farmer was instructed to follow the feeding during medication days and register any pigs that did not eat normally. In herd 4, the daily dose was given to the pigs through a sophisticated automated feeding system. Each pen had an automatic feeder, which identified each individual pig by its transponder device and delivered individual daily feed rations in several small portions during the day. The feeder had a dispenser capable of measuring small amounts of feed components. The dispenser measured, mixed and dosed the ketoprofen or placebo medication for each pig in the first feed portion in the morning. The feeder also measured the amount of feed eaten by each individual pig during the whole day.

The researchers had no possibility of deciding the antimicrobial medication given to the affected animals; only ketoprofen and placebo could be added in each herd. In herd #1, all pigs were treated with intramuscular injections of long-acting tetracycline (20 mg/kg) on DAYs 0, 2 and 4. In herd #2, intramuscular tetracycline injections (10 mg/kg) were given daily for 5 days to the pigs with clinical signs of respiratory disease. Unfortunately, the farmer had no exact records of the treated animals, but approximately 30% of all pigs in the room were treated and most of the representative pigs were likely to be included in the group of animals receiving tetracycline. In herd #3, all pigs were given intramuscular injections of tetracycline 3 and 1 days before the first farm visit (DAYs − 1 and − 3) and the treatment was continued per os (20 mg/kg) starting on DAY -1 for five days. In herd #4, no antibiotics were used because of mild clinical signs.

Laboratory analyses

Blood samples were transported to the laboratory during the day of the farm visits and centrifuged (3000 rpm, 10 min) there. The sera were stored at − 18 °C until analysis. The EDTA samples were investigated on the day of sampling. The haemoglobin concentration (HGB), haematocrit (HCR), red blood cell count (RBC), white blood cell count (WBC), and platelet count (PLT) were measured for samples taken on DAY 0 and DAY 3 using an Animal Blood Counter Veterinary machine (ABX Diagnostics, Montpellier, France) in the Saari Laboratory, Faculty of Veterinary Medicine, Department of Production Animal Medicine, University of Helsinki.

For aerobic pathogen detection, the lung tissue samples were cultivated on bovine blood agar and incubated at 37 °C. In addition, for possible APP biotype 1 and *Haemophilus parasuis* isolation, the samples were cultivated on bovine blood agar with a *Staphylococcus aureus* streak and incubated under a 5% CO_2 atmosphere at 37 °C. The small colonies showing enhanced growth around the *S. aureus* streak were isolated and confirmed by a positive Camp reaction. They were tested using multiplex PCR, which identified the species and APP serotypes 2, 5 and 6. The non-haemolytic NAD-dependent isolates with a negative CAMP reaction were further tested for *Haemophilus parasuis* using biochemical tests (oxidase, catalase, urease, fermentation of xylose, mannitol, inulin, trehalose and xylose supplemented with NAD and horse serum).

Serum Hp was analysed from samples taken on DAY 0, 3 and 30 using a modified haemoglobin-binding assay developed for cows [24], in which tetramethylbenzidine was used as a substrate [25] and 5 µl of sample volume (originally 20 µl). The assay was adapted for microtitration plates and optical densities of the wells were read at 450 nm using a spectrophotometer (Multiskan MS,

Labsystems Oy, Vantaa, Finland). Pooled and lyophilized aliquots of porcine acute phase serum were used to create standard curves by serial dilutions. The standard curve range was 181–2900 mg/L. Samples with higher results than the standard range were diluted and re-assayed. The assay was calibrated using a porcine serum sample of known Hp concentration provided by the European Commission Concerted Action Project (number QLK5-CT-1999-0153). Serum SAA was analysed from samples taken on DAY 0, 3 and 30 with a commercial sandwich ELISA according to the manufacturer's instructions for porcine serum (Phase SAA assay, Tridelta Development Ltd., Maynooth, Co. Kildare, Ireland).

Serum concentrations of both ketoprofen enantiomers (S- and R-ketoprofen) were determined for all DAY 3 samples from animals in the ketoprofen treatment group. In addition, eight samples taken on day 0 (before treatment) and eight from DAY 3 from the placebo-treated animals were analysed. Chiral high-performance liquid chromatography (HPLC) combined with UV detection was used for the quantitative analysis of ketoprofen enantiomers in pig serum. The analysis method was modified from a previously published description [26]. Samples were prepared by mixing 300 µl of serum, 50 µl of internal standard solution (S-(+)-naproxen, 100 µg/ml) and 650 µl of 0.4% formic acid in water:propanol (96:4). Solid-phase extraction cartridges were conditioned with 1.2 ml of 1% acetic acid in propanol and 1 ml of water. Samples (1 ml) were passed through the cartridges, which were then washed with 1.5 ml of 0.4% formic acid in water:propanol (96:4), followed by 1 ml of water. Solutes were eluted with 1.2 ml of 1% acetic acid in propanol. The solvent was evaporated to dryness in a stream of nitrogen. The residue was redissolved in mobile phase A and transferred into autosampler vials for HPLC analysis. The chromatography system consisted of a Waters Alliance 2695 Separations module and a Waters 2487 Dual λ absorbance detector. The analytical column was an Ultron ES-OVM chiral column (4.6 × 150 mm) preceded by a Ultron ES-OVM chiral guard column (4.0 × 10 mm), both from Shinwa Chemical Industries Ltd. (Kyoto, Japan). The mobile phase was an isocratic mixture of A: 16 mM phosphate buffer (pH 3.0) and B: acetonitrile (93:7). The flow rate was 1.0 ml/min. The UV detector was set at 254 nm. The chromatograms were processed using Empower 3 software (Waters). The linear concentration range was from 0.1 µg/ml to 20.0 µg/ml. Calibration curves were weighted by $1/x^2$ and yielded coefficients of determination (R^2) of 0,997–1000 and 0,997–0,999 for S-ketoprofen and R-ketoprofen. The inter-assay accuracy of the quality control samples (at three different

concentration levels, 0.3, 7.5 and 15.0 µg/ml) ranged from 94.9% to 104.4% for S-ketoprofen and from 94.1% to 103.7% for R-ketoprofen.

The samples from the 15 pigs (out of 20 sampled animals) having paired serum samples available after sample taking and processing, in sampling order, both from DAY 0 and DAY 30 were used for APP serology. APP antibodies were measured using two commercial test kits: IDEXX APP-ApxIV ELISA (IDEXX, Liebefeld-Bern, Switzerland) to detect antibodies against ApxIV toxin, which is produced by all known APP serotypes and IDvet ID Screen APP 2 indirect ELISA (IDvet, Grabels, France) to detect antibodies against LPS specific to APP serotype 2. Both tests were performed according to the manufacturer's instructions. The absorbance results were interpreted as negative or unclear (score 0), or positive with scores ranging from 1 to 5. Seroconversion was defined as an increase in the score by at least one number, e.g. from negative to 1, or from 3 to 4, between DAY 0 and DAY 30. If both the first and the second sample showed the highest antibody level 5, the pig was also defined as seroconverted.

Similarly, the 15 animals from each herd having paired sera available from DAY 0 and DAY 30 were used for SIV serology. All blood samples were tested with influenza A antibody ELISA (ID Screen® Influenza A Antibody Competition, IdVet, Grabels, France) according to the instructions of the kit manufacturer. If at least one pig tested unclear or positive in influenza A ELISA on DAY 0 or 30, blood samples of that herd were further analysed using a haemagglutination inhibition (HI) test according to the operating procedure of the European Surveillance of Influenza in Swine with the antigens H1N1 (SW/Best/96), H1N2 (SW/Gent/7625/99) and H3N2 (SW/St. Oedenrode/96). All the antigens were provided by GD Animal Health Service (Deventer, NL). A sample was considered HI positive if the HI titre was ≥1:20. Seroconversion was defined as an increase in the HI titre between DAY 0 and DAY 30.

Statistical analysis
A required sample size of 80 pigs per group was calculated for the main outcome (daily weight gain) with power 0.8 and confidence level 0.95 assuming equal variances and adjusted for clustering at pen level (assuming cluster size 11, intra cluster correlation 0.1 and coefficient of variation of cluster sizes of 0.1) and assuming a 100-g difference in daily weight gain between the treatment groups.

Descriptive statistics were calculated for daily weight gain, blood parameters, concentrations of S- and R-ketoprofen and for clinical signs and behaviour. An animal was used as the observational unit and results are presented as means and standard deviations (sd) for both treatment groups for all other data except behavioural variables. Mean occurrence (as a proportion of a total of 24 observations per pig) of each behaviour of the five pigs in each pen per observation day were calculated and pen mean was used in the statistical analyses. Because of different baseline levels of body temperature, weight, Hp and SAA concentrations on DAY 0 between the treatment groups, the changes in these variables between DAY 0 vs. DAY 3 within each treatment group were calculated by subtracting the value on DAY 0 from the value on DAY 3.

Descriptive statistics were compared within the treatment groups (ketoprofen/placebo) across different days by paired t-tests for body temperature, all blood parameters (except SAA values), weight and daily weight gain, by McNemar's test for clinical signs, by a repeated measures general linear model for differences in behavioural variables, including farm as a fixed factor, and by Wilcoxon's signed rank non-parametric test for SAA values. Effect of treatment on the magnitude of change in behaviour was tested with univariate models, including farm as fixed factor.

Drinking behaviour was very rare as was also 'other behaviour'. These parameters were therefore not included when analysing the data. Due to technical errors during the observations, no records for activities were available for two of the pens on one farm.

Crude associations between outcome variables and treatment (ketoprofen/placebo) and other explanatory variables (sex) were evaluated using a liberal p-value (0.2) or strong suspicion of biological causal connection. Linear regression was used for that purpose for daily weight gain, body temperature and blood parameters excluding SAA values on DAY 0 and 3. Wilcoxon rank-sum non-parametric testing was used for SAA values on DAY 0 and 3. Logistic regression was used for variables related to clinical signs. Crude associations were not tested for behavioural variables.

Finally, multivariate models were built for the variables evaluated as significant in the crude association analysis and for the behavioural variables. A multilevel mixed-effects linear regression model was fitted for the outcomes weight and daily weigth gain, body temperature and change in body temperature as well as for the Hp and change in Hp and SAA concentrations, containing pen and farm as random intercepts and treatment and sex as fixed effects. Use of antimicrobial treatment in the herd to manage this respiratory outbreak (yes/no) was included as a fixed effect in the multilevel mixed-effects linear regression models for daily weight gain from DAY 0 to DAY 30 and for body temperature for DAY 3. In all other models, antimicrobial treatment did

not remain significant and did not act as a confounder. A repeated measures general linear model with treatment and farm as fixed factors was fitted for behaviour variables. Because of marked variability of actualized interval of DAY 0 and DAY 30 herd visits, the number of days between the first and third herd visits was included in appropriate models. The level of significance was set to 0.05.

For brief model diagnostics, the basic assumptions of linear models were inspected with regard to the data structure and nature of the outcome variables. In addition, residuals were scrutinized. No serious breaches of the underlying assumptions were detected.

The results for Hp and SAA regarding third blood sampling (DAY 30) are presented only in the annex. The serum blood sample on DAY 30 was mainly taken for serology and acute phase proteins were analysed as the samples were readily available. However, it is unlikely that the ketoprofen medication used on DAY 1–3 had any effect on acute phase proteins on DAY 30.

Statistical analysis for all other outcomes than behaviour was made with STATA 14.2 program and the analysis of behavioural data was made with SPSS 21 statistical software.

Results

Data consisted of 160 representative pigs for the herd condition from four farms: 75 (46.9%) castrated boars, 20 (20.5%) intact boars and 65 (40.6%) gilts, altogether 80 finishers in both the ketoprofen and placebo groups. In three herds, there were only castrated boars and females, which were distributed evenly in each herd. Intact boars were present on one farm, where they constituted half of the animals. All three sexes were divided evenly between the ketoprofen and placebo groups.

Behaviour analysis

The results of the behavioural data for different treatment groups are presented in Table 2. Several behavioural differences are presented in the ketoprofen-treated pigs on DAY 3 as compared to DAY 0 based on repeated measures general linear model. On DAY 3, they were observed to stand, walk and lie more often on sternum and less often on flank and more often alone (not in contact with other pigs) than on DAY 0. In addition, the ketoprofen-treated pigs were more active and showed more nosing on DAY 3. Correspondingly, fewer observations of passive behaviour were recorded on DAY 3. In the placebo-treated pigs, the only observed change in behaviour from DAY 0 to DAY 3 was a decrease in lying on sternum. Figure 2a and b present the magnitude of these changes in the ketoprofen- and placebo-treated pigs.

Table 2 Behaviour of representative pigs in a group having a respiratory infection presented as proportion of observations mean ± sd out of 24 observations in two hours before treatment (DAY 0) and on the last day of treatment (DAY 3). The pigs were given ketoprofen or placebo on DAY 1–3

Behaviour	Treatment group	N of pens	DAY 0 Mean ± sd	N of pens	DAY 3 Mean ± sd
Lie flank	Placebo	16	0.32 ± 0.17^{A}	16	0.37 ± 0.12^{A}
	Ketoprofen	16	$0.43 \pm 0.19^{a,B}$	16	$0.23 \pm 0.11^{b,B}$
Lie sternum	Placebo	16	0.52 ± 0.17^{a}	16	$0.44 \pm 0.11^{b,A}$
	Ketoprofen	16	0.43 ± 0.13^{a}	16	$0.51 \pm 0.10^{b,B}$
Sit	Placebo	16	0.03 ± 0.02	16	0.04 ± 0.02
	Ketoprofen	16	0.02 ± 0.02	16	0.03 ± 0.02
Stand	Placebo	16	0.09 ± 0.07	16	0.10 ± 0.05^{A}
	Ketoprofen	16	0.09 ± 0.08^{a}	16	$0.17 \pm 0.08^{b,B}$
Walk	Placebo	16	0.04 ± 0.01	16	0.05 ± 0.05
	Ketoprofen	16	0.03 ± 0.03^{a}	16	0.07 ± 0.04^{b}
Lie alone	Placebo	16	0.09 ± 0.09	16	0.09 ± 0.06
	Ketoprofen	16	0.09 ± 0.10^{a}	16	0.14 ± 0.11^{b}
Active	Placebo	14	0.16 ± 0.10	14	0.20 ± 0.16
	Ketoprofen	14	0.11 ± 0.09^{a}	14	0.21 ± 0.14^{b}
Passive	Placebo	14	0.69 ± 0.14	14	0.67 ± 0.16
	Ketoprofen	14	0.80 ± 0.16^{a}	14	0.60 ± 0.13^{b}
Eat	Placebo	14	0.03 ± 0.03	14	0.03 ± 0.02
	Ketoprofen	14	0.03 ± 0.03	14	0.04 ± 0.04
Nosing	Placebo	14	0.10 ± 0.07	14	0.10 ± 0.07^{A}
	Ketoprofen	14	0.05 ± 0.06^{a}	14	$0.15 \pm 0.11^{b,B}$

[a,b]Values with different superscripts within the same row differ significantly, $p \leq 0.05$
[A,B] Values with different superscripts within the same column differ significantly, $p \leq 0.05$

Clinical signs and rectal temperature

The summary of clinical signs and rectal temperature of study animals during the clinical examination is presented in Table 3. Within the groups, the body temperature and number of coughing pigs decreased in both the ketoprofen- and placebo-treated pigs from the time of acute disease towards the end of the study when animals recovered from clinical disease. There was no treatment effect on any clinical signs based on results from single variable logistic regression models.

According to the mixed model, rectal temperature tended to be somewhat lower (by 0.23 °C) on DAY 0 in the placebo group compared to the ketoprofen-treated group ($p = 0.07$). On DAY 3, pigs receiving the placebo had significantly higher (by 0.26 °C) rectal temperature than those treated with ketoprofen ($p = 0.01$). The pigs in the three herds with antimicrobial treatment did have 0.4 °C lower body temperature on DAY 3 than the pigs in the herd not receiving antibiotic treatment ($p < 0.01$). No difference was detected in body temperature on DAY 30. The rectal temperature change from DAY 0 to DAY 3 was affected by the ketoprofen treatment ($p < 0.001$). The body temperature of the placebo-treated pigs decreased less (on the average by 0.3 °C from DAY 0 to

DAY 3) than that of ketoprofen-treated pigs (by 0.8 °C). There was no difference in temperature change between DAY 0 and 30 between the treatment groups.

Acute phase proteins

Haptoglobin serum concentrations were measured for 77 ketoprofen-treated animals on DAY 0 and 75 for DAY 3 and for placebo-treated animals 79 and 77, respectively. Serum amyloid A concentrations were measured for 77 ketoprofen-treated animals on DAY 0 and 75 for DAY 3 and for placebo-treated animals 79 and 78, respectively.

Hp serum concentrations were higher on DAY 0 compared to DAY 3 in both treatment groups ($p < 0.01$ for ketoprofen group and $p = 0.01$ for placebo group). Based on a mixed model, there was no difference in Hp concentrations between the treatment groups before treatment (DAY 0). The treatment was associated with Hp levels on DAY 3. Pigs in the placebo group had, on the average, 268 mg/l higher haptoglobin concentrations in serum than the pigs in the ketoprofen-treated group ($p = 0.01$). The Hp concentration change from DAY 0 to DAY 3 (calculated by subtracting Hp on DAY 0 from Hp on DAY 3) was not associated with the treatment.

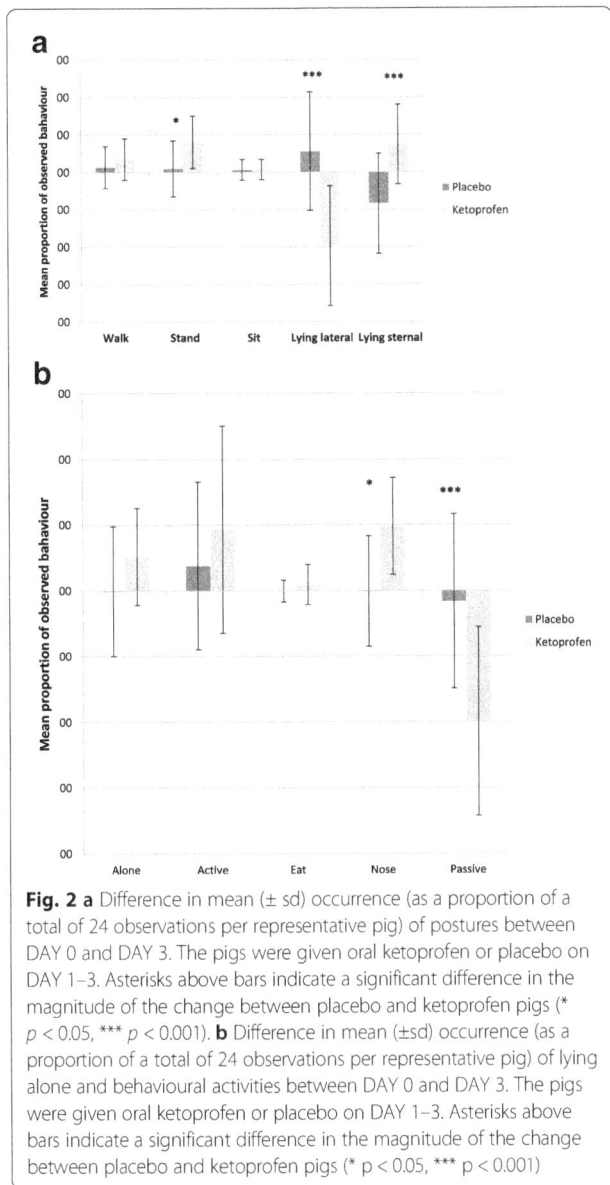

Fig. 2 a Difference in mean (± sd) occurrence (as a proportion of a total of 24 observations per representative pig) of postures between DAY 0 and DAY 3. The pigs were given oral ketoprofen or placebo on DAY 1–3. Asterisks above bars indicate a significant difference in the magnitude of the change between placebo and ketoprofen pigs (* $p < 0.05$, *** $p < 0.001$). **b** Difference in mean (±sd) occurrence (as a proportion of a total of 24 observations per representative pig) of lying alone and behavioural activities between DAY 0 and DAY 3. The pigs were given oral ketoprofen or placebo on DAY 1–3. Asterisks above bars indicate a significant difference in the magnitude of the change between placebo and ketoprofen pigs (* $p < 0.05$, *** $p < 0.001$)

Figure 3 presents Hp concentrations of pigs in the keto-profen- and placebo-treated groups.

SAA concentrations were higher on DAY 0 compared to DAY 3 in both treatment groups ($p < 0.01$ for both treatment groups). Based on Wilcoxon's rank-sum non-parametric test, there was no statistically significant difference between the treatment groups in SAA concentrations on DAY 0 or DAY3. The SAA concentration change from DAY 0 to DAY 3 (calculated by subtracting SAA on DAY 0 from SAA on DAY 3) was not affected by the treatment. Figure 4 presents SAA concentrations of pigs in both groups.

Clinical blood parameters

Table 4 contains detailed results for complete blood count parameters. Treatment was not associated with any of the blood parameters analysed.

Body weight, daily weight gain

The farmers reported three (2.5%) animals that did not eat normally during the medication days on the three farms having long troughs. On the fourth farm with the automated feeding system measuring the amount of feed eaten by each individual pig, all pigs included in the study ate the medicated feed portion by noon. The pigs in the placebo and ketoprofen groups ate similar and increasing amounts of feed from DAY 0 to DAY 3 on this farm.

Body weights were not statistically significantly different between the treatment groups on DAY 0 or DAY 3, even if the pigs in the placebo group tended to be somewhat lighter than those receiving ketoprofen. Based on mixed model, daily weight gain between DAY 0–3 was not significantly associated with the treatment, but pigs in the placebo group showed better daily weight gain (by 104 g per day) from DAY 0 to DAY 30 ($p = 0.01$) than the ketoprofen group. The pigs in the herds with anti-microbial treatment had 169 g less daily weight gain from DAY 0 to DAY 30 compared to the pigs in the herd not receiving antimicrobials ($p = 0.01$). However, antimicrobial treatment did not confound the ketoprofen treatment effect during the same time period. Table 5 shows all body weight-related results.

Ketoprofen concentrations

No samples collected from the placebo-treated pigs or collected from the ketoprofen-treated pigs before treatment start (baseline samples) contained detectable amounts of S- or R-ketoprofen. Serum S-ketoprofen concentrations were above the validated lower limit of quantification (LLOQ; 0.1 µg/ml) in 76 out of the 79 (96%) samples taken from ketoprofen-treated pigs on the last day of treatment. The remaining three pigs had serum S-ketoprofen concentrations just below the LLOQ. For R-ketoprofen, serum concentrations were above the LLOQ in 47 samples (60%). The mean (+sd) serum concentrations of S- and R-ketoprofen on DAY 3 were 1.41 ± 1.58 and 0.22 ± 0.20 µg/ml. The concentration frequency distributions of S- and R-ketoprofen on DAY 3 are presented in Fig. 5a and b. The blood samples for ketoprofen analysis were taken on DAY 3, on the average 324 ± 35 min after administration of the medicine mixed in feed.

Pathogens involved in the respiratory infection

Based on the results from the autopsies and serology, all herds had an acute respiratory outbreak caused by APP and in one herd, also swine influenza virus may have been involved. At least one pig out of three autopsied per herd revealed an acute lung infection, where APP could be cultured and diagnosed as APP serotype 2. No other APP serotypes were discovered. In one individual

Table 3 Summary of clinical signs and rectal temperature of representative pigs in a group with respiratory infection

		DAY 0		DAY 3		DAY 30	
Variable	Treatment group						
		N	N (%) of animals	N	N (%) of animals	N	N (%) of animals
Cough	Placebo	80	9 (11.3)[a]	80	0 (0)[b]	50	0 (0)[b]
	Ketoprofen	80	7 (8.8)[a]	79	0 (0)[b]	50	0 (0)
Tear staining	Placebo	80	41 (51.2)	80	46 (56.3)	50	29 (58)
	Ketoprofen	80	42 (52.5)	79	42 (53.2)	50	34 (68)
Bitten tail	Placebo	80	20 (25)	80	13 (16.3)[b]	50	15 (30)[c]
	Ketoprofen	80	16 (20)	79	18 (22.8)	50	14 (28)
		°C mean ± sd		°C mean ± sd		°C mean ± sd	
Rectal temperature	Placebo	80	39.8 ± 0.6[a]	80	39.4 ± 0.4[b,A]	80	39.3 ± 0.2[b]
	Ketoprofen	80	40.0 ± 0.8[a]	80	39.1 ± 0.4[b,B]	80	39.3 ± 0.3[c]

Pigs were given oral ketoprofen (3 mg/day) or a placebo during DAY 1–3. The clinical inspections were performed before treatment (DAY 0), on the last day of treatment (DAY 3) and on DAY 30
[a,b,c]Values with different superscripts within the same row differ significantly, p ≤ 0.05
[A,B]Values with different superscripts within the same column differ significantly, p = 0.01

animal, the pathological examination showed a mixed bacterial infection, where in addition to APP, *Pasteurella multocida* could be cultured. None of the autopsies revealed signs of other respiratory pathogens.

All four herds had pigs with seroconversion of APP antibodies in their paired serum samples. On the average, 67% and 45% of the pigs seroconverted between DAY 0 and DAY 30 based on either ApxIV toxin or APP2 LPS serological tests. In addition, in one herd, 13% of the animals had rising antibodies against SIV in their paired samples between DAY 0 and DAY 30.

Discussion

The aim was to evaluate possible effects of NSAID medication administered in feed to finishing pigs during acute respiratory disease outbreaks in field conditions.

Drug exposure was documented by concentration analysis in serum. Ketoprofen had the expected antipyretic effect and reduced behavioural signs of sickness. However, no statistically significant differences were noted between the ketoprofen- and placebo-treated animals in clinical signs, short-term weight gain or blood parameters. Unexpectedly, the animals of the placebo group showed better daily weight gain during the 30-day observation period after the medication than the ketoprofen-treated animals.

Behaviour

The increase in activity and postures related to higher activity levels (standing, walking, lying on sternum) of the ketoprofen-treated pigs on DAY 3 compared to

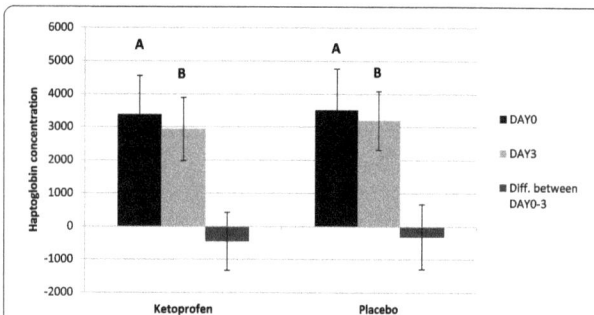

Fig. 3 Haptoglobin concentrations (mg/l, mean and sd) for finishing pigs in herds having a respiratory disease outbreak. The pigs were given oral ketoprofen during DAY 1–3 and sampled before treatment (DAY 0) and on the last day of treatment (DAY 3). Bars marked with different letters (A, B) differ significantly from each other (p < 0.05), the comparison is valid only within treatment group (ketoprofen/placebo)

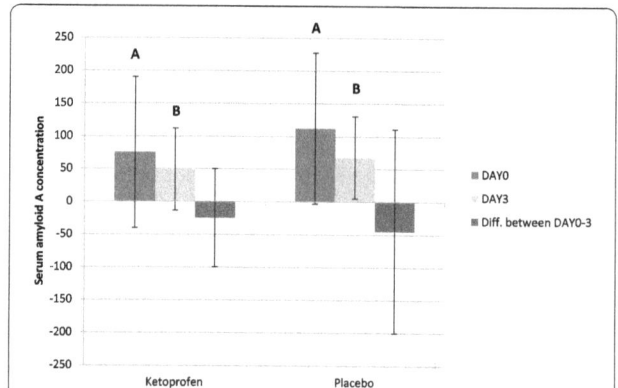

Fig. 4 Serum amyloid A concentrations (mg/l, mean and sd) for finishing pigs in herds with a respiratory disease outbreak. The pigs were given oral ketoprofen or placebo during DAY 1–3 and sampled before treatment (DAY 0), on the last day of treatment (DAY 3) and on DAY 30. Bars marked with different letters differ significantly from each other (p < 0.01)

Table 4 Clinical blood parameters (mean and standard deviation, sd) of representative pigs in a group of finishing pigs with respiratory clinical signs

Variable	Treatment group	DAY 0		DAY 3	
		N	(Mean ± sd)	N	(Mean ± sd)
WBC (10^9)	Placebo	74	24.4 ± 6.4	74	25.1 ± 6.3
	Ketoprofen	75	23.1 ± 5.6	78	23.9 ± 5.3
HB (g/l)	Placebo	74	112.6 ± 10.0	74	110.9 ± 11.1
	Ketoprofen	75	110.5 ± 12.1	78	112.0 ± 11.0
HCT (%)	Placebo	74	34.5 ± 4.5	74	34.6 ± 3.9
	Ketoprofen	75	34.5 ± 4.2	78	34.7 ± 3.7
PLT (1000/µl)	Placebo	74	394.8 ± 127.3	74	411.6 ± 112.3
	Ketoprofen	75	368.0 ± 115.3[a]	78	414.3 ± 90.2[b]

The pigs were given oral ketoprofen (3 mg/kg) or placebo during DAY 1–3 and sampled before treatment (DAY 0) and on the last day of treatment (DAY 3)
White blood cell count = WBC, haemoglobin = HG, haematocrit = HCT, platelet count = PLT
[a,b]Values with different superscripts within the same row differ significantly, p ≤ 0.05

DAY 0 all indicate a decrease in behavioural signs of sickness [27], which was not apparent in the placebo-treated pigs. In our study, the pigs had only mild clinical signs and none of the animals was clearly dyspnoeic. Thus, we did not interpret sitting, or lying in a sternal position to be signs of pigs trying to ease their respiration. Instead, we interpreted lying in a sternal position as a sign of a more active behaviour compared to lying on the flank, which was further supported in the ketoprofen-treated pigs by increased nosing, which is a form of exploratory behaviour. Exploration has been reported to be reduced as a result of sickness [27]. The increase in lying alone in the ketoprofen group was interpreted as a sign of improved control of body temperature, as pigs are known to huddle when they experience a colder ambient temperature.

The only observed difference in frequency of behaviours on DAY 0 between treatment groups was in the lying in a flank position. We are unable to give any causal explanation for this difference. We suppose it to be coincidental especially because any other behaviours did not have baseline differences.

Altogether, the behavioural changes reported here are in line with changes seen in pigs experimentally infected with viral respiratory disease [2, 6]. Recently, ketoprofen has been shown to prevent the development of sickness behaviour, including depression caused by lipopolysaccharide-induced inflammation, which is in agreement with the observed higher activity levels observed in the current study [22].

Clinical signs and rectal temperature

Before treatment, both groups had elevated rectal temperatures because they had been suffering from an acute respiratory infection for one or two days. On the last day of treatment, the body temperature had gone down in both treatment groups. The decline was, however, more pronounced in the ketoprofen group. This effect is understandable as ketoprofen has a good antipyretic effect in swine given in drinking water [15]. We show here that an antipyretic effect can also be achieved by giving ketoprofen in feed in clinical conditions.

We did not observe a treatment effect on any clinical signs (cough, tear staining, bitten tail) evaluated. Most previous studies reported an improvement in clinical signs on NSAID treated animals compared to the non-treated controls suffering from respiratory infection [14, 15]. In our study, some animals had already been treated with antimicrobial agents before the first visit, which may have lowered the severity of the clinical signs and made the possible differences in clinical signs pre- and post-medication smaller and thus less likely to be detected. Respiratory disease outbreaks were quite mild, as approximately only 10% of study pigs were coughing before the treatment. Furthermore, none of the pigs were coughing any longer at the second and third study visits, and dyspnea was not observed during the whole study period, which confirms the acute nature of the clinical respiratory disease in our study herds. On the other

Table 5 Body weight and daily weight gain of representative pigs in a group of finishing pigs with respiratory clinical signs

Variable	Treatment group	N	DAY 0 Mean ± sd	N	DAY 3 Mean ± sd	N	DAY 30 Mean ± sd
Body weight, kg	Placebo	60	40.1 ± 7.1[a]	60	43.1 ± 7.5[a]	50	70.9 ± 9.5[b]
	Ketoprofen	60	43.4 ± 8.8[a]	60	46.3 ± 9.1[a]	50	71.1 ± 12.2[b]
			DAY0–DAY 3		DAY 0–DAY 30		
Daily weight gain, g	Placebo	60	1046 ± 719	50	992.5 ± 145[A]		
	Ketoprofen	60	1235 ± 721 [a]	50	886.8 ± 197[b,B]		

The pigs were given oral ketoprofen (3 mg/kg) or placebo during DAY 1–3 and weighed before treatment (DAY 0), on the last day of treatment (DAY 3) and on DAY 30
[a,b]Values with different superscripts within the same row differ significantly, p ≤ 0.05
[A,B]Values with different superscripts within the same column differ significantly, p = 0.01

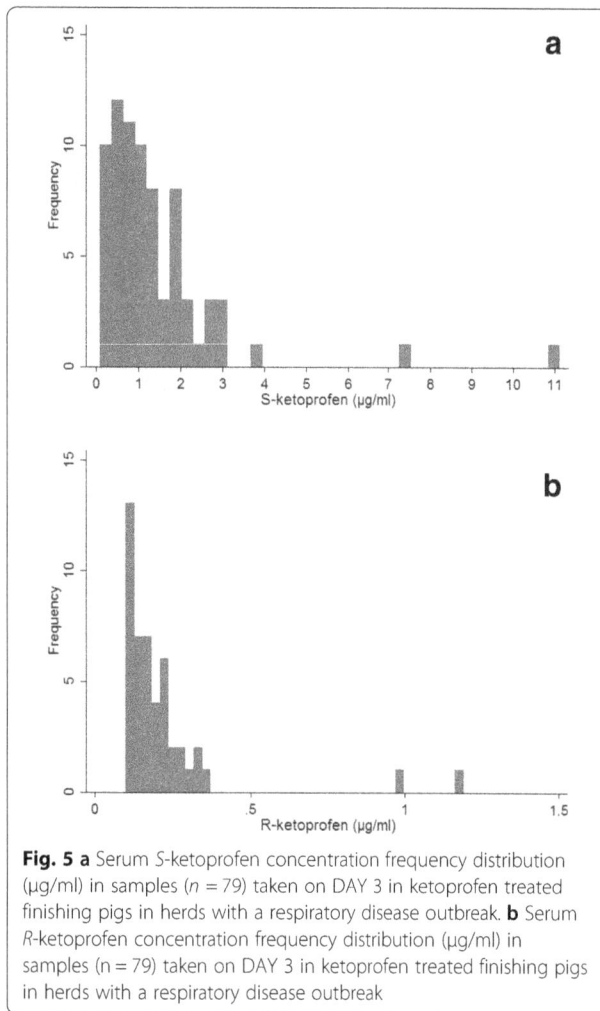

Fig. 5 a Serum S-ketoprofen concentration frequency distribution (μg/ml) in samples (n = 79) taken on DAY 3 in ketoprofen treated finishing pigs in herds with a respiratory disease outbreak. **b** Serum R-ketoprofen concentration frequency distribution (μg/ml) in samples (n = 79) taken on DAY 3 in ketoprofen treated finishing pigs in herds with a respiratory disease outbreak

sampling days, the Hp concentrations in both treatment groups were higher than the reference range (10–1310 mg/l) measured in a healthy boar herd [29]. A very similar range of Hp concentrations (2000–4000 mg/l) has been reported in pigs experimentally infected with APP or swine influenza virus [10, 13] and in pigs infected with several respiratory pathogens in clinical conditions [11]. However, it should be kept in mind that Hp concentration variation between herds could be notable depending on the overall health status and management of the herd, and Hp concentration comparisons between farms may not be very informative [30–32]. The magnitude of change in Hp concentrations from DAY 0 to DAY 3 was not affected by the treatment. Similar results of NSAID having no effect on Hp levels in endotoxin-challenged pigs have been obtained earlier [20].

SAA concentrations measured in specific pathogen free pigs are usually below 15 mg/l [11]. Compared to this reference value, SAA concentrations in this study before treatment in both treatment groups was clearly elevated and indicative of a positive acute phase response. Infected animals reach peak SAA concentrations within 1–2 days post infection and SAA seems to remain elevated at least 4 days post infection [10, 13, 28]. Our observed concentrations were in a similar range (40–60 mg/l) as those in swine influenza virus (SIV) infected pigs two days post infection [29]. In pigs experimentally infected with APP, even higher SAA concentrations (400–600 mg/l) were found 2–4 days post infection [10]. In co-infection with SIV and *Pasteurella multocida*, the peak level of SAA was observed as 155 μg/ml [13]. We did not find an effect of ketoprofen on SAA levels in pigs suffering from respiratory infection. Unfortunately, there is no previous knowledge regarding the effect of ketoprofen on SAA levels in infected pigs. In young calves, ketoprofen alone is able to decrease SAA concentrations after lipopolysaccaride challenge [33]. As the observed difference between the treatment groups in the change in SAA values from DAY 0 to DAY 3 was substantial, it might be that our study lacked sufficient power to detect a statistically significant treatment effect.

Other blood parameters

The white blood cell count (WBC) was slightly elevated on DAY 0 and DAY 3 in pigs in both treatment groups compared to species specific reference values [34]. All other blood parameters in study pigs were within normal limits, as expected. There was no treatment effect on WBC which is in agreement with an older study where pigs were infected with APP [3]. The lack of treatment effect may be due to the overall mild clinical signs observed. On the other hand, very little is known about WBC alterations in pigs during respiratory disease or associated with NSAID treatment. It might be that they are not very sensitive markers of infection or

hand, as all pigs recovered swiftly, it may be that we missed the most acute phase of the disease episode. In case of an acute respiratory disease, the time elapsed after the beginning of the outbreak and the first herd visit may have been too long.

There were numerous missing values in the data regarding the clinical observations made on DAY 30, which may have led to observation bias. However, the missing values were distributed evenly to all herds and both treatment groups, which makes this bias unlikely.

Haptoglobin and serum amyloid a

Regardless the treatment group, serum Hp concentration was elevated on DAY 0 compared to DAY 3 or DAY 30. Our samples were taken approximately two and five days post infection, even though there might be notable variation as we do not know the exact day of onset of clinical signs. As Hp reaches its peak concentration 2–3 days post infection and stays elevated up to 7 or more days post infection [10, 13, 28] it is likely that we had a good chance to detect elevated Hp serum concentrations. On all three effectiveness of NSAID treatment in pigs. Other researchers have also suspected that comparison to reference values is complicated by a number of factors, especially in pigs. For example, the values may not be applicable for modern pig breeds [35].

Daily weight gain

There was no treatment effect on daily weight gain during the treatment from DAY 0 to DAY 3. In a previous study, no effect of ketoprofen on daily weight gain was seen during ten days of medication, when the drug was administered in drinking water to pigs suffering from porcine respiratory disease complex [15]. As already stated, the medication may have been started too late after the onset of an acute disease. If started earlier during the most acute phase of the disease, the medication may have had better possibilities to have the desired effect. As the observed difference between the treatment groups in weight gain from DAY 0 to DAY 3 was substantial, it might be that our study again lacked sufficient power to detect a statistically significant treatment effect.

We did observe approximately 100 g/day better average daily weight gain in the placebo group from DAY 0 to DAY 30 compared to the ketoprofen-treated group. Although unlikely, it cannot be ruled out that the three-day ketoprofen medication could have had a long-lasting effect on weight gain. The issue should be investigated further and biological explanations sought. The animals of the placebo group were by chance slightly smaller at the beginning of the trial than those allocated to the ketoprofen treatment, even if the difference was not statistically significant. We suspected that the observed difference in daily weight gain was at least to some extent due to compensatory growth of the smaller pigs in the placebo group. However, when this possible biological explanation was investigated further with analysis of covariance (results not shown), this was not the case.

No perceived difficulties occurred in administering the ketoprofen product per os mixed with regular pig feed. Pigs in three of the herds were on restrictive feeding where feed was available only at certain times and in limited amounts. Probably the restricted feeding made it easier to ascertain the intake of medicated feed, which was offered just before the regular feeding when the pigs were hungry. However, also in one of the herds with an automatic feeder, the pigs consumed the medicated feed with no problems. We did not observe treatment effect on appetite of pigs during the treatment, while the feed consumption increased steadily each day after DAY 0 (results not shown). In another study, NSAID treatment has been reported to lessen the decrease in feed consumption in infected pigs compared to non-medicated animals [3].

Possible negative effects of NSAID medication

Even though NSAID medication may be helpful in inflammatory conditions, it should be kept in mind that negative effects have been reported in humans following NSAID consumption. Gastric ulceration is a well-known side-effect of NSAIDs in human medicine [36]. In the context of respiratory diseases, the frequency of severe bacterial infections after exposure to NSAIDs has been observed to be elevated in children [37]. Most studies on ketoprofen medication in pigs do not mention the possibility of negative effects. Such absence of information should not be interpreted as absence of possible drawbacks. However, in one study experimentally infected pigs were treated with NSAIDs, euthanized 48 h after the challenge and autopsied. None of the animals showed macroscopic kidney lesions or recent gastric ulcers [3]. In the current study, no negative effects were observed by the farm personnel during the three days of double-blinded medication with ketoprofen or placebo. However, it should be admitted that minor side effects, if present, might have gone unnoticed in the clinical setting. As already discussed earlier, 3-day treatment with ketoprofen was in our study associated with lower body weight gain during the subsequent 30-day observation period, but in the absence of a plausible biological explanation for such an adverse effect on growth, causality should not be assumed.

When per os medication is given to pigs in a group, the treatment is difficult, even impossible, to restrict only to certain animals in a group. In our study, ketoprofen (or placebo) was given to all animals in the same pen where the representative pigs were housed as this was considered to be the most feasible way to manage oral medication in most commercial piggeries. It is likely that some pigs received the medication even if they were healthy, thus exposing them to possible negative effects without any possible benefit. However, in case of respiratory diseases, the outbreak usually concerns the entire compartment. In addition to this, some animals might be subclinically infected and in need of medication. Thus, we suggest that making medication decisions on a pen-level would be accurate enough in the case of acute infectious respiratory disease in pigs.

Ketoprofen concentrations

Medication mixed in feed of pigs comes with substantial risks of under- or overdosing. Our study shows that the pigs ate their ketoprofen dose voluntarily, because the total mean serum concentration was 1.6 µg/ml at six hours after feeding. In the ketoprofen concentration values of individual pigs, there was only one clearly higher (11.1 µg/ml) value. Based on this information, it is not likely that individual animals should have consumed the majority of medicated feed and possibly ingested significant overdoses of ketoprofen. Ketoprofen was administered as a racemic mixture of two enantiomers, *S*- and *R*-ketoprofen. Only *S*-ketoprofen is pharmacologically active. While both enantiomers have approximately similar pharmacokinetic properties in humans [38], they are handled in significantly different fashion in several animal species, including pigs [39]. Very marked chiral conversion of *R*-ketoprofen to *S*-ketoprofen has been observed, resulting in much faster clearance of *R*-ketoprofen compared to the *S*-form, and low exposure to *R*-ketoprofen [38, 40]. Our results are in line with these observations. The oral bioavailability of *S*-ketoprofen has been reported to be approximately 80%, when 3 mg/kg oral and intravenous doses have been compared in pigs [39]. The concentrations of *S*-ketoprofen in the serum samples collected approximately 6 h after administration of the drug mixed in feed were close to what has previously been reported after controlled oral administration of similar doses [39]. The maximum concentration of ketoprofen (measured as S- and R-ketoprofen or racemic ketoprofen) in serum is usually recorded 1–2 h after controlled oral administration by gavage [16, 41]. It has been reported that the mean racemic ketoprofen concentration in plasma was at least 1 µg/ml for about 10 h after oral administration at a dosage of 3 mg/kg in experimental settings, and this was theoretically considered as an effective dose [41]. Low total plasma racemic ketoprofen concentrations in pigs (0.1–2.09 µg/ml, depending on the dose given) have anti-inflammatory effects [17]. Very low half maximal inhibitory concentrations (IC_{50} 0.0003–0.003 µg/ml) of *S*-ketoprofen regarding inflammatory cytokine synthesis have been reported in the goat [42]. In this study, mean serum concentrations, derived from single blood samples, of S-ketoprofen and total racemic ketoprofen were 1.4 µg/ml and 1.55 µg/ml. Based on current, partly insufficient knowledge of required therapeutic levels for ketoprofen in pigs, the S-ketoprofen concentrations in our study should be estimated as adequate.

Conclusions

The results indicate that ketoprofen administered in feed at approximately 3 mg/kg body weight reduced behavioural signs of sickness and had an antipyretic effect. As there were no effects of ketoprofen on clinical signs, feed intake or blood parameters, it can be assumed that the effect of ketoprofen mainly affected the welfare of the pigs, while the effect on recovery was less pronounced. However, the medication in this study was perhaps started only after the most severe clinical phase of the respiratory disease was over, and this delay might have hampered the evaluation of treatment effects. A possible adverse effect on production cannot be excluded, as the ketoprofen-treated animals showed lesser average growth over the 30-day observation period than the placebo-treated animals. Clinically significant drug exposure was achieved by administering ketoprofen per os mixed with regular pig feed in regular farm conditions in commercial herds.

Acknowledgements
We thank the farmers for letting us collect these results with their herds. We would like also to thank the following experts for analyzing the samples in the laboratories of Finnish Food Safety Authority Evira: Taina Laine (pathological examinations), Kirsti Pelkola (bacteriology), Mirja Raunio-Saarnisto and Sinikka Pelkonen (APP serology) and Tiina Nokireki (SIV serology).

Funding
This work was partly funded by the ESNIP3 Consortium (European Surveillance Network for Influenza in Pigs 3, grant #259949, FP7-Influenza-2010). Funding was also obtained for this study from the Ministry of Agriculture and Forestry of Finland (Makera-funding), Vetcare Ltd. and three slaughterhouses (Atria, HK Scan and Snellman).

Authors' contributions
Outi Hälli (OH) wrote the draft of the manuscript. Minna Haimi-Hakala, Tapio Laurila, Claudio Oliviero and Mari Heinonen did the herd visits. Toomas Orro took care of the laboratory analyses for acute phase proteins. Mika Scheinin and Saija Sirén performed the ketoprofen analyses. OH made statistical analyses except for behavioural data, which were analysed by Anna Valros. All authors took an active part in planning the study and commenting the data analysis and the manuscript. All authors read and approved the final manuscript.

Competing interests
M. Scheinin has been engaged in contract research for Vetcare Ltd., not associated with this study. The other authors declare that they have no competing interests.

Author details
[1]Faculty of Veterinary Medicine, University of Helsinki, Paroninkuja 20, 04920 Saarentaus, FI, Finland. [2]Department of Clinical Veterinary Medicine, Estonian University of Life Sciences, Kreutzwaldi 62, 51014 Tartu, EE, Estonia. [3]Faculty of Veterinary Medicine, University of Helsinki, P.O. Box 57, 00014 Helsinki, FI, Finland. [4]Institute of Biomedicine, University of Turku, and Unit of Clinical Pharmacology, Turku University Hospital, 20014 Turku, FI, Finland.

References
1. Christensen C, Sørensen V, Mousing J. Diseases Of the respiratory system. In: Straw BE, D'Allaire S, Mengeling WL, Taylor DJ, editors. Diseases of swine. 8th ed: Iowa State University press; 1999. p. 913–40.
2. Sutherland MA, Niekamp SR, Johnson RW, Van Alstine WG, Salak-Johnson JL. Heat and social rank impact behaviour and physiology of PRRS-virus-infected pigs. Physiol Behav. 2007;90:73–81.

3. Swinkels JM, Piipers A, Venooy JC, Van Nes A, Verheijden JH. Effects of ketoprofen and flunixin in pigs experimentally infected with Actinobacillus pleuropneumoniae. J Vet Pharmacol Ther. 1994;17:299–303.

4. van Leengoed A, Kamp EM. Endobrochial inoculation of various doses of Haemophilus (Actinobacillus) pleuropneumoniae in pigs. Am J Vet Res. 1989;50:2054–9.

5. Bailey M, Engler H, Hunzeker J, Sheridan JF. The hypothalamic-pituitary-adrenal axis and viral infection. Viral Immunol. 2003;16:141–57.

6. Escobar J, Van Alstine WG, Baker DH, Johnson RW. Behaviour of pigs with viral and bacterial pneumonia. Appl Anim Behav Sci. 2007;105:42–50.

7. Lampreave F, Gonzáles-Ramón N, Martinez-Avensa S, Hernández MA, Lorenzo HK, Garcia-Gil A, Piñeiro A. Characterization of the acute phase serum protein response in pigs. Electrophoresis. 1994;15:672–6.

8. Eckersall PD, Saini PK, McComb C. The acute phase response of acid soluble glycoprotein, α-acid glycoprotein, ceruloplasmin, haptoglobin an C-reactive protein, in the pig. Vet Immunol Immunopathol. 1996;51:377–85.

9. PMH H, Klausen J, Nielsen JP, Gonzáles-Ramón N, Piñeiro M, Lampreave F, Alava MA. The porcine acuten phase response to infection with Actinobacillus pleuropneumoniae. Haptoglobin, C-reactive protein, major acute phase protein and serum amyloid a protein are sensitive indicators of infection. Comp Biochem Physiol. 1998;119B:365–73.

10. Hultén C, Johansson E, Fossum C, Wallgren P. Interleukin 6, serum amyloid a and haptoglobin as markers of treatment efficacy in pigs experimentally infected with Actinobacillus pleuropneumoniae. Vet Microbiol. 2003;95:75–89.

11. Parra MD, Fuentes P, Tecles F, Martinez-Subiela S, Martinez JS, Munõs A, Cerón JJ. Porcine acute phase protein concentrations in different disease in field conditions. J Vet Med B Infect Dis Vet Public Health. 2006;53:488–93.

12. Petersen HH, Dideriksen D, Christiansen BM, Nielsen JP. Serum haptoglobin concentrations as a marker of clinical signs in finishing pigs. Vet Rec. 2002;151:85–9.

13. Pomorska-Mól M, Markowska-Daniel I, Kwit K, Czyzewska E, Dors A, Rachubik J, Pejsak Z. Immune and inflammatory response in pigs during acute influenza caused by H1N1 swine influenza virus. Arch Virol. 2014;159:2605–14.

14. Mackinnon JD. The proper use and benefits of veterinary antimicrobial agents in swine practice. Vet Microbiol. 1993;35:357–67.

15. Salichs M, Sabaté D, Homedes J. Efficacy of ketoprofen administered in drinking water at a low dose for the treatment of porcine respiratory disease complex. J Anim Sci. 2013;91:4469–75.

16. Mustonen K, Niemi A, Raekallio M, Heinonen M, Peltoniemi OA, Palviainen M, Siven M, Peltoniemi M, Vainio O. Enantiospecific ketoprofen concentrations in plasma after oral and intramuscular administrations in growing pigs. Acta Vet Scand. 2012a;54:55.

17. Mustonen K, Banting A, Raekallio M, Heinonen M, Peltoniemi OA, Vainio O. Dose-response investigation of oral ketoprofen in pigs challenged with Escherichia Coli endotoxin. Vet Rec. 2012b;171:70.

18. Sabate D, Salichs M, Salichs M, Homedes J. Efficacy trial of ketoprofen based oral solution as adjunctive therapy to antibacterial treatment of porcine respiratory disease. J Vet Pharmacol Ther. 2012;35(suppl.3):137–78.

19. Salichs M, Sabaté D, Ciervo O, Homedes J. Comparison of the antipyretic efficacy of ketoprofen, acetylsalicylic acid, and paracetamol, orally administered to swine. J Vet Pharmacol Ther. 2012;35:198–201.

20. Friton GM, Schmidt H, Schrödl W. Clinical and anti-inflammatory effects of treating endotoxin-challenged pigs with meloxicam. Vet Rec. 2006;159:552–7.

21. Swinkels JM, Pijpers A, Veernoy JCM, Van Nes A, Verheijden JHM. Effects of ketoprofen and flunixin in pigs experimentally infected with Actinobacillus pleuropneumoniae. J Vet Pharmacol Ther 1994;17:299–303.

22. Wyns H, Meyer E, Plessers E, Watteyn A, van Bergen T, Schauvliege S, De Baers S, Devresse M, De Backer P, Greubels S. Modulation by gamithromycin and ketoprofen of in vitro and in vivo porcine lipopolysaccharide-induced inflammation. Vet Immunology and Immunopathol. 2015;168:211–22.

23. Haimi-Hakala M, Hälli O, Laurila T, Raunio-Saarnisto M, Nokireki T, Laine T, Nykäsenoja S, Pelkola K, Segales J, Sibila M, Oliviero C, Peltoniemi O, Pelkonen S, Heinonen M. Etiology of acute respiratory disease in fattening pigs in Finland. Porcine Health Manag. 2017;3:19. https://doi.org/10.1186/s40813-017-0065-2.

24. Makimura S, Suzuki N. Quantitative determination of bovine serum Haptoglobin and its elevation in some inflammatory diseases. Nihon Juigaku Zasshi. 1982;44:15–21.

25. Alsemgeest SP, Kalsbeek HC, Wensing T, Koeman JP, van Ederen AM, Gruys E. Concentrations of serum amyloid-a (SAA) and haptoglobin (HP) as parameters of inflammatory diseases in cattle. Vet Q. 1994;16:21–3.

26. Menzel-Soglowek S, Geisslinger G, Brune K. Stereoselective high-performance liquid chromatographic determination of ketoprofen, ibuprofen and fenoprofen in plasma using a chiral alpha 1-acid glycoprotein column. J Chromatogr. 1990;532:295–303.

27. Weary DM, Huzzey JM, von Keyserlingk MA. Board-invited review: using behavior to predict and identify ill health in animals. J Anim Sci. 2009;87:770–7.

28. Pomorska-Mól M, Markowska-Daniel I, Kwit K, Stepaniewska K, Pejsak Z. C-reactive protein, haptoglobin, serum amyloid a and pig major acute phase protein response in pigs simultaneously infected with H1N1 swinw influenza virus and Pasteurella multocida. BMC Vet Res. 2013;9:14.

29. Diack AB, Gladney CD, Mellencamp MA, Stear MJ, Eckersall PD. Characterisation of plasma acute phase protein concentrations in a high health boar herd. Vet Immunol Immunopathol. 2011;139:107–12.

30. Chen HH, Lin JH, Fung HP, Ho LL, Yang PC, Lee WC, Lee YP, Chu RM. Serum acute phase proteins and swine health status. The Canadian J Vet Res. 2003;67:283–90.

31. Amory JR, Mackenzie AM, Eckersall PD, Stear MJ, Pearce GP. Influence of rearing conditions and respiratory disease on haptoglobin levels in the pig at slaughter. Res Vet Sci. 2007;83:428–35.

32. Pig-MAP and haptoglobin concentration reference values in swine form commercial farms, Piñeiro C, Piñeiro M, Morales J, Andrés M, Lorenzo E, Pozo MD, Alava MA, Lampreave F. Vet J. 2009;179:78–84.

33. Plessers E, Wyns H, Watteyn A, Pardon B, Baere SD, Sys SU, Backer PD, Croubels S. Immunomodulatory properties of gamithromycin and ketoprofen in lipopolysaccharide-challenged calves with emphasis on the acute-phase response. Vet Immunol Immunopathol. 2016;171:28–37.

34. Fielder SE. In: the Merck veterinary manual. Hematologic reference ranges 2016. http://www.merckvetmanual.com/appendixes/reference-guides/hematologic-reference-ranges. Accessed 17 Dec 2016.

35. Lumsden JH. "Normal" or reference values: questions and comments. Vet Clin Pathol. 1998;27:102–6.

36. Hawkey CJ. Non-steroidal anti-inflammatory drug gastropathy: causes and treatment. Scand J Gastroenterol Suppl. 1996;220:124–7.

37. Leroy S, Marc E, Bavoux F, Tréluyer JM, Gendrel D, Bréart G, Pons G, Chalumeau M. Hospitalization for severe bacterial infections in children after exposure to NSAIDs: a prospective adverse drug reaction reporting study. Clin Drug Investig. 2010;30:179–85.

38. Jamali F, Brocks DR. Clinical Pharmacokinetics of ketoprofen and itsenantiomers. Clin Pharmacokinet. 1990;1:197–217.

39. Neirinckx E, Croubels S, De Boever S, Remon JP, Bosmans T, Daminet S, De Backer P, Vervaet C. Species comparison of enantioselective oral bioavailability and pharmacokinetics of ketoprofen. Res V et Sci. 2011; 91:415–21.

40. Neirinckx E, Croubels S, Remon JP, Devreese M, De Backer P, Vervaet C. Chiral inversion of R(−) to S(+) ketoprofen in pigs. Vet J. 2011;190(2):290.

41. Raekallio MR, Mustonen KM, Heinonen ML, Peltoniemi OA, Säkkinen MS, Peltoniemi SM, Honkavaara JM, Vainio OM. Evaluation of bioequivalence after oral, intramuscular, and intravenous administration of racemic ketoprofen in pigs. Am J Vet. 2008;69:108–13.

42. Arifah AK, Landoni MF, Lees P. Pharmacodynamics, chiral pharmacokinetics and PK-PD modelling of ketoprofen in the goat. J Vet Pharmacol Ther. 2003; 26:139–50.

8

Effect of antimicrobials administered via liquid feed on the occurrence of sulphonamide and trimethoprim resistant Enterobacteriaceae

Oliver Heller[1,4], Roger Stephan[2], Sophie Thanner[4], Michael Hässig[3], Giuseppe Bee[4], Andreas Gutzwiller[4] and Xaver Sidler[1*]

Abstract

Background: Drugs for the treatment of groups of pigs receiving liquid feed are frequently mixed into the feed and administered via the pipelines of the feeding installations. In-feed antimicrobials may select antimicrobial resistant strains among the bacteria which form the biofilm of these pipelines and are shed into the liquid feed.

Objective and methods: In order to evaluate the risk of selecting antimicrobial resistant bacteria in the biofilm of liquid feeding installations, the effect of the administration of antimicrobials via the pipelines on the occurrence of antimicrobial resistance in the feed was examined in a case-control study. A premix containing either sulphonamide plus trimethoprim or sulphonamide plus chlortetracycline plus tylosin or chlortetracycline was administered via the pipelines to each batch of bought-in fattening pigs in 7, 3 and 3 case farms respectively, whereas antimicrobials had not been administered via the liquid feeding installation for at least 2 years in the 14 control farms. Enterobacteriaceae and sulphonamide-trimethoprim resistant Enterobacteriaceae were counted in twelve and eight feed samples collected in each case and in each control farm respectively during one fattening period. The semiparametric Generalized Estimating Equations (GEE) method was used for the statistical data analysis.

Results: The ratio of sulphonamide and trimethoprim resistant to total Enterobacteriaceae was higher in the feed of the case farms compared to the control farms ($P < 0.001$) and did not decrease after treatment during the fattening period.

Conclusion: The administration of antimicrobials via the liquid feeding installation selects antibiotic resistant bacteria in the biofilm lining the pipelines, which may contaminate the liquid feed for extended periods and transmit their resistance genes to the gastrointestinal flora of the pigs. Alternatives to the administration of antimicrobials via pipelines of liquid feeding installations for group treatment should be developed.

Keywords: Antimicrobial resistance, Oral group therapy, Sulphonamide, Trimethoprim, Enterobacteriaceae, Liquid feeding, Fattening pigs

* Correspondence: xsidler@vetclinics.uzh.ch
[1]Department for Farm Animals, Division of Swine Medicine, University of Zurich, Winterthurerstrasse 260, 8057 Zurich, Switzerland
Full list of author information is available at the end of the article

Background

Because a high antimicrobial use is associated with high levels of antimicrobial resistance (AMR) [1], the prudent and reduced use of antimicrobials in farm animals has become an important goal. Between 2008 and 2014, the annual amount of antimicrobials used for disease prevention and treatment in Swiss farm animals decreased by almost a third, from 71 to 48 tons [2]. In 2014, antimicrobial premixes for in-feed use accounted for 60% of the total amount of antimicrobials used in farm animals. Among pigs, newly weaned pigs and pigs entering a fattening unit are the two groups that are most frequently treated with antimicrobials [3]. Although the routine prophylactic use of antimicrobials is strongly discouraged [4], oral group treatment for disease prevention is still the main indication (79%) for antimicrobial use in fattening pigs in Switzerland [5], followed by oral group therapy in disease outbreaks (18%) and individual treatment of sick animals (3%). In Switzerland, the most commonly used antimicrobial drug for oral group treatment contains sulphathiazole, sulphadimidine and trimethoprim, being followed by a combination containing chlortetracycline, sulphadimidine and tylosin, and drugs containing either chlortetracycline or colistin.

"In Switzerland, by-products of the food industry, in particular whey, a by-product of the cheese production, are part of most pig fattening rations. The most economical way to use these by-products is to mix them on the farm with commercial complementary feeds and administer the mixed feeds via liquid feeding installations." Dry feed and liquid (usually whey or water) are mixed in the mixing tank and pumped through a ring line to the drop pipes and into the feed troughs. In these liquid feeding installations, the liquid feed inside the ring line remains there between two feeding times, being diluted with water in some farms, and is pumped back into the mixing tank during the next mixing process. The lines of liquid feeding systems are coated with a biofilm, consisting of a community of microorganisms which stick together and produce a slime composed of extracellular polymeric substances. The administration of antimicrobials via liquid feeding installations poses a risk of selecting antimicrobial resistant bacteria in the biofilm. The latter may therefore be regarded as a potential reservoir of resistant bacteria. At any time, parts of the biofilm can be detached by mechanical forces or various biological processes [6] and disperse in the liquid feed. Antibiotic resistant bacteria originating from the biofilm are therefore ingested by pigs, thus adding further AMR genes to the AMR gene pool already present in the pig gut. According to the WHO [7], major gaps exist in the surveillance related to the emergence of AMR in foodborne bacteria. The effect of antimicrobials administered via liquid feeding installations on the AMR prevalence in the liquid feed has to our knowledge not been studied yet. The aim of this case-control-study was to assess the effect of the administration of three different antimicrobial drug formulations via liquid feeding installations on the prevalence of sulphonamide + trimethoprim resistant Enterobacteriaceae used as indicator bacteria in the liquid feed for pigs.

Methods

Study design, farm management investigation and sample collection

A total of 27 pig fattening farms located in different regions of Switzerland which used computer-assisted liquid feeding installations were included in the case-control study. In the 13 case farms, antimicrobials had been administered in-feed via the feed pipeline in every fattening period lasting about 3 months for at least the last 2 years prior to the study. In the 14 control farms, antimicrobials had not been administered via the pipeline for at least 2 years prior to the study. The type of the prescribed drug used as well as the esFigurlished feeding and cleaning protocols in each farm were not changed in the study period. Every farmer was interviewed about management practices such as animal movement and animal treatments using antimicrobials, the construction and functioning of the liquid feeding installation and the routine for its cleaning and disinfection, the ingredients (concentrate, whey or water) of the liquid feed and the use of acidifying feed additives.

Between April and December 2015, feed samples were collected at six time points in the case and at four time points in the control farms. In the case farms, the first sampling was done before treatment, which began within a few days after the pigs weighing 25 to 30 kg entered the fattening unit, in order to know the resistance situation before antimicrobial administration. The remaining five sampling points in time were scheduled on day 6 (i.e. during medication), 12, 18, 36 and 76 after the start of the antimicrobial group treatment. In the control farms, where no short term variation of the antimicrobial resistance situation was to be expected, the second, third and fourth sampling times were fixed on day 8, 14 and 78 after the first sampling. Two samples were collected at each point in time. One sample was collected at the end of the ring line, which is situated right over the mixing tank, when the feed remaining in the ring line between two feeding periods was pumped into the mixing tank at the next feeding. The other sample was collected at the opening of the drop pipe above the feeding trough which was furthest away from the mixing tank. The outflowing liquid feed was collected in a sterile container. As liquid feed in all farms remained in the ring line between feeding times, the feed samples were collected at the morning feeding, thus ensuring to obtain samples of liquid feed that had interacted with the biofilm during the longest time period between two feeding times (11–16 h).

Microbiological analyses

All feed samples were kept cool during transport and were processed immediately upon arrival in the laboratory. Their pH value was determined using a pH meter (Orion 525, Hügli, Abtwil), and their mould and yeast count was determined according to ISO 21527–1:2008. The number of Enterobacteriaceae and of Enterobacteriaceae which were resistant to sulphonamide and to trimethoprim was determined by means of two serial dilutions with a detection limit of 10 colony forming units/ml (cfu/ml) each. MacConkey agar (Oxoid, Hampshire, UK) and MacConkey agar supplemented with 152 µg/ml sulphamethoxazole (Sigma-Aldrich, St. Louis, USA) and 8 µg/ml trimethoprim (Sigma-Aldrich, St. Louis, USA) were used for the detection of all and of resistant Enterobacteriaceae. The colonies were counted after anaerobic incubation at 37 °C during 24 h. The antimicrobial resistance of the isolated colonies was verified by subculturing one morphologically distinct resistant colony on a MacConkey agar supplemented with 152 µg/ml sulphamethoxazole and 8 µg/ml trimethoprim as described above.

In order to detect resistant Enterobacteriaceae below the detection limit of the quantitative assessment, the two samples collected at the first sampling in every case farm and the two samples collected at the last sampling in every control farm were enriched for Enterobacteriaceae using 10 ml of liquid feed and 90 ml of Enterobacteriaceae Enrichment broth (BD, Franklin Lakes, USA), and the Enterobacteriaceae were subcultured as described above.

Data processing and statistical analysis

The microbial counts were log10 transformed after adding one to the counts to adjust for zero values in the data. The ratio of resistant/all Enterobacteriaceae was calculated using the untransformed counts. Since most

variables did not meet the assumption of normal distribution of residuals even after log transformation, the semiparametric Generalized Estimating Equations (GEE) method was used for the statistical analysis. For multiple comparisons, Tukey contrasts were calculated, using the single step method in order to adjust the P values for family-wise error rate. The data were analysed using the open access statistical package R geepack [8].

Three statistical data analyses were made, taking into account all data, the case data only and the control data only. For the statistical evaluation of the combined case and control data, the model contained the fixed factors group affiliation (case, control), sampling time (case: 1, 4, 5, 6; control: 1, 2, 3, 4) and sampling location (ring line, drop pipe), and the random factor farm as well as the interactions group affiliation × sampling location and group affiliation × sampling time. The model for the case data evaluation contained the fixed factors sulphonamide administration (yes, no), chlortetracycline administration (yes, no), sampling time (1, 2, 3, 4, 5, 6), feed acidification (yes, no) and sampling location (ring line, drop pipe), and the random factor farm as well as the interactions sulphonamide × sampling location and chlortetracycline × sampling location. The model for the control case data evaluation contained the fixed factors feed acidification (yes, no), liquid feed component (whey, water), sampling time (1, 2, 3, 4), sampling location (circuit line, drop line) and the random factor farm plus the interaction acidification × liquid feed component.

Results
Farm characteristics

All-in, all-out was practised in all case farms and in one control farm, whereas there was a continuous flow of animals in 13 control farms. In seven case farms a sulphonamide-trimethoprim combination was used, whereas a sulphonamide-chlortetracycline-tylosin combination was administered in three farms and chlortetracycline alone was used in three farms. (Table 1). The daily dose per kg body weight recommended by the drug manufacturers was 40 mg sulphonamide, 8 mg

Table 1 Administered drugs, cleaning and feeding protocols in the case and control farms

Farms	drug	Additive for cleaning[a]	Feed acidification[b]	Liquid feed component
Case farms (n = 13)	drug1: 7 drug2: 3 drug3: 3	Acid[b]: 4 Soda[c]: 8 No: 1	Yes: 3 No: 10	Whey[d]: 3 Water: 10
Control farms (n = 14)	no drug	Acid[b]: 4 Soda[c]: 4 Other: 2 (No cleaning: 4)	Yes: 5 No: 9	Whey[d]: 5 Water: 9

Drug 1: sulphonamide + trimethoprim; drug 2: chlortetracycline + sulphonamide + tylosin; drug 3: chlortetracycline
[a]addition to water for circuit pipeline cleaning or flushing after cleaning
[b]organic acids
[c]caustic soda alone or with sodium hypochlorite
[d]the whey was acidified in two case and in two control farms

trimethoprim and 3.6 mg tylosin. In the mono-drug and in the antimicrobial combination premix the recommended dose of chlortetracycline was 20–30 and 21 mg/kg body weight, respectively. In two farms each the administered dose was one third below and one fourth above the recommended dose respectively. The length of the antimicrobial group therapy varied between 6 and 10 days. The antimicrobial premixes were added to the feed in the mixing tank. The daily dose was administered in five farms at one feeding in the morning, in six farms at two feedings, one in the morning and one in the afternoon or evening, and in two farms at three feedings. In all case farms the amount of liquid feed offered was initially restricted to 50 to 60% of the nutrient requirements and was then gradually increased to 100% of the requirements (corresponding to about 4 l per animal weighing 25 to 30 kg). The gradual increase occurred within 8 to 10 days, in order to ensure the complete drug intake from the first treatment day on. In the farms where sulphonamide and trimethoprim were administered at the recommended dose, the estimated antimicrobial content per ml liquid feed was 500 μg sulphonamide and 100 μg trimethoprim at the beginning and 250 μg sulphonamide and 50 μg trimethoprim towards the end of the treatment period, under the condition that the drug was administered in the whole daily ration.

The ring lines were cleaned after treatment in four farms and at the end of each fattening period in all case farms. The ring line cleaning interval was about 1 week, 3 months and 6 to 12 months in two, five and three control farms, respectively, while in four control farms the ring lines had not been cleaned for years. In most farms, organic acids or soda were added to the water used for flushing the ring lines (Table 1).

Evaluation of the case and control farm data

Enterobacteriaceae resistant to sulphonamide and trimethoprim could be isolated without prior enrichment from the feed of all 13 case farms and from the feed of 5 control farms. After enrichment of the 28 samples collected in the control farms, 12 samples of feed flowing from the drop pipe into the feed trough and 8 samples collected at the end of the ring line tested positive for resistant Enterobacteriaceae. In summary, resistant Enterobacteriaceae were detected either without or after enrichment in all farms with the exception of 2 control farms.

In comparison to the control farms, the feed of the case farms contained higher numbers of Enterobacteriaceae ($P < 0.01$), of resistant Enterobacteriaceae ($P < 0.001$) and of moulds ($P < 0.01$), while the yeast count and the pH did not differ between the farms ($P > 0.05$; Table 2). Thirty and 0.02% of the Enterobacteriaceae isolated in the samples of the case and the control farms, respectively, were resistant to sulphonamides and to trimethoprim ($P < 0.001$).

Feed collected from the drop pipes had higher counts of Enterobacteriaceae ($P < 0.001$), of resistant Enterobacteriaceae ($P < 0.001$) and of moulds ($P < 0.01$), and had a higher pH ($P < 0.001$) compared to feed collected at the end of the ring line, whereas the yeast count did not differ ($P > 0.05$) between the two locations (Table 2).

Case farm data evaluation

There was no difference in the Enterobacteriaceae count, the resistant Enterobacteriaceae count and the ratio of resistant to total Enterobacteriaceae in the feed between the 10 farms were sulphonamides were administered and the three farms were chlortetracycline only was used ($P > 0.05$). The total number and the number of resistant Enterobacteriaceae, which showed a similar variation over time (Fig. 1) were high in the first sample collected at both sampling sites, but then decreased and remained rather constant until the last sampling point in time. The ratio of resistant to total Enterobacteriaceae did not differ between the sampling points in time ($P > 0.05$).

Feed acidification was associated with lower counts of total and of resistant Enterobacteriaceae ($P < 0.001$). Feed collected at the opening of the drop pipes was more heavily contaminated with both total and resistant Enerobacteriaceae ($P < 0.001$) than feed collected at the end of the ring line.

Table 2 Enterobacteriaceae (EB), moulds and yeast (log 10 cfu/ml; arithmetic means, standard errors SE in brackets), the proportion of Enterobacteriaceae resistant to sulphonamide and trimethoprim (STrEB), and the pH in the feed. Case vs. control farms and drop pipes vs. ring lines

	Case		Control		P	Drop pipes		Ring lines		P
EB	2.37	(0.14)	1.37	(0.14)	0.001	2.38	(0.15)	1.53	(0.14)	0.001
STrEB	1.60	(0.14)	0.15	(0.05)	<0.001	1.26	(0.14)	0.74	(0.12)	<0.001
%STrEB	30.0	(3.3)	0.02	(0.01)	<0.001	21.2	(3.3)	17.6	(3.6)	0.93
Moulds	1.55	(0.10)	0.86	(0.11)	0.004	1.56	(0.12)	0.97	(0.10)	0.002
Yeast	5.23	(0.09)	5.81	(0.09)	0.10	5.59	(0.08)	5.36	(0.11)	0.76
pH	5.18	(0.05)	5.03	(0.04)	0.42	5.32	(0.04)	4.93	(0.05)	<0.001

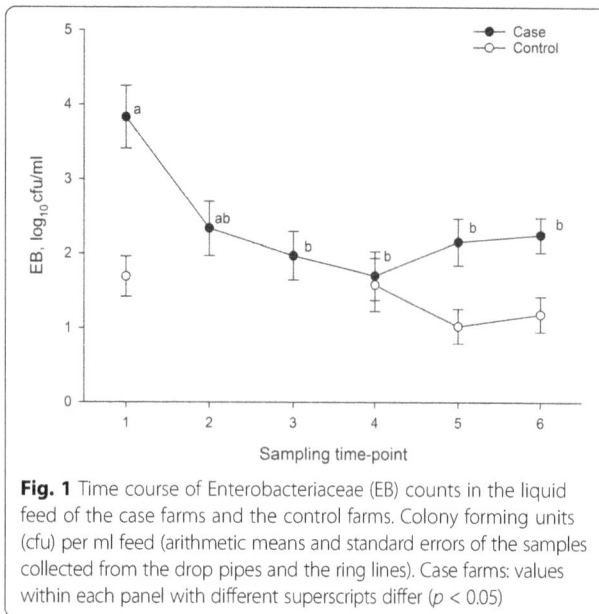

Fig. 1 Time course of Enterobacteriaceae (EB) counts in the liquid feed of the case farms and the control farms. Colony forming units (cfu) per ml feed (arithmetic means and standard errors of the samples collected from the drop pipes and the ring lines). Case farms: values within each panel with different superscripts differ ($p < 0.05$)

Control farm data evaluation

Neither the liquid component of the diet (whey vs. water) nor the sampling point in time (Fig. 2) influenced the count of total and of resistant Enterobacteriaceae. As in the case farms, feed acidification was associated with a lower Enterobacteriaceae count ($P < 0.001$), and feed collected from the drop pipes contained more Enterobacteriaceae ($P < 0.001$) than the samples collected at the end of the ring line.

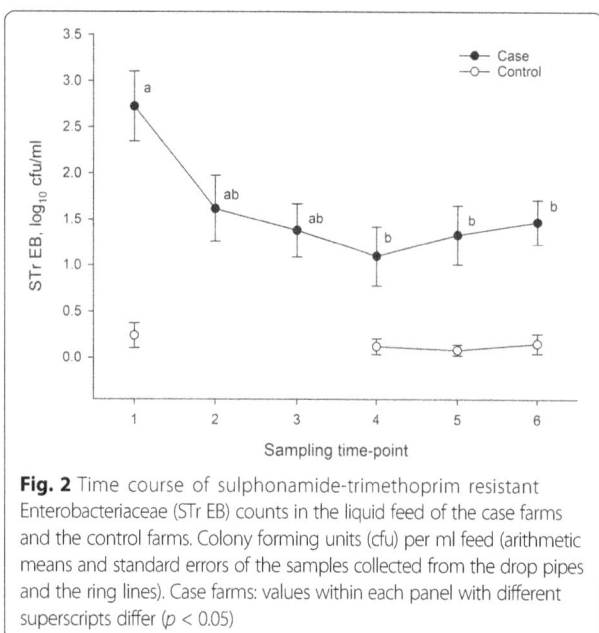

Fig. 2 Time course of sulphonamide-trimethoprim resistant Enterobacteriaceae (STr EB) counts in the liquid feed of the case farms and the control farms. Colony forming units (cfu) per ml feed (arithmetic means and standard errors of the samples collected from the drop pipes and the ring lines). Case farms: values within each panel with different superscripts differ ($p < 0.05$)

Discussion

In the case farms, which all had an all-in, all-out management with feeding installations temporarily not in use between lots of pigs, the pipelines of the liquid feeding system were cleaned more regularly, and alkalising soda was used more frequently than in the control farms. These management practices are probably the principal reason for the higher Enterobacteriaceae and mould counts in the feed of the case farms. The high initial Enterobacteriaceae counts in the feed samples collected in the case farms in particular, which are close to the acceptable upper limit of 10^4 cfu/ml [9], may be a consequence of the Enterobacteriaceae proliferation which commonly occurs during the first days of liquid feeding after a thorough cleaning and disinfection of the feeding installation [10]. The disinfection of the pipelines with alkalising products is known to supress the lacto-bacteria and to favour the growth of Enterobacteriaceae [10, 11]. The aerobic conditions in the drop pipes, which do not contain feed between feeding times, are the most probable cause of the higher Enterobacteriaceae and mould counts and the higher pH in the samples collected above the feed troughs compared to those collected at the end of the ring line.

Because the Enterobacteriaceae count differed between the feed of the case and the control farms for reasons, which are probably not associated with the use of antimicrobials, higher counts of resistant Enterobacteriaceae would be detected in the case farms even in case antimicrobials had not caused a shift in the bacterial population towards resistant Enterobacteriaceae. The differences in the ratio of resistant to total Enterobacteriaceae between the case and the control farms is therefore the relevant criterion by which the effect of the temporary presence of antimicrobials in the pipelines on the prevalence of resistant bacteria in the feed has to be evaluated.

The higher proportion of resistant Enterobacteriaceae in the feed samples of the case farms compared to those from control farms shows that the repeated short-term administration of antimicrobials via the liquid feeding installation is associated with a quantitative shift from a predominantly susceptible towards a sulphonamide and trimethoprim resistant Enterobacteriaceae population. This finding is in accordance with results of studies that link the use of antimicrobials with an increased frequency of resistant bacteria in the environment [12, 13]. However, the difference between the case and the control farms was more pronounced than expected, given the extensive use of sulphonamides and tetracyclines in farm animals over the last 50 years, the frequent occurrence of resistance to these antimicrobials in pathogenic as well as in commensal bacteria [14] and the persistence of the resistance in environmental bacteria [15].

The finding that resistant Enterobacteriaceae could be isolated in the feed of 25 of the 27 farms, although in nine control farms only after enrichment, shows that resistance to sulphonamides plus trimethoprim is widespread in Swiss pig farms. The number of resistant Enterobacteriaceae in the feed would therefore probably rapidly increase if one of the three drugs used in the case farms were administered via the liquid feeding installations of the control farms.

The number of resistant Enterobacteriaceae and the ratio of resistant to total Enterobacteriaceae were not lower in the three case farms where the pigs were treated with the chlortetracycline mono-drug premix compared to the ten farms where sulphonamides were administered. Co-selection, i.e. the selection by chlortetracycline of bacteria which show resistance to sulphonamide and trimethoprim in addition to tetracycline resistance, is the most probable cause for that finding. Wu et al. [16] investigated the prevalence of the sulphonamide resistance genes (sul1, sul2 and sul3) in E. coli isolated from pig faeces, pig carcasses and human stools and conducted conjugation experiments with a subset of the isolates. They showed that tetracycline resistance genes could be co-transferred with sul1 and/or sul2 resistance genes. Gibbons et al. [17] identified the use of antimicrobial combinations containing sulphonamide and trimethoprim as a risk factor for the occurrence of E. coli showing resistance to tetracycline in the faeces of pigs. Heller et al. [18] reported that Enterobacteriaceae showing resistance to tetracycline were more prevalent in the feed of farms where sulphonamides and trimethoprim were administered via the liquid feeding installations than in farms where the feeding installations were not used for antimicrobial administration.

The selection process of AMR in a liquid feeding system can potentially occur in antimicrobial containing liquid feed that remains in the circuit pipeline after the feeding or in the biofilm coating the lines of the liquid feeding installation. Whereas bacteria in the liquid feed remaining in the circuit pipeline between feeding cycles are almost completely flushed out during the next feeding, bacteria embedded in the biofilm are very persistant. Because of their high concentration in the feed, in-feed antimicrobials will exert a selective pressure at least on the bacteria near the biofilm-feed interface. Compared to their planktonic counterparts, bacteria enclosed in biofilms profit from a variety of advantages when exposed to antimicrobials, as the extracellular polymeric substances confer, among other things, protection against antimicrobial agents such as antibiotics and disinfectants, and facilitate horizontal gene transfer, i.e. the exchange of mobile genetic elements, which may carry AMR genes, between bacteria [19–23]. Bacteria embedded in a biofilm may be 10 to 1000 times more resistant to antimicrobials than planktonic bacteria [22, 24],

suggesting that antimicrobial concentrations may be sub-inhibitory within a biofilm. The use of antimicrobials at sub-inhibitory doses is known to promote the emergence, selection and spread of resistant bacteria [25–27]. The biofilm coating the lines of the liquid feeding system may thus enhance the selection, the persistence and the spread of resistant bacteria, which may be transferred into the liquid feed. The suggested role of the biofilm as a permanent source of resistant bacteria is supported by our finding that the ratio of resistant to total Enterobacteriaceae remained constant during the whole sampling period.

Although the mean number of resistant Enterobacteriaceae at the end of the drop pipes ($< 10^2$ cfu/ml) was barely above the detection limit even in the case farms, the fattening pigs, which consumed several litres of liquid feed per day, ingested approximately 10^5 to 10^6 resistant Enterobacteriaceae per day. As lactic acid bacteria usually dominate the bacterial flora of liquid feed [11], whose resistance to sulphonamide and trimethoprim was not investigated in this study, the impact of the administration of antimicrobials via the liquid feeding system on the reservoir of sulphonamide and trimethoprim resistance genes and thus the potential of AMR spread among bacteria in the liquid feed was likely to be underestimated. Corpet [28] studied the effect of eating sterilised food on the level of tetracycline resistance among Enterobacteriaceae in human faeces and showed that the ingestion of sterile food leads to a reduction of tetracycline resistance by a factor of 1000. This experiment demonstrated the distinct effect of ingesting commensal food-borne bacteria on the level of AMR in the gut without the oral application of any antimicrobials. This study also suggests that the reduction of the microbial count of animal feed containing a high proportion of resistant bacteria may mitigate the negative effect of such feed on the AMR of the animals' gastrointestinal bacteria. The addition of organic acids to liquid feed, which have been shown to reduce the number of Enterobacteriaceae and of lactic acid bacteria under experimental conditions [29] and which were associated with reduced Enterobacteriaceae counts in the present study, may help to reduce the number of ingested resistant bacteria in addition to their well-documented beneficial effects on the animals' intestinal health.

This case-control study has several limitations. Resistance to sulphonamide and trimethoprim was not determined in the individual components of the analysed liquid feed (water, whey, dry feed). It was therefore not possible to assess the proportion of resistant bacteria introduced from outside into the liquid feeding system. The higher cleaning frequency, the more frequent use of alkalising disinfectants and the temporary non-use of the feeding installations in the case farms contributed without doubt to the higher Enterobacteriaceae count in the feed collected in the case farms. Although it would have been preferable to include only farms using the all-in, all-out management system in the study, this was not possible because of the limited number of farms which could be recruited for the study. The authors' intention was to detect the influence of antimicrobial administration via the liquid feeding installation on the level of resistance to sulphonamide and trimethoprim in average Swiss pig fattening farms. Observational studies including farms with differing management practices have the advantage of being representative of the farming community, allowing the generalisation of the results. On the other hand, it cannot be ruled out that unidentified confounders may have biased the outcome.

Conclusions

Under the current liquid feeding system management conditions, in-feed antimicrobials which are transported through the lines of liquid feeding installations are selecting resistant bacteria in the biofilm of the lining, which becomes a reservoir of AMR. Resistance to antimicrobials may thus be transmitted via the feed to future batches of fattening pigs even if these are no longer treated with the antimicrobials which have caused AMR in the bacteria colonizing the pipelines. While our findings may not be used to directly link the use of antimicrobials via the liquid feeding system to the emergence of resistant bacteria in the human gut, they should nonetheless, together with the constantly growing body of evidence for the transfer of resistant bacteria from farm animals to humans, and based on the precautionary principle [30], prompt farmers and veterinarians alike to further decrease the amount of antimicrobials used in farm animals. In particular the administration of antimicrobials via liquid feeding systems which are colonised by biofilms have to be avoided unless efficient procedures to reduce the number of resistant bacteria in these linings will be developed.

Abbreviations
AMR: Antimicrobial resistance; Cfu: Colony forming unit; EB: Enterobacteriaceae; STr: Resistant against sulphonamides and trimethoprim

Acknowledgments
We thank K. Zurfluh for her technical assistance in the lab and all the farmers who participated in this study for their valuable support.

Funding
This study is a part of the research programme REDYMO (reduction and dynamics of antibiotic resistant and persistent microorganisms along food chains, www.agroscope.admin.ch/redymo) and was funded by Agroscope.

Authors' contributions
ST, GB, AG, and XS initiated and supervised the project. ST wrote the original project proposal. RS delivered his expertise on microbiology and antimicrobial sensitivity testing and had a profound influence on the elaboration of the definitive project design. OH selected the study farms, collected the samples, conducted the lab works and did part of the statistical analysis, and was therefore the main investigator. In addition, he was the head writer of the manuscript. ST, GB, AG and MH advised OH on the statistical analysis. All authors read and approved the final manuscript.

Competing interests
The authors declare that they have no competing interests.

Author details
[1]Department for Farm Animals, Division of Swine Medicine, University of Zurich, Winterthurerstrasse 260, 8057 Zurich, Switzerland. [2]Institute for Food Safety and Hygiene, University of Zurich, Winterthurerstrasse 272, 8057 Zurich, Switzerland. [3]Department for Farm Animals, Section for Ambulatory Service and Herd Health, University of Zurich, Winterthurerstrasse 260, 8057 Zurich, Switzerland. [4]Institute for Livestock Sciences, Agroscope, Tioleyre 4, 1725 Posieux, Switzerland.

References
1. Chantziaras I, Boyen F, Callens B, Dewulf J. Correlation between veterinary antimicrobial use and antimicrobial resistance in food-producing animals: a report on seven countries. J Antimicrob Chemother. 2013;69(3):827–34.
2. ARCH-Vet Gesamtbericht. Bericht über den Vertrieb von Antibiotika in der Veterinärmedizin und das Antibiotikaresistenzmonitoring bei Nutztieren in der Schweiz. Köniz: Hrsg. Bundesamt für Lebensmittelsicherheit und Veterinärwesen (BLV); 2014. http://www.blv.admin.ch/dokumentation/04506/04518/index.html. Accessed 01 May 2016
3. Müntener CR, Stebler R, Horisberger U, Althaus FR, Gassner B. Berechnung der Therapieintensität bei Ferkeln und Mastschweinen beim Einsatz von Antibiotika in Fütterungsarzneimitteln. Schweiz Arch Tierheilkd. 2013;155(6): 365–72.
4. http://ec.europa.eu/health/antimicrobial_resistance/docs/2015_prudent_use_guidelines_en.pdf Accessed 6 June 2016.
5. Riklin A. Antibitotikumeinsatz in Schweizer Schweinemastbetrieben. Doctoral thesis: University of Zurich; 2015. http://www.vet.uzh.ch/dissertationen/diss_anzeige.php?ID=1063&sprache=e. Accessed 01 May 2016
6. Karatan E, Watnick P. Signals, regulatory networks, and materials that build and break bacterial biofilms. Microbiol Mol Biol Rev. 2009;73(2):310–47.
7. World Health Organization. Antimicrobial resistance: global report on surveillance. Geneva: World Health organization; 2014.
8. Halekoh U, Hojsgaard S, Yan J. The R package geepack for generalized estimating equations. J Stat Softw. 2006;15(2):1–11.
9. Kamphues J, Coenen M, Iben C, Kienzle E, Pallauf J, Simon O, Wanner M, Zentek J. Supplemente zu Vorlesungen und Übungen in der Tierernährung. 11th ed. Hannover: M. Schaper; 2009.
10. Hansen ID, Mortensen B. Pipe-cleaners beware. Pig Int. 1989;19(11):8–10.
11. Brooks PH, Beal JD, Niven S. Liquid feeding of pigs: potential for reducing environmental impact and for improving productivity and food safety. Rec Adv Anim Nutr Austr. 2001;13:49–63.
12. Andersson DI, Hughes D. Persistence of antibiotic resistance in bacterial populations. FEMS Microbiol Rev. 2011;35:901–11.
13. Aminov RI. The role of antibiotics and antibiotic resistance in nature. Environ Microbiol. 2009;11(12):2970–88.
14. Pruden A, Arabi M. Quantifying anthropogenic impacts on environmental reservoirs of antibiotic resistance. In: Keen P, Montforts H, editors. Antimicrobial resistance in the environment. Hoboken: Wiley and Sons; 2012. p. 173–201.
15. Ghosh S, LaPara T. The effects of subtherapeutic antibiotic use in farm animals on the proliferation and persistence of antibiotic resistance among soil bacteria. ISME J. 2007;1:191–203.

16. Wu S, Dalsgaard A, Hammerum AM, Porsbo LJ, Jensen LB. Prevalence and characterization of plasmids carrying sulfonamide resistance genes among *Escherichia coli* from pigs, pig carcasses and human. Acta Vet Scand. 2010; 52:47.

17. Gibbons JF, Boland F, Egan J, Fanning S, Markey BK, Leonard FC. Antimicrobial resistance of faecal *Escherichia coli* isolates from pig farms with different durations of in-feed antimicrobial use. Zoonoses Public Health. 2015; doi:10.1111/zph.12225.

18. Heller O, Sidler X, Hässig M, Thanner S, Bee G, Gutzwiller A, Stephan R. The effect of the administration of three different antimicrobial premix formulations via the liquid feeding system on the occurrence of Enterobacteriaceae resistant to tetracycline in the liquid feed for pigs. Schweiz Arch Tierheilkd. 2016;158:411–22.

19. Flemming H-C, Wingender J. The biofilm matrix. Nat Rev Microbiol. 2010;8: 623–33.

20. Donlan RM, Costerton JW. Biofilms: survival mechanisms of clinically relevant microorganisms. Clin Microbiol Rev. 2002;15(2):167–93.

21. Molin S, Tolker-Nielsen T. Gene transfer occurs with enhanced efficiency in biofilms and induces enhanced stabilisation of the biofilm structure. Curr Opin Biotechnol. 2003;14:255–61.

22. Høiby N, Bjarnsholt T, Givskov M, Molin S, Ciofu O. Antibiotic resistance of bacterial biofilms. Int J Antimicrob Ag. 2010;35(4):322–32.

23. Kovaleva J, Degener JE, van der Mei HC. Mimicking disinfection and drying of biofilms in contaminated endoscopes. J Hosp Infect. 2010;76:345–50.

24. Kaplan JB. Antibiotic-induced biofilm formation. Int J Artif Organs. 2011; 34(9):737–51.

25. Barbosa TM, Levy SB. The impact of antibiotic use on resistance development and persistence. Drug Resist Updat. 2000;3:303–11.

26. Stine OC, Johnson JA, Keefer-Norris A, Perry KL, Tigno J, Qaiyumi S, Stine MS, Morris JG Jr. Widespread distribution of tetracycline resistance genes in a confined animal feeding facility. Int J Antimicrob Ag. 2007;29(3):348–52.

27. Marshall BM, Levy SB. Food animals and antimicrobials: impacts on human health. Clin Microbiol Rev. 2011;24(4):718–33.

28. Corpet DE. Antibiotic resistance from food. N Engl J Med. 1988;318:1206–7.

29. Canibe N, Miettinen H, Jensen BB. Effect of adding lactobacillus plantarum or a formic acid containing product to fermented liquid feed on gastrointestinal ecology and growth performance of piglets. Livest Sci. 2008;114:251–62.

30. Kriebel D, Tickner J, Epstein P, Lemons J, Levins R, Loechler EL, Quinn M, Rudel R, Schettler T, Stoto M. The precautionary principle in environmental science. Environ Health Perspect. 2001;109(9):871–6.

9

Factors associated with the growing-finishing performances of swine herds: an exploratory study on serological and herd level indicators

C. Fablet[1,5*], N. Rose[1,5], B. Grasland[2,5], N. Robert[3], E. Lewandowski[3] and M. Gosselin[4]

Abstract

Background: Growing and finishing performances of pigs strongly influence farm efficiency and profitability. The performances of the pigs rely on the herd health status and also on several non-infectious factors. Many recommendations for the improvement of the technical performances of a herd are based on the results of studies assessing the effect of one or a limited number of infections or environmental factors. Few studies investigated jointly the influence of both type of factors on swine herd performances. This work aimed at identifying infectious and non-infectious factors associated with the growing and finishing performances of 41 French swine herds.

Results: Two groups of herds were identified using a clustering analysis: a cluster of 24 herds with the highest technical performance values (mean average daily gain = 781.1 g/day +/− 26.3; mean feed conversion ratio = 2.5 kg/kg +/− 0.1; mean mortality rate = 4.1% +/− 0.9; and mean carcass slaughter weight = 121.2 kg +/− 5.2) and a cluster of 17 herds with the lowest performance values (mean average daily gain =715.8 g/day +/− 26.5; mean feed conversion ratio = 2.6 kg/kg +/− 0.1; mean mortality rate = 6.8% +/− 2.0; and mean carcass slaughter weight = 117. 7 kg +/− 3.6). Multiple correspondence analysis was used to identify factors associated with the level of technical performance. Infection with the porcine reproductive and respiratory syndrome virus and the porcine circovirus type 2 were infectious factors associated with the cluster having the lowest performance values. This cluster also featured farrow-to-finish type herds, a short interval between successive batches of pigs (≤3 weeks) and mixing of pigs from different batches in the growing or/and finishing steps. Inconsistency between nursery and fattening building management was another factor associated with the low-performance cluster. The odds of a herd showing low growing-finishing performance was significantly increased when infected by PRRS virus in the growing-finishing steps (OR = 8.8, 95% confidence interval [95% CI]: 1.8–41.7) and belonging to a farrow-to-finish type herd (OR = 5.1, 95% CI = 1.1–23.8).

Conclusions: Herd management and viral infections significantly influenced the performance levels of the swine herds included in this study.

Keywords: Herd technical performance, Management, PRRS, PCV2

* Correspondence: christelle.fablet@anses.fr
[1]Agence Nationale de Sécurité Sanitaire de l'alimentation, de
l'environnement et du travail (Anses), Laboratoire de Ploufragan/Plouzané,
Unité Epidémiologie et Bien-Etre du Porc, B.P. 53, 22440 Ploufragan, France
[5]Université Bretagne-Loire, Cité internationale 1 place Paul Ricoeur CS 54417,
35044 Rennes, France
Full list of author information is available at the end of the article

Background

Swine farm profitability and efficiency rely in part on technical performance, which in turn depends on pig health and welfare. Several infectious respiratory or digestive pathogens can reduce swine performance during the growing-finishing steps. The porcine reproductive and respiratory syndrome virus (PRRSV), porcine circovirus type 2 (PCV2), swine influenza A viruses (swIAV), *Mycoplasma hyopneumoniae* (*M. hyopneumoniae*) and *Lawsonia intracellularis* (*L. intracellularis*) are among the main infectious pathogens causing, alone or in combination, marked economic losses to the swine industry throughout the world [1–4]. *Mycoplasma hyopneumoniae* is the aetiological cause of enzootic pneumonia and is considered to be one of the primary pathogens involved in the porcine respiratory disease complex (PRDC) together with PRRSV, PCV2 and/or swIAV [3, 5]. PCV2 also contributes to other syndromes collectively known as porcine circovirus-associated diseases [6], whereas PRRSV alone is responsible for reproductive failures in pregnant sows, high pre-weaning mortality in piglets infected in utero and respiratory signs in growers and finishers [7–9]. Proliferative enteropathy caused by *L. intracellularis* is another current disease – but targets the digestive tract – having considerable impact on pig production and herd economics [10].

Non-infectious factors also directly drive herd performance through diet and climatic conditions, or indirectly by affecting the occurrence and severity of diseases [11, 12]. Non-infectious environmental factors act on the pathogen load (i.e. the amount of micro-organisms to which the pig is exposed), the intensity and frequency of pathogen exposition, and on the pig, by modulating the defence mechanisms through which the pig handles the pathogen challenge [13]. Disease outcome in turn depends on the balance between the pathogen pressure and the pig's ability to cope with them. In modern swine production systems, multiple environmental factors may interfere with this delicate balance and need to be considered and adapted to reduce disease incidence and severity and thus enhance farm profitability.

Many recommendations for the improvement of the technical performances of a herd are based on the results of studies assessing the effect of one or a limited number of pathogens or environmental factors. To date, few studies have simultaneously investigated both types of factor on swine herd performance. This situation may be related to the difficulty of running studies obtaining valid findings. Effective and valuable recommendations indeed rely on valid results that allow inference about the associations to the target population. Obtaining reliable data is a crucial and challenging issue that needs to be properly considered in observational studies. Data collection should be designed in order to reduce potential bias and ensure the validity of the measures. Questionnaires are one of the most commonly used tools for collecting data, particularly related to environmental factors, in veterinary epidemiology [14]. The information validity of data obtained by questionnaire should be assessed whenever possible [15]. Hence, in questionnaire-based survey, it is advised to combine interviews with people working on farm with direct observation during an on-farm visit so as to decrease misclassification bias. Compliance with the reported measures is another tricky point that may lead to information bias and which is the hardest to assess [16]. Dealing with diagnostic tests used to describe infectious factors, imperfect diagnostic procedures could also represent a source of bias. The assays should have previously been assessed and validated under experimental and field conditions in order to adjust the results according to the diagnostic performances and to control misclassification bias. The aim of our study was to identify infectious and non-infectious factors associated with the technical performance of the growing-finishing steps in a sample of 41 herds.

Methods

Study design

Data and sera used were collected from 41 French pig farms involved in a study on the course of PCV2 infection (western France 2014–2015). The study was carried out in subclinically PCV2-infected herds without piglet vaccination against this virus. The herds were provided by the veterinarians at 'Univet santé élevage' and 'Cybelvet' veterinary clinics. Blood was sampled from 20 pigs selected at random from two batches in each herd (10 pigs 10–12 weeks old and 10 pigs at least 22 weeks old). Data on management, biosecurity and farm practices were collected via a questionnaire that was filled out with the farmer. The questionnaire is available upon request (in French, 26 closed or semi-closed questions). The main technical performance values of the growing-finishing steps (average daily weight gain from 8 to 115 kg [ADG], feed conversion ratio from 8 to 115 kg [FCR], mortality from 8 to 115 kg [MORT] and carcass slaughter weight [CSW] in 2014) were obtained from the technical-economic database managed by the French Pork and Pig Institute (IFIP).

Laboratory analyses

Serum samples from all pigs were tested for antibodies against *L. intracellularis* (SVANOVIR L.intracellularis/Ileitis-Ab, Boehringer Ingelheim Svanova, Sweden, successor of the bioScreen Ileitis Antibody ELISA with sensitivity (Se) ranging from 72 to 96.5% and specificity (Sp) from 83 to 100%; [17–19]), *M. hyopneumoniae* (*Mycoplasma hyopneumoniae* ELISA, OXOID Ltd., UK; formely DAKO

ELISA; with Sp = 100% and Se ranging from 49% to 100% according to experimental trials [20–23]) and PCV2 (SER-ELISA® PCV2 Ab Mono Blocking, Synbiotics Europe, France, Se = 86% and Sp = 85% [24]). A serum sample was considered positive for *L. intracellularis* antibodies if the percentage inhibition was ≥30% [18]. Any serum sample presenting a percentage inhibition was > 50% was considered positive for *M. hyopneumoniae* antibodies [22, 23]. A serum sample was classified as positive for PCV2 antibodies if the SERELISA® titer was > 170 ELISA units [24].

Pools of 5 samples were constituted and analysed to detect PRRSV antibodies (IDEXX PRRS X3 Ab Test, IDEXX, USA, Se = 97.5% and Sp = 100% of pool of 5 serum samples from growing-finishing pigs [25]). A pool was considered positive when the sample to positive control (S/P) optical density ratio was ≥0.4. Antibodies against swIAV were detected in the serum samples of the oldest pigs (*n* = 6 samples/herd) using a commercial ELISA kit (ID Screen® Influenza A antibody competition, IDVet, France, Se = 69% and Sp = 89%, [26]). A serum sample was classified positive for swIAV antibodies if the percentage inhibition was ≥60% [27].

Statistical analysis
Definition of the outcome (the level of herd growing-finishing performances) and explanatory variables
Associations between the four parameters describing the technical performance (ADG, FCR, MORT, CSW) of the growing-finishing pigs in the sampled herds were investigated using principal component analysis. The main objective in principal component analysis is to detect associations within a set of continuous variables in a small number of dimensions and to provide a low-dimensional (often two-dimensional) graphical representation of these associations [28]. Each variable is represented by an arrow (eigenvector) inside a correlation circle, the longer the length of the arrow, the higher the contribution of the variable to the inertia. The angle between arrows indicates the degree of correlation between the variables; the smaller the angle, the higher the correlation. An angle of 90° indicates that the two variables are independent and an angle of 180° shows a negative correlation.

The parameters describing technical performance were then included in a clustering analysis to identify the groups differing in performance. This classification process leads to clusters of herds based on the degree of similarity between the samples with regard to the variables. Two groups of herds were formed. A *t*-test was used to compare ADG and CSW between the two groups (*p* < 0.05) and a Kruskal-Wallis test was used to compare FCR and MORT between the groups (p < 0.05). These two groups were thereafter used as a dichotomous outcome variable to assess the relationships between

infectious and non-infectious factors associated with the level of growing-finishing performance of the herds.

All the explanatory variables related to the infectious agents were classified into two or more categories according to the frequency of pigs positive for a given pathogen per age category and/or at the herd level when applicable. The cut-off points were determined according to the distribution of variables. The serological status of the batch and/or the herd to a given pathogen was also considered when relevant. A unit (herd or batch) was classified as positive when at least one sample tested positive. Regarding PCV2, the laboratory analyses leading to semi-quantitative results, i.e. titer expressed as ELISA units [29], the frequency of pigs with high antibody titers was also calculated and categorized. For all variables, the number of categories was limited to ensure minimal category frequencies of 10%. Since PRRS natural infection were known to occur in PRRS vaccinated herds (data from veterinarians in charge of the herd health management, personal communications), vaccinated herds were considered as PRRS-seropositive herds. Description of these explanatory variables is given Table 1. All the variables related to non-infectious factors were categorical variables.

Associations between the level of growing-finishing performances and the infectious and non-infectious factors
A two-step procedure was used to assess the relationships between the explanatory variables and the level of herd growing-finishing performance. The first step was based on a univariable analysis relating the outcome variable to each explanatory variable. Only factors associated with the level of growing-finishing performance (likelihood ratio χ^2-test, *p* < 0.15) were selected for a multivariable analysis.

The second step involved a multiple correspondence analysis that included all factors that had passed the first screening step. The main objective in multiple correspondence analysis is to detect the associations within a set of categorical variables in a small number of dimensions and to provide a low-dimensional (often two-dimensional) graphical representation of these associations [30, 31]. The FactoMineR package for R was used [32]. The effects of the explanatory factors on the level of technical performances were then quantified by performing a logistic-regression analysis. All selected explanatory variables were checked for multicolinearity (χ^2-test, *p* < 0.05), and those most strongly associated with the outcome variable and having biological relevance were selected. The logistic regression was performed according to the method described in Hosmer and Lemeshow [33] (PROC LOGISTIC, SAS 9.1, SAS Inst., Cary, NC, USA). A backward stepwise procedure was used to select the variables that were significantly

Table 1 Description of the categorical explanatory variables related to the serological status to bacterial and viral pathogens

Definition of the variables	% herds per level
% of pigs seropositive to *Lawsonia intracellularis* after 16 weeks of age	
< 60%	26.83
≥ 60%	73.17
Pigs seropositive to *Lawsonia intracellularis*	
before 16 weeks of age	51.22
after 16 weeks of age	48.78
% of finishing pigs seropositive to *Lawsonia intracellularis*	
< 50%	60.98
≥ 50%	39.02
Serological status to *Mycoplasma hyopneumoniae*	
Negative	55
Positive (at least one positive sample)	45
Serological profile to *Mycoplasma hyopneumoniae*	
Negative	55
Positive before 16 weeks of age (at least one positive sample)	37.5
Positive after 16 weeks of age (at least one positive sample)	7.5
% of pigs with antibodies against *Mycoplasma hyopneumoniae* before 16 weeks of age	
≤ 20%	80.49
> 20%	19.51
% of pigs with antibodies against *Mycoplasma hyopneumoniae* before 16 weeks of age	
≤ 10%	73.17
> 10%	26.83
% of pigs with antibodies against *Mycoplasma hyopneumoniae* after 16 weeks of age	
≤ 10%	80.49
> 10%	19.51
% of pigs with antibodies against *Mycoplasma hyopneumoniae* during the finishing phase	
≤ 10%	78.05
> 10%	21.95
% of pigs with antibodies against swine Influenza A virus	
≤ 20%	56.1
> 20%	43.9
% of pigs with antibodies against swine Influenza A virus	
≤ 80%	70.73
> 80%	29.27
Serological status to swine Influenza A virus	
Negative	46.34
Positive (at least one positive sample)	53.66

Table 1 Description of the categorical explanatory variables related to the serological status to bacterial and viral pathogens *(Continued)*

Definition of the variables	% herds per level
Antibodies against PRRSV before 16 weeks of age	
No	80.49
Yes (at least one positive pool)	19.51
Antibodies against PRRSV after 16 weeks of age	
No	56.1
Yes (at least one positive pool)	43.9
Serological status to PRRSV	
Negative	56.1
Positive (at least one positive pool)	43.9
Serological profile to PRRSV	
Negative	56.1
Positive before 16 weeks of age (at least one positive pool)	19.51
Positive after 16 weeks of age (at least one positive pool)	24.39
% of pigs with antibodies against Porcine Circovirus Type 2 (PCV2) before 16 weeks of age	
≤ 50%	29.27
> 50%	70.73
% of pigs with antibodies against Porcine PCV2 after 16 weeks of age	
≤ 70%	19.51
> 70%	80.49
Anti-PCV2 IgG antibody titers > 5000 ELISA units before 16 weeks of age	
No	85.37
Yes (at least one pig)	14.63
Anti-PCV2 IgG antibody titers > 5000 ELISA units after 16 weeks of age	
No	31.71
Yes (at least one pig)	68.29
Anti-PCV2 IgG antibody titers > 5000 ELISA units during the fattening phase	
No	31.71
Yes (at least one pig)	68.29
> 10% of pigs with a SERELISA® titer > 5000 ELISA Units for antibodies against PCV2	
No	41.46
Yes	58.54
> 20% of pigs with a SERELISA® titer > 5000 ELISA Units for antibodies against PCV2	
No	51.22
Yes	48.78

($p < 0.05$) associated with the outcome variable. At each step, the variable with the highest p-value was removed from the model. This procedure was continued until all variables were significant ($p < 0.05$). The odds ratio and 95% confidence intervals were calculated from the final logistic model. Goodness-of-fit for the final model was assessed using the Pearson χ^2, deviance and Hosmer-Lemeshow goodness-of-fit [33].

Results
Features of the study sample
The herds were located in western France. In all, 20 herds were farrow-to-finish with on average 217 sows (standard deviation [SD]: 149 sows) and 21 herds were weaning-to-finishing farms (on average 3769 pigs, SD = 1413 pigs). Replacement stock and sows were vaccinated against PCV2 in 31.7% of the herds and 24.4% of the herds only vaccinated gilts against this virus. Growing pigs were not vaccinated against swIAV or PCV2 in any of the herds. In 73.2% and 19.5% of the herds, piglets were vaccinated against *M. hyopneumoniae* or PRRS respectively.

Relationships between the technical parameters
The principal component analysis revealed one group of positively correlated variables (right side of the map) describing the feed conversion ratio from 8 to 115 kg and the mortality from 8 to 115 kg (Fig. 1). These variables were negatively correlated with average daily gain from 8 to 115 kg. The carcass slaughter weight was not correlated with the other three variables.

Clusters of herds related to growing-finishing performance
Two groups of herds were identified by the clustering analysis: a cluster of 24 herds with the highest technical performance values (group 1) and a cluster of 17 herds with the lowest performance values (group 2) (Table 2).

Factors associated with the levels of growing-finishing performance
The variables included in the study are presented in Additional file 1. In the univariable analysis, 14 variables were associated ($p < 0.15$) with the level of herd growing-finishing performance (Additional file 1). Of these variables, 6 were included in the final multiple correspondence analysis (Fig. 2). PRRSV infection and a frequency of pigs with high antibody titers (> 5000 ELISA units) > 10% were associated with the cluster having the lowest performance values (group 2). This cluster was also characterised by farrow-to-finish-type herds and a short interval between successive batches of pigs (≤3 weeks). Mixing the pigs in the growing or/and finishing steps and inconsistency between the nursery and the fattening building management (the size of the fattening rooms do not fit well with the size of the batch of piglets coming from the nursery to follow a strict all-in-all-out management at the fattening room level, i.e. without mingling pigs from different batches in the same area) were other features of this low-performance

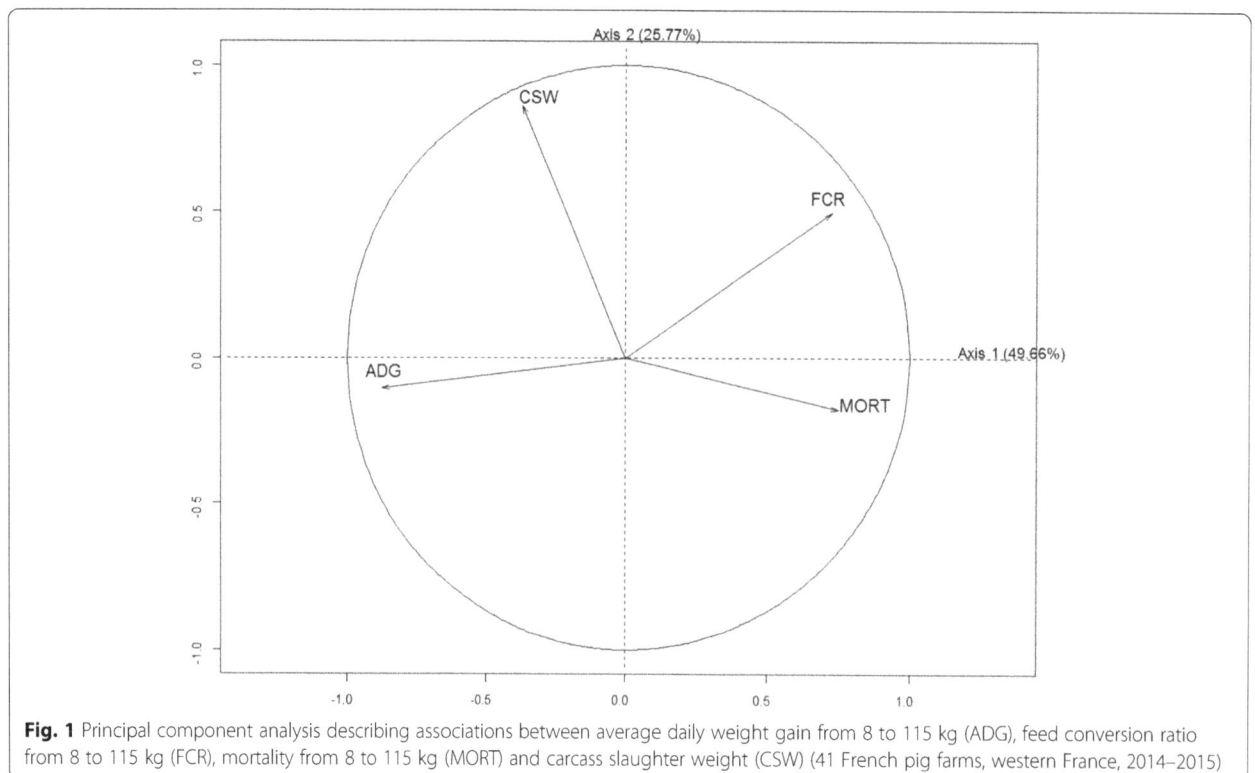

Fig. 1 Principal component analysis describing associations between average daily weight gain from 8 to 115 kg (ADG), feed conversion ratio from 8 to 115 kg (FCR), mortality from 8 to 115 kg (MORT) and carcass slaughter weight (CSW) (41 French pig farms, western France, 2014–2015)

Table 2 Technical characteristics of the whole sample and the two identified groups with different levels of growing-finishing performance as defined by the hierarchical cluster analysis (mean and standard deviation [sd])

	Overall sample (41 herds)		Group 1 (24 herds)		Group 2 (17 herds)		p-value[a]
	mean	sd	mean	sd	Mean	sd	
Average daily weight gain from 8 to 115 kg (g/day)	754.00	41.61	781.08	26.28	715.76	26.50	< 0.01
Feed conversion ratio from 8 to 115 kg (kg/kg)	2.53	0.13	2.48	0.08	2.60	0.14	< 0.01
Mortality from 8 to 115 kg (%)	5.21	1.99	4.09	0.93	6.79	2.03	< 0.01
Carcass slaughter weight (kg)	119.78	4.91	121.22	5.21	117.75	3.58	< 0.01

[a]Comparison between group 1 and group 2, Kruskal-Wallis test, $p < 0.05$

cluster. In the logistic regression analysis, two factors significantly increased the odds of a herd showing low performance (group 2) (Table 3): PRRSV infection in the growing-finishing steps and being a farrow-to-finish-type herd. The Pearson χ^2 ($p = 0.72$), deviance ($p = 0.72$) and Hosmer-Lemeshow ($p = 0.94$) goodness-of-fit tests indicated a good fit between the model and the observations.

Discussion

In the present study, the herds were classified according to four technical parameters: average daily weight gain, feed conversion ratio, mortality rate and carcass weight of slaughtered pigs. Feed-conversion efficiency, daily weight gain and mortality are recognized as the most important production-performance factors on fattening farms [34]. All these parameters were therefore used to describe the herds according to their technical performance. Carcass slaughter weight was also taken into account because of the potential economic impact of this parameter on farmer income: farmers being partly paid according to the carcass weight. Growth performances were negatively correlated with the feed conversion ratio and mortality rate in our study. Pig growth and feed conversion efficiency have previously been shown to be correlated [34].

The study was carried out in a non-negligible, but limited, number of herds without piglet vaccination against PCV2 and without clinical signs related to PCV2-associated diseases. The results of the study may therefore only apply to this kind of herd; furthermore, our herds cannot be considered representative of this population because they were not selected at random. However, the present survey serves as an exploratory study to help design future large-scale studies, providing

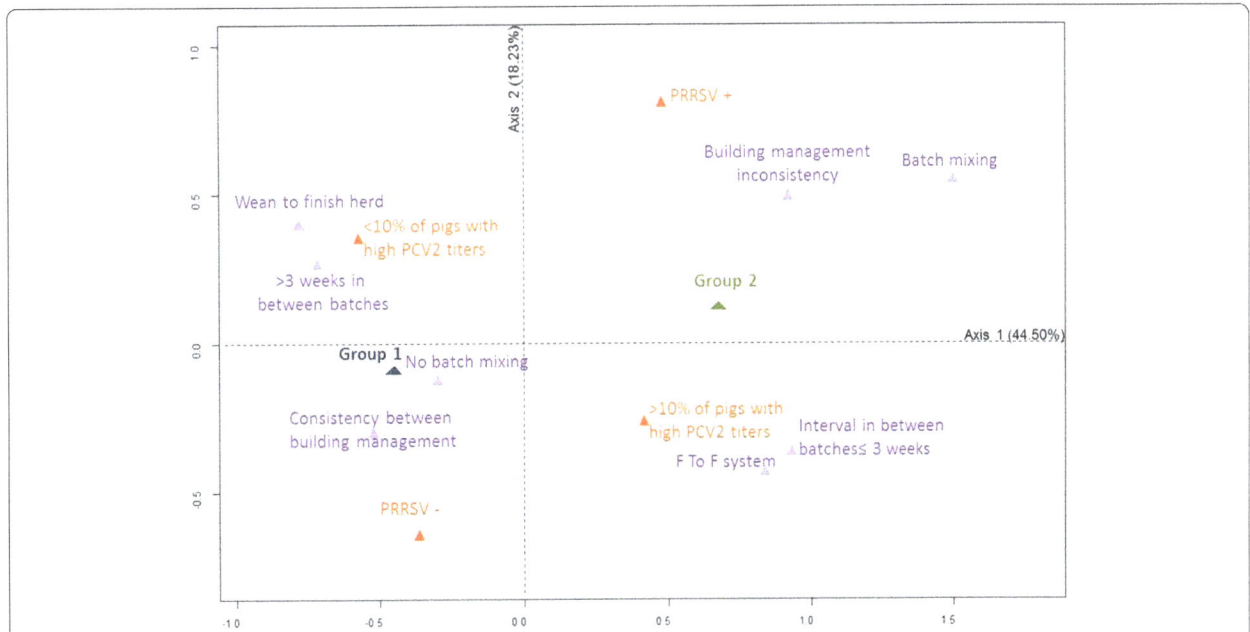

Fig. 2 Multiple correspondence analysis describing associations between the level of growing-finishing performance and infectious and non-infectious factors (41 herds, western France, 2013–2014). Group 1: Herds having the highest growing-finishing performance values; Group 2: herds having the lowest growing-finishing performance values; PRRSV -: PRRSV seronegative infection status of growers and finishers; PRRSV +: PRRSV seropositive infection status of growers and finishers; %PCV2 titers low: < 10% of pigs with a SERELISA® titer> 5000 ELISA Units for antibodies against PCV2; %PCV2 titers high: > 10% of pigs with a SERELISA® titer > 5000 ELISA Units for antibodies against PCV2; F To F system: Farrow-to-finish herds

Table 3 Final logistic regression model for factors associated with low growing-finishing performance (41 herds, odds ratio (OR) with 95% confidence interval (CI))

Variables	% of herds identified as low performers (Group 2)	OR	95% CI	p
Herd type				0.04
Farrow-to-finish	65.0	5.1	1.1–23.8	
Wean-to-finish	19.1	–		
PRRSV serological status of growers and finishers				0.01
Negative	26.1	–		
Positive	61.1	8.8	1.8–41.7	

insight into factors associated with reduced herd performance in the growing-finishing steps in herds without obvious clinical signs of PCVD and without PCV2 vaccination of piglets. These factors can be further investigated in prospective observational studies to assess the time sequence of events. In cross-sectional studies, the outcome and potential risk factors are measured at one particular time point, making the temporality and the separation of cause and effects difficult to ascertain. In the present study, data on the technical performance as well as non-infectious factors were collected in the year prior to data collection on the infectious variables, all assayed at one time point. This study design is well-suited for examining invariable characteristics (factors that are consistent in time and not influenced by the presence or absence of the disease) [35, 36], and, accordingly, our data were mainly related to herd management, hygiene and biosecurity measures, which are believed to be relatively constant over time [37]. All data were collected by the veterinarians in charge of the herd health management plan, against which the farmer's answers to the questionnaire could be compared. The infectious status of the herds regarding several respiratory or digestive pathogens was established by laboratory analysis performed on the samples collected during the study. The results were compared with the veterinarians' knowledge of the herd health status and discrepancies were checked and corrected when needed if recent infections had occurred. Misclassification bias of infectious status was thus reduced.

Serology is an efficient tool widely used to describe exposure to pathogens in swine field studies [3, 38–41]. Most of the assays being generally imperfects, association of different tests such as serological and molecular techniques is recommended to increase diagnostic accuracy [3]. We solely used ELISAs in our exploratory study to determine the infectious status of the batches and herds. The ability to accurately identify associations between infectious pathogens and herd performance in growing finishing steps may thus have been reduced. On

the other hand, imperfect diagnostic procedures could also represent a source of information bias. Most of the ELISAs used showed reasonable to high diagnostic performances which may have limited incorrect classification of infectious statuses. However, the results should be considered as preliminary risk indicators that pave the way for future large scale studies combining different diagnostic tests to further assess the infectious and immune statuses of the animals in regards to the growing and finishing performance.

Vaccination may impair the interpretation of serological results when the test does not differentiate antibodies against natural infection from those induced by commercial vaccines. In our study, most of the herds vaccinated against *M. hyopneumoniae* and in a fewer extent against PRRS. For *M. hyopneumoniae*, antibodies detectable in the serum of fattening pigs were found to be indicative of a recent infection independently from vaccination history, thus validating the usefulness of *M. hyopneumoniae* ELISA in our study limited to the fattening step [42, 43]. Herds where piglets were vaccinated against PRRS were considered as positive in the analyses in order to avoid a reduction in study power and because veterinarians in charge of the herd health management plan confirm that field strains were circulating.

Here, viral infections, particularly PRRSV and PCV2 infections were associated with decreased growing-finishing performance. Both viruses may be responsible, alone or in association with other infectious pathogens, for reduced technical and economical performances of infected herds having clinical or subclinical signs associated with these infections. Decreased performance is generally due to higher mortality and/or feed conversion efficiency and/or reduced daily weight gain [44, 45]. Infections by these viruses are also involved in the porcine respiratory disease complex (PRDC), one of the most costly diseases for the swine industry worldwide. Nevertheless, in our study, only PRRSV infection significantly increased the odds of reduced performance. This infection may therefore have a stronger impact on growing-finishing performance in herds without clinical signs of PCVD in western France than the PCV2 infection.

Even though earlier studies showed that growth performance of pigs subclinically infected with *L. intracellularis* is poor [46], the level of infection by *L. intracellularis* was not associated with lower herd performance in our study. Several other pathogens may disturb the gut health, particularly at the weaning age. Further studies involving the main frequent digestive pathogens in growers and finishers are needed to better assess the impact of these infections on the herd performances.

M. hyopneumoniae is the primary pathogen of enzo-otic pneumonia, a chronic respiratory disease in pigs leading to decreased performance [3]. However *M. hyopneumoniae* was not found as a main infectious pathogen associated with the cluster of lower performance. In herds clinically affected by *M. hyopneumoniae*, the sero-prevalence level is generally high in the fattening unit [39, 47]. The frequency of seropositive pigs was quite low in our study suggesting a low incidence of *M. hyopneumoniae* infection in the sampled herds and a limited impact of *M. hyopneumoniae* infection on the growing and finishing performance. However, serological results alone lack of sensitivity for the diagnosis of *M. hyopneumoniae*. They have to be combined with a second parameter as clinical signs or detection of the micro-organism from samples. The detection of *M. hyopneumoniae* by PCR techniques from a variety of samples is seen as a highly sensitive tool [3]. It should thus be used in combination with serological assays in further large scale study assessing the impact of *M. hyopneumoniae* infection on growing-finishing performance.

Non-infectious factors related to farm characteristics and management practices also influenced the level of herd performance. A farrow-to-finish-type herd, a short interval in between batches, inconsistency in building management between nursery and finishing steps and mixing pigs from different batches were all factors associated with decreased performance in the growing-finishing steps, with herd type being the only factor significantly increasing the odds of having reduced herd performance. The effects of these non-infectious factors may be linked to their impact on swine health and pathogen transmission.

The type of herd has commonly been identified as a risk factor for respiratory diseases and is also found to be associated with PRRSV seropositivity [12, 48]. However, results are not always consistent across the studies. A negative effect of the finishing system, when observed, is often associated with purchasing growing pigs from multiple sources, with little attention to disease entry and control measures. In our study, wean-to-finish herds – a feature of the high performing herd group – were associated with a single or a limited number of sources, using all-in-all-out procedures. Similarly, Cleveland-Nielsen et al. [49] showed that herd type was highly correlated with management factors, suggesting that the protective effect associated with a finishing herd may be attributable to the all-in-all-out system of production. The main explanations for the greater risk in farrow-to-finish farms generally involve the often continuous movement of animals and the close contact between sows and their offspring. Sows may be reservoirs of infectious pathogens [50, 51] and the purchase of breeding stock may lead to the introduction of pathogenic micro-

organisms [52]. Furthermore, the spread of infection within the herd is favoured by the probability of contact between animals of different ages and with different immune status. Infection spread is enhanced by the continuous movement of pigs inherent in this production system, which is often coupled with poor building design and layout [53]. The multi-site production technique was in part developed to circumvent the negative impacts of one-site production rearing systems. Multi-site rearing systems are defined as any farm in which the stages of production or age groups are reared on separate sites and locations [54]. All-in-all-out management rather than continuous pig flow is required in such a system. By combining strict all-in-all-out management policies and geographical separation of the production sites, the multi-site rearing system allows to reduce or even to avoid pathogens transmission from sows to piglets and as a consequence to enhance pig performance [54]. Interestingly, rearing single-source isowean piglets in multi-site production systems was found to be beneficial for the production performance rather than rearing pigs originating from multiple sources [54].

Herd type and management practices are interrelated and their specific effects are not always easy to identify and evaluate. In our study, herd type was strongly associated with other management practices such as the interval between successive batches and mixing pigs from different batches as well as inconsistency in building management between nursery and finishing steps. Even though the logistic regression models quantified the effect of the explanatory factors on the outcome, this method cannot incorporate highly correlated factors. Multiple correspondence analysis helps overcome this limitation, even though the strength of association between each explanatory factor and the outcome is not directly quantified [55]. We thus combined both types of analysis to better describe the underlying relationships of strongly correlated explanatory variables and expand on the number of parameters that farmers and their herd health advisors can adjust. The effect of herd-type included in the final regression model may thus be considered given its relationship with other management factors and their interactions.

The effect of the interval between successive batches is a singular result of our study. Similarly, Fablet et al. [56] showed that a short interval between successive batches of pigs is a risk factor for pneumonia severity, suggesting that increasing the time interval between successive batches of pigs reduces animal movement frequency and prevents mixing pigs from successive batches with different infectious and immune statuses. Reducing the frequency of animal movements may thus lead to a more stable overall immune status of the herd than a management system with continuous animal movements. We may speculate that all management practices limiting the spread of pathogens within the herd are more likely to contribute to higher technical performance.

The effect of inconsistency in building design between the nursery and finishing steps on herd performances was identified for the first time. Inconsistency in building design between the successive growing steps is generally associated with mixing pigs from different pens within a batch and/or mixing pigs between batches in the same room or even pens. In our study, mixing pigs between batches was positively correlated with inconsistency between building management. Several studies indicate that the lack of all-in-all-out management and mixing pigs during the production stages negatively affect the respiratory health or favoured respiratory infections [49, 57, 58]. On the other hand, movements are usually associated with the practice of regrouping pigs and hierarchical fights generally occur after mingling. All these conditions are sources of stress for the pigs [59], which may then weaken immune response and increase disease susceptibility. Regrouping also enhances the probability of pathogen transmission and frequent movements in subsequent facilities increases the opportunities for exposure to residual infectious agents. Ultimately, the intermingled non-infectious factors related to management practices and herd type strongly influence disease transmission pattern and severity and, in turn, herd performance.

Conclusions

Risky herd profiles were hereby identified in regard to the technical performance of swine herds. Herd management and viral infections significantly influenced the performance levels of the swine herds included in this study. Areas for improvement related to management practices are available for farmers and those involved in herd health management and performance. Improvement of management practices and reduction in the occurrence of viral infections should significantly contribute to higher herd performance levels and thus farm profitability.

Abbreviations
95% CI: 95% Confidence interval; ADG: Average daily weight gain; CSW: Carcass slaughter weight; FCR: Feed conversion ratio; MORT: % of mortality from 8 to 115 kg; OR: Odds-ratio; PCV2: Porcine circovirus type 2; PRRSV: Porcine Reproductive and Respiratory Syndrome Virus

Acknowledgements
The authors are grateful to Dr. Sophie Brilland, Dr. Nathalie Deville, Dr. Patrick Gambade, Dr. Sébastien Lopez and Dr. Yohan Piel for their help and support in data collection.

Funding
This study received a financial support from Boehringer Ingelheim.

Authors' contributions
MG contributed to the design of the study and the practical work. EL, NR and BG assisted in designing the study. CF performed the statistical analysis and wrote the first draft of the manuscript. All authors reviewed and completed the draft, and read and approved the final manuscript.

Competing interests
The authors declare that they have no competing interests.

Author details
[1]Agence Nationale de Sécurité Sanitaire de l'alimentation, de l'environnement et du travail (Anses), Laboratoire de Ploufragan/Plouzané, Unité Epidémiologie et Bien-Etre du Porc, B.P. 53, 22440 Ploufragan, France. [2]Agence Nationale de Sécurité Sanitaire de l'alimentation, de l'environnement et du travail (Anses), Laboratoire de Ploufragan/Plouzané, Unité Génétique Virale et Biosécurité, B.P. 53, 22440 Ploufragan, France. [3]Boehringer Ingelheim France - Santé Animale, Les Jardins de la Teillais, 3 allée de la grande Egalonne, 35740 Pacé, France. [4]Univet Santé Elevage, rue Monge, 22600 Loudéac, France. [5]Université Bretagne-Loire, Cité internationale 1 place Paul Ricoeur CS 54417, 35044 Rennes, France.

References
1. Mc Orist S, Gebhart C. Proliferative enteropathy, in Diseases of Swine. In: J. J. Zimmerman, et al., Editors. West Sussex: John Wiley and Sons; 2012. p. 811–20.
2. Neumann EJ, Kliebenstein JB, Johnson CD, Mabry JW, Bush EJ, Seitzinger AH, Green AL, Zimmerman JJ. Assessment of the economic impact of porcine reproductive and respiratory syndrome on swine production in the United States. J Am Vet Med Assoc. 2005;227:385–92.
3. Thacker, E. and F.C. Minion, Mycoplasmosis, in Diseases of swine, J.J. Zimmerman, et al., Editors. 2012, John Wiley and Sons. p. 779–797.
4. Nathues H, Alarcon P, Rushton J, Jolie R, Fiebig K, Jimenez M, Geurts V, Nathues C. Cost of porcine reproductive and respiratory syndrome virus at individual farm level – an economic disease model. Prev Vet Med. 2017;142: 16–29.
5. Opriessnig T, Gimenez-Lirola LG, Halbur PG. Polymicrobial respiratory disease in pigs. Anim Health Res Rev. 2012;12:133–48.
6. Segalés J. Porcine circovirus type 2 (PCV2) infections: clinical signs, pathology and laboratory diagnosis. Virus Res. 2012;164:10–9.
7. Done SH, Paton DJ, White MEG. Porcine reproductive and respiratory syndrome (PRRS): a review, with emphasis on pathological, virological and diagnostic aspects. Br Vet J. 1996;152:153–74.
8. Rossow KD. Porcine reproductive and respiratory syndrome. Vet Pathol. 1998;35:1–20.

9.   Kranker S, Nielsen J, Bille-Hansen V, Bøtner A. Experimental inoculation of swine at various stages of gestation with a Danish isolate of porcine reproductive and respiratory syndrome virus (PRRSV). Vet Microbiol. 1998;61: 21–31.

10. Jacobson M, Fellström C, Jensen-Waern M. Porcine proliferative enteropathy: an important disease with questions remaining to be solved. Vet J. 2010; 184:264–8.

11. Myers AJ, Goodband RD, Tokach MD, Dritz SS, DeRouchey JM, Nelssen JL. The effects of diet form and feeder design on the growth performance of finishing pigs. J Anim Sci. 2013;91:3420–8.

12. Fablet, C., An overview of the impact of the environment on enzootic respiratory diseases in pigs, in Sustainable animal production, A. Aland and F. Madec, Editors. 2009, Wageningen academic publishers: Wageningen, The Netherlands p 269–290.

13. Gonyou, H.W., S.P. Lemay, and Y. Zhang, Effects of the environment on productivity and disease, in Diseases of Swine, 9th edition, B. Straw, et al., Editors. 2006, Iowa State University press: Ames, Iowa p 1027-1038.

14. Dohoo, I.R., W. Martin, and H. Stryhn, Veterinary epidemiologic research. 2003, Prince Edward Island, Canada: Atlantic Veterinary College Inc., University of Prince Edward Island, Charlottetown. 706.

15. Scholl DT, Farver TB, Dobbelaar P, Brand A, Brouwer F, Maas M. Repeatability evaluation of a dairy farm management questionnaire. Prev Vet Med. 1994; 18:129–43.

16. Racicot M, Venne D, Durivage A, Vaillancourt J-P. Evaluation of strategies to enhance biosecurity compliance on poultry farms in Québec: effect of audits and cameras. Prev Vet Med. 2012;103:208–18.

17. Collins A, Gonsalves J, Fell S, Barchia I. Comparison of a commercial ELISA with an indirect fluorescent antibody test to detect antibodies to Lawsonia Intracellularis in experimentally challenged pigs. Aust Vet J. 2012;90:97–9.

18. Magtoto RL, Vegi A, Wang C, Johnson JK, Ramamoorthy S. Evaluation and use of a serological assay for the detection of antibodies to Lawsonia Intracellularis in swine. Int J Vet Sci Med. 2014;2:109–13.

19. Jacobson M, Wallgren P, Nordengrahn A, Merza M, Emanuelson U. Evaluation of a blocking ELISA for the detection of antibodies against Lawsonia Intracellularis in pig sera. Acta Vet Scand. 2011;53:23.

20. Sørensen V, Ahrens P, Barfod K, Feenstra AA, Feld NC, Friis NF, Bille-Hansen V, Jensen NE, Pedersen MW. Mycoplasma hyopneumoniae infection in pigs: duration of the disease and evaluation of four diagnostic assays. Vet Microbiol. 1997;54:23–34.

21. Erlandson KR, Evans RB, Thacker BJ. Evaluation of three serum antibody enzyme-linked immunosorbent assays for mycoplasma hyopneumoniae. J Swine Health Prod. 2005;13:198–203.

22. Ameri-Mahabadi M, Zhou E-M, Hsu WH. Comparison of two swine mycoplasma Hyopneumoniae enzyme-linked immunosorbent assays for detection of antibodies from vaccinated pigs and field serum samples. J Vet Diagn Investig. 2005;17:61–4.

23. Marois C, Dory D, Fablet C, Madec F, Kobisch M. Development of a quantitative real-time TaqMan PCR assay for determination of the minimal dose of mycoplasma hyopneumoniae strain 116 required to induce pneumonia in SPF pigs. J Appl Microbiol. 2010;108:1523–33.

24. Fablet C, Rose N, Bernard C, Messager I, Piel Y, Grasland B. Estimation of the diagnostic performance of two ELISAs to detect PCV2 antibodies in pig sera using a Bayesian method. J Virol Methods. 2017;249:121–5.

25. Fablet C, Renson P, Pol F, Dorenlor V, Mahe S, Eono F, Eveno E, Le Dimna M, Liegard-Vanhecke D, Eudier S, Rose N, Bourry O. Oral fluid versus blood sampling in group-housed sows and finishing pigs: feasibility and performance of antibody detection for porcine reproductive and respiratory syndrome virus (PRRSV). Vet Microbiol. 2017;204:25–34.

26. Tse M, Kim M, Chan CH, Ho PL, Ma SK, Guan Y, Peiris JSM. Evaluation of three commercially available influenza a type-specific blocking enzyme-linked immunosorbent assays for seroepidemiological studies of influenza a virus infection in pigs. Clin Vacc Immunol. 2012;19:334–7.

27. Lange E, Kalthoff D, Blohm U, Teifke JP, Breithaupt A, Maresch C, Starick E, Fereidouni S, Hoffmann B, Mettenleiter TC, Beer M, Vahlenkamp TW. Pathogenesis and transmission of the novel swine-origin influenza virus a/ H1N1 after experimental infection of pigs. J Gen Virol. 2009;90:2119–23.

28. Joliffe, I., Principal component analysis. 2nd edition, ed. S.S.i. Statistics. 2002, New York, USA: Springer 487.

29. Guillossou S, Lebon E, Mieli L, Bonnard M, Thomsen C. Development of a quantification method to specific anti-ORF2 antibody using a blocking ELISA. in 20th International Pig Veterinary Congress. 2008. Durban, South Africa: 22 to 26 June p.402.

30. Benzecri JP. Correspondence Analysis Handbook, ed. M. Dekker. 1992, New York 688. ISBN: 0-8247-8437-5.

31. Greenacre M. Correspondence Analysis in Practice. 2nd edn. Ed. London: Chapman&Hall/CRC; 2007.

32. R Development Core Team. R: A language and environment for statistical Computing 2008; Availabele from: http://www.R-project.org.

33. Hosmer DW, Lemeshow S. In: Wiley, editor. Applied logistic regression. New York: Wiley; 1989. p. 307.

34. Heinonen M, Grohn YT, Saloniemi H, Eskola E, Tuovinen VK. The effects of health classification and housing and management of feeder pigs on performance and meat inspection findings of all-in-all-out swine-finishing herds. Prev Vet Med. 2001;49:41–54.

35. Stegeman A, Elbers ARW, van Oirschot JT, Hunneman WA, Kimman TG, Tielen MJM. A retrospective study into characteristics associated with the seroprevalence of pseudorabies virus-infected breeding pigs in vaccinated herds in the southern Netherlands. Prev Vet Med. 1995;22:273–83.

36. Maes D, Deluyker H, Verdonck M, Cartryck F, Miry C, Vrijens B, De Kruif A. Risk indicators for the seroprevalence of mycoplasma hyopneumoniae, porcine influenza viruses and Aujeszky's disease virus in slaughter pigs from fattening pig herds. J Veterinary Med Ser B. 1999;46:341–52.

37. Stärk KDC, Pfeiffer DU, Morris RS. Risk factors for respiratory diseases in New Zealand pig herds. New Zeal Vet J. 1998;46:3–10.

38. Rose N, Larour G, Le Diguerher G, Eveno E, Jolly JP, Blanchard P, Oger A, Le Dimna M, Jestin A, Madec F. Risk factors for porcine post-weaning multisystemic wasting syndrome (PMWS) in 149 French farrow-to-finish herds. Prev Vet Med. 2003;61:209–25.

39. Nathues H, Chang YM, Wieland B, Rechter G, Spergser J, Rosengarten R, Kreienbrock L, Grosse Beilage E. Herd-level risk factors for the seropositivity to mycoplasma hyopneumoniae and the occurrence of enzootic pneumonia among fattening pigs in areas of endemic infection and high pig density. Transbound Emerg Dis. 2014;61:316–28.

40. Resende, T.P., C.E.R. Pereira, M.d.P. Gabardo, J.P.A. Haddad, Z.I.P. Lobato, and R.M.C. Guedes, Serological profile, seroprevalence and risk factors related to Lawsonia Intracellularis infection in swine herds from Minas Gerais state, Brazil. BMC Vet Res 2015; 11: 306.

41. Fablet C, Marois-Créhan C, Simon G, Grasland B, Jestin A, Kobisch M, Madec F, Rose N. Infectious agents associated with respiratory diseases in 125 farrow-to-finish pig herds: a cross-sectional study. Vet Microbiol. 2012;157:152–63.

42. Maes D, Deluyker H, Verdonck M, Castryck F, Miry C, Lein A, Vrijens B, de Kruif A. Effect of vaccination against mycoplasma hyopneumoniae in pig herds with a continuous production system. J Veterinary Med Ser B. 1998; 45:495–505.

43. Maes D, Deluyker H, Verdonck M, Castryck F, Miry C, Vrijens B, Verbeke W, Viaene J, de Kruif A. Effect of vaccination against mycoplasma hyopneumoniae in pig herds with an all-in/all-out production system. Vaccine. 1999;17:1024–34.

44. Holtkamp DJ, Kliebenstein JB, Neumann E, Zimmerman J, Rotto HF, Yoder TK, Wang C, Ueske PE, Mowrer CL, Haley CA. Assessment of the economic impact of porcine reproductive and respiratory syndrome virus on the United States pork producers. J Swine Health Prod. 2013;21:72–84.

45. Alarcon P, Rushton J, Nathues H, Wieland B. Economic efficiency analysis of different strategies to control post-weaning multi-systemic wasting syndrome and porcine circovirus type 2 subclinical infection in 3-weekly batch system farms. Prev Vet Med. 2013;110:103–18.

46. Guedes R. Update on epidemiology and diagnosis of porcine proliferative enteropathy. J Swine Health Prod. 2004;12:134–8.

47. Nathues H, Spergser J, Rosengarten R, Kreienbrock L, grosse Beilage E. Value of the clinical examination in diagnosing enzootic pneumonia in fattening pigs. Vet J. 2012;193:443–7.

48. Mousing J, Permin A, Mortensen S, Bøtner A, Willeberg P. A case-control questionnaire survey of risk factors for porcine reproductive and respiratory syndrome (PRRS) seropositivity in Danish swine herds. Vet Microbiol. 1997; 55:323–8.

49. Cleveland-Nielsen A, Nielsen EO, Ersboll AK. Chronic pleuritis in Danish slaughter pig herds. Prev Vet Med. 2002;55:121–35.

50. Calsamiglia M, Pijoan C. Colonisation state and colostral immunity to mycoplasma hyopneumoniae of different parity sows. Vet Rec. 2000; 146:530–2.

51. Desrosiers R. A review of some aspects of the epidemiology, diagnosis, and control of mycoplasma hyopneumoniae infections. J Swine Health Prod. 2001;9:233–7.

52. Maes D, Deluyker H, Verdonck M, Castryck F, Miry C, Vrijens B, De Kruif A. Herd factors associated with the seroprevalences of four major respiratory pathogens in slaughter pigs from farrow-to-finish pig herds. Vet Res. 2000; 31:313–27.

53. Sibila M, Calsamiglia M, Vidal D, Badiella L, Aldaz A, Jensen JC. Dynamics of mycoplasma hyopneumoniae infection in 12 farms with different production systems. Can J Vet Res. 2004;68:12–8.

54. Harris DL. Multi-site pig production. Ames: Iowa State University Press; 2000. p. 228.

55. Dohoo IR, Ducrot C, Fourichon C, Donald A, Hurnik D. An overview of techniques for dealing with large numbers of independent variables in epidemiologic studies. Prev Vet Med. 1996;29:221–39.

56. Fablet C, Dorenlor V, Eono F, Eveno E, Jolly JP, Portier F, Bidan F, Madec F, Rose N. Noninfectious factors associated with pneumonia and pleuritis in slaughtered pigs from 143 farrow-to-finish pig farms. Prev Vet Med. 2012; 104:271–80.

57. Fablet C, Simon G, Dorenlor V, Eono F, Eveno E, Gorin S, Quéguiner S, Madec F, Rose N. Different herd level factors associated with H1N1 or H1N2 influenza virus infections in fattening pigs. Prev Vet Med. 2013;112:257–65.

58. Fablet C, Marois-Crehan C, Grasland B, Simon G, Rose N. Factors associated with herd-level PRRSV infection and age-time to seroconversion in farrow-to-finish herds. Vet Microbiol. 2016;192:10–20.

59. Blecha F, Pollman DS, Nichols DA. Immunological reactions of pigs regrouped at or near weaning. Am J Vet Res. 1985;46:1934–7.

10

Zinc oxide enriched peat influence *Escherichia coli* infection related diarrhea, growth rates, serum and tissue zinc levels in Norwegian piglets around weaning: five case herd trials

M. Oropeza-Moe[1]* , C.A. Grøntvedt[2], C.J. Phythian[1], H. Sørum[3], A.K. Fauske[3] and T. Framstad[4]

Abstract

Background: Zinc oxide (ZnO), commonly used to control post-weaning diarrhea in piglets, has been highlighted as of potential concern from an environmental perspective. The aim of this field trial was to examine effects of different sources and levels of ZnO added to peat on average daily weight gain (ADG), fecal score in pens and serum and tissue zinc (Zn) levels around time of weaning in order to reduce the environmental impact without loss of the beneficial effect of ZnO on intestinal health and growth. Five case herds with enterotoxic colibacillosis challenges were included. The piglets entered the study aged three or five weeks. All piglets received a commercial diet containing <150 mg Zn/ per kg of complete feed. Four treatment groups received commercial peat added A: uncoated ZnO, B: lipid microencapsulated ZnO, C: solely commercial peat or D: no peat (Farms 2 and 3).

Results: At Farms 1, 2 and 3, a significant effect of treatment was identified for fecal score ($P < 0.05$). Treatment A led to lower fecal scores compared to treatments C ($P < 0.05$) and D ($P < 0.01$). At Farms 2 and 3, there was a significant difference in individual average daily weight gain (iADG) between treatment A and D ($P < 0.05$). The iADG of piglets receiving treatment B did not differ significantly from treatment A.

Conclusions: In 2016, The European Medicines Agency's Committee on Veterinary Medicinal Products concluded that the benefits of ZnO for the prevention of diarrhea in pigs do not outweigh the risks to the environment. Effective alternative measures to reduce the accumulation of Zn in the environment have not been identified. Our results imply that peat added low concentration of both coated and uncoated ZnO influences the gut health of weaned piglets reflected by enhanced weight gain and reduced occurrence of diarrhea. This preventive approach certainly represents a favourable alternative in the "One Health" perspective. It will also contribute to reduced antibiotic use in pig farming while diminishing the environmental consequences caused by ZnO.

Keywords: Piglet, ZnO enriched peat, Coated ZnO, Diarrhea, Growth rates, Serum ZnO, One Health

* Correspondence: marianne.oropeza-moe@nmbu.no
[1]Department of Production Animal Clinical Sciences, Norwegian University of Life Sciences (NMBU) Faculty of Veterinary Medicine, Campus Sandnes, Sandnes, Norway
Full list of author information is available at the end of the article

Background

Piglets are vulnerable to *Escherichia coli* (*E. coli*) infections around weaning since circulating plasma antibodies are low and passive intestinal immunity provided by antibodies in the sow's milk (IgA) is lost when the sow and piglets are separated [1, 2]. The separation from the sow, a different environment, commingling with unfamiliar piglets, hierarchy establishment through fighting and abrupt change in nutrition, are major changes that show a negative influence on immune functions and may result in *E. coli* associated post-weaning diarrhea (PWD) or edema disease (ED) [3–7].

E. coli causing PWD or ED enter the organism by ingestion and colonize the small intestine after attaching to porcine receptors on the enterocytes with fimbrial adhesins. The degree of colonization determines whether clinical manifestations occur or not. Fimbriae-designated *E. coli* F18$^+$ and F4$^+$ are typical pathogens involed in ED and PWD, *E. coli* F5$^+$, F6$^+$ and F41$^+$ can occur in suckling pigs [8, 9]. Enterotoxigenic *E. coli* (ETEC) strains cause watery diarrhea and systemic disease in piglets due to their ability to colonize the intestine through expression of adhesins and the ability to produce the toxins heat labile (LT) or heat stable (ST) enterotoxins as well as Shigatoxin 2e (STx2e) [10–12]. The ED causing hemolytic *E. coli* F18ab$^+$ produce Stx2e [13].

Since 2006, the use of antibiotic growth promoters in piglets has been banned in Europe [14]. As a consequence, there has been an increase in some uses of 'therapeutic' antibiotics and possibly switches to different and more modern antibiotics [15]. Therefore, AR development in production animals remain a serious problem in consumer health protection. Various natural materials such e.g. organic acids or zinc (Zn) have been tested as alternatives to antibiotics.

Zinc oxide (ZnO) at therapeutic concentrations (2000 ppm or more) has been widely used to prevent porcine colibacillosis, improve suboptimal weight gain and feed efficiency. The small-intestinal mucosa is altered by feeding of 3000 ppm Zn for 14 days [16], thus potentially increasing the absorptive capacity of the small intestine and consequently improving growth. Dietary treatment with ZnO has been associated with significant differences in the transcript abundance of several genes. Dietary ZnO supplementation influence metallothionein mRNA expression in the intestine and liver, enhances expression of the tight junction genes occludin and ZO-1 both at mRNA and protein levels and further enhances small intestinal IGF-I and IGF-I receptor gene expression, which can explain improved intestinal health [16–18]. An influence on the gastrointestinal microbiota in weaned piglets has been described [19–21]. Reduced fermentation of digestible nutrients in the proximal part of the gastrointestinal tract may render more available energy for the host and contribute to the growth-promoting effect of high dietary ZnO doses [20].

ZnO tend to dissociate after uptake in the low pH environment of the anterior gastrointestinal tract, allowing interaction with other nutrient and ingredient potentially leading to impaired absorption, and thus decreased bioavailability [22]. Long term use of pharmacological ZnO concentrations (2000 to 4000 mg Zn/ kg) to pigs feed, increases the concentration of Zn in the pig manure and results in Zn accumulation of arable land [23, 24]. Accumulation of Zn in soils may impose a toxicity risk on plants and micro-organisms [25]. Therefore, European feed legislation limits total dietary Zn in complete feed to 150 ppm [26]. Recent studies also support the assertion that Zn in feed may favour or select for AR [27–32].

Microencapsulated ZnO products are available on today's market. According to the manufacturers, lipid microencapsulation avoids ionization of the active component in the animal stomach. Therefore biological properties are preserved and the biological effects are excerted in the animals' small intestine [33, 34]. Studies have stated that coated ZnO at inclusion levels between 100 and 200 ppm in basal diets show similar effects as uncoated ZnO on growth promotion, reduced incidence of diarrhea and microbiota composition regulation [33–36].

A different approach to prevent intestinal disease in weaned piglets is peat supplementation, which has been associated with beneficial effects on health status, growth and mortality rates [37–39]. Peat contain humic substances including humic acids showing detoxifying properties because of chelate formation with potentially toxic substances such as heavy metals [40, 41], stimulation of digestion [42] and anti-inflammatory and antiviral effects [43, 44]. Due to its low pH (3.0 to 5.5) peat causes a reduction of the pH of the intestinal contents with subsequent reduced growth of *Enterobacteriaceae* [38]. Humic and fulvic acids have shown to improve nutrient uptake in suckling piglets [45]. Limited literature is available regarding the optimal dosage of peat preparations to piglets. An inclusion level of 0,5% humic substances to dietary treatments may improve ADG in weaned piglets [46]. Independent studies have stated that the effects of batches containing dietary humic substances are variable, warranting further investigation [39, 46]. An important prerequisite when applying peat supplementation to animals, is the monitoring of potentially pathogenic mycobacteria sometimes present in batches of peat preparations [47, 48]. These case herd trials aimed to explore the effects of different ZnO sources and ZnO levels in peat preparations on pre- and post-weaning fecal consistency and weight gain. Additionally, initial and final Zn-serum concentrations, liver and kidney Zn levels were examined at two of the farms.

A feed additive consisting of peat and uncoated or coated ZnO was produced. We anticipated that this preparation would show both peat and ZnO derived beneficial effects and therefore low ZnO levels added to peat should show the same effects as pharmacological ZnO levels added to feed. We hypothesized that low level ZnO enriched peat would improve piglet average daily weight gain (ADG) and reduce fecal score.

Methods

Preparation and quality control of Zn oxide enriched peat

Commercial peat (Pluss Avvenningstorv, Felleskjøpet, Norway) was used as the peat substrate in treatments A, B and C. It contained 31.1% dry matter and <5 mg Zn/ kg at a pH of 5.3. The contents of molds and yeasts were below 100 CFU/ g, no *Salmonella spp.* were detected and bacterial colony counts (30 °C) were 9000 CFU/ g. The commercial peat was analyzed by Alcontrol Laboratories (Stjørdal, Norway) by employing standard methods (Dir152/2009/ EU [49], ISO 6869 [50], NMKL 98 [51], NordVal no: 014 [52], Tecra [53], NS-EN ISO 10523:2012 [54]).

Zn sources used to prepare the peat supplements included uncoated Normin Sink®, (8% Zn, Normin, Hønefoss, Norway) and lipid microencapsulated Zincoret® S (0.3% Zn, Vetagro S.p.A, Reggio Emilia, Italy). ZnO enriched peat was prepared by Fossli AS (Frosta, Norway). Peat A was commercial peat added 2819 mg/L uncoated ZnO (2255 mg Zn/L). Peat B was commercial peat added 321 mg/L coated ZnO (257 mg Zn/L). Peat C was commercial peat without ZnO-additives. Uncoated or coated ZnO was added to a batch of peat and transported in sacks of 80 L. The farmers and veterinarians (authors) were double-blinded to the composition of the treatment groups. The Zn content in peat preparations was analyzed prior to the start of the trial by standard methods at an accredited laboratory (Labnett Laboratories, Stjørdal, Norway) [55]. Peat was analyzed at the Norwegian Veterinary Institute in Oslo by a polymerase chain reaction to identify strains of *Mycobacterium avium* with specific primers (IS901-IS902) [56, 57]. No pathogenic *Mycobacteria avium* were detected by applying IS901-IS902 specific primers on samples isolated from the peat preparation.

Case herds

Five Norwegian commercial pig herds with a documented history of clinical disease associated with *E. coli* infections were recruited (Table 1). Fecal samples from the case herds were submitted to serological testing (agglutination in microtiterplates with boiled antigen and single O-antisera) or PCR analyses conducted at the Norwegian Veterinary Institute or at the Norwegian School of Veterinary Science, respectively. At Farm 1, diarrhea occurred repeatedly around 3 weeks of age. At

Table 1 Documented virotypes and serotypes of *E. coli* causing ETEC and STEC at the case herds 1 to 5 prior to performing trials

Farm	Piglet genotype	Pathotype	Virotype	O serogroups
1	LYLL	ETEC	F4	
2	LYHH	ETEC		O149
3	LYLL	ETEC		O138
4	LYLD	ETEC	LT:STb	
5	LYHH	STEC	Stx2e:F18	O139

The pathotypes, virotypes and O serogroups verified at the case herds 1 to 5 prior to recruitment for the trials are listed. Strains of *E.coli* isolated from fecal samples of piglets after post mortem examination were either forwarded by the veterinarian in charge to the Norwegian Veterinary Institute for serotype determination (agglutination in microtiterplates with boiled antigen and single O-antisera) or to the Norwegian School of Veterinary Science in Oslo for virulence pattern determination (PCR analysis). The pathotype Enterotoxigenic *E. coli* (ETEC) was found at Farms 1 to 4 while Shiga-toxigenic *E. coli* (STEC) was found at Farm 5. Virotypes at Farms 1, 4 and 5 were F4, LT:STb and Stx2e:F18, respectively. The O serogroups O149, O138 and O139 were identified at Farms 2, 3 and 5, respectively. Genetic combinations of piglets included Landrace x Yorkshire (LY) x Landrace x Landrace (LL) (LYLL) at Farm 1. At Farm 2, LY x Hampshire/Hampshire (HH) (LYHH) were used. At Farm 3, LYLL piglets were utilized. LY x Landrace/Duroc (LYLD) and LYHH were used at Farms 4 to 5, respectively

Farms 2–4, PWD was observed regularly. At Farm 5, ED had caused significant losses across multiple batches.

All dams were vaccinated against *E. coli* (recombinant adhesin F4 (F4ab, F4 ac, F4ad), recombinant adhesin F5, field strain adhesins F6 and F41) for passive transfer of lactogenic immunity in the suckling piglets.

Animal management and measurements

The trials began with piglets aged two weeks on Farm 1 whilst on Farms 2–5, piglets close to five weeks (the average weaning age in Norway) of age were enrolled in the trials. Across all farms, piglets (females and castrated males) were weaned at 32 to 33 days of age (10.16 ± 1.80 kg of bodyweight (BW)). Digital thermometers were used to monitor the room temperatures at Farms 1 to 3. At Farm 1, room temperature was 18 °C ± 2 °C and the temperature on the piglet creep floor, measured with a handheld laser device, was 24–25 °C. At Farms 2 and 3, room temperature showed fluctuations (day and night) between 23 and 21 °C at initiation of the trials. The room temperature was gradually reduced (0.5 °C per day) and set to 18 °C. At Farms 4 and 5, the temperature was set to 22 °C at initiation of the trials and reduced gradually to 18 °C. The light (L): dark (D) periods were 16 L:8D. At Farm 1, the piglets were fed their basic feed on the floor. Restrictive feeding was conducted at Farms 2 and 3 while Farms 4 and 5 practiced ad libitum feeding. The pigs had free access to drinking water. Natural wood shawings were used as bedding material at all farms.

Concentrate feed used at all five trial farms was a standard starter feed (Table 2). Pens of 10 to 12 piglets were allocated to one of three treatments (A to D). A

Table 2 Composition of basal feed at trial farms

Farm:	Farm 1	Farm 2	Farm 3	Farm 4	Farm 5
Production stage:	PrW[a]	PoW[b]	PoW	PoW	PoW
	Feed composition				
Crude protein (%)	16.00	19.60	18.30	18.00	18.10
Dry matter (%)	88.00	88.20	86.90	87.40	88.00
Lysine (%)	1.23	1.39	1.20	1.20	1.28
Crude fat (%)	3.00	6.00	5.10	5.30	4.90
Crude ash (%)	5.00	4.70	5.00	4.50	5.20
Vit. A (IU)	10,000	8000	10,000	8000	10,000
Vit. D (IU)	1500	1300	1000	1500	1500
Vit. E (mg)	200	180	150	150	200
Copper sulphate (mg/kg)	15	26	15	32	15
Sodium selenite (mg/kg)	0.20	0.10	0.30	0.40	0.20
6-phytase (FYT/kg)	500	500	1500	703	500
Zn (mg/kg)	120	141	120	141	120

Composition of basal feed fed at the five trial farms. The levels of crude protein varied between 16% (Farm 1, preweaning phase) and 19.6% (Farm 2, postweaning phase). Vitamin levels were comparable. Sodium selenite levels varied between 0.1 and 0.4 mg/kg
[a]PrW: Pre-weaning
[b]PoW: Post-weaning

farmers consent to include a control group (treatment D) was attained at Farms 2 and 3.

The treatment duration at each case farm was decided based on known challenges with *E. coli* infections and the expected duration of clinical cases based on the farmers previous experiences. *E. coli* associated diarrhea in suckling piglets from 2 to 4 weeks of age was a documented herd health problem at Farm 1. Therefore, treatments A to C were provided from 2 weeks of age until weaning. One liter of peat A, B or C was provided to each pen twice a day. At Farms 2, 3 and 4, experiencing repeated cases of *E. coli* associated PWD, treatments with 1 L peat/ pen twice a day were initiated at weaning (day 0) and continued for 14 to 17 days.

Farm 5 struggled with repeated cases of *E. coli* associated ED. Due to the known presence of a highly 'aggressive' *E. coli* strain, animals received 2 L daily of treatments A, B or C starting one week before weaning (day −7). The next 2 weeks, the animals received twice the amount of peat compared to Farms 1, 2 and 3; 4 L daily of treatments A, B or C (day 0–14). The last week, these animals again received 2 L daily of treatments A, B or C (day 15 to 21 after weaning) as the abrupt withdrawal of ZnO supplementation may favour the growth of Shiga-toxigenic *E. coli* (STEC).

BW was registered and blood samples were collected from randomly selected and ear tagged piglets at Farms 2 (*n* = 12) and 3 (*n* = 6) via the external jugular vein prior to study entry at weaning (day 0). The same piglets were bled and weighed individually at termination of the trials.

On Farm 1, all piglets in one farrowing unit were ear tagged and the body weight was registered on study entry, at two weeks of age (– day 21, three weeks before weaning) and day 0 (weaning day). On Farms 2 to 5, group weights of pigs within the same pens were recorded on day 0 and on the last day of the trial (day 14–21). Each trial pen was evaluated for clinical signs of disease (depression, signs of dehydration and perineal staining) and fecal consistency scores by the same veterinarian at each farm. Clinical signs of disease were not scored. A standardized four-point categorical fecal scoring system was used (score 1: firm, 2: pasty, 3: loose and 4: liquid feces). Observation of a pen with liquid feces (category 4) was scored as diarrhea, irrespective of the number of piglets affected. Rectal swabs on charcoal transport medium were taken from all piglets with fecal score 4 for bacteriological culture. No antibiotic treatment was applied at the case farms during the trials.

On Farm 2, three animals (*n* = 3) from each group A, B, C and D were euthanized by captive bolt gun and exsanguination on days 7 and 15 of the trial for collection of totally 24 fresh liver and 24 kidney samples.

Serum and tissue Zn analysis

Blood samples were collected in 9 ml serum collection tubes coated with clot activator (Vacuette®, Med-Kjemi AS, Norway). All samples were directly transported to the laboratory within a maximum of 120 min following sample collection without any prior chilling. Samples were analysed to determine the following parameters: iron (Fe), inorganic phosphate (P), copper (Cu), zinc (Zn), calcium (Ca), magnesium (Mg) and ceruloplasmin (Cp) levels. Levels of Fe and P were assessed by a colorimetric method (ABX Pentra 400 Analyzer, Horiba). Cu, Zn, Ca, Mg and Cp were determined by Atomic absorption spectrometry (AAnalyst 300 Perkin Elmer). Due to limited financial resources, blood sampling was restricted to Farms 2 and 3.

Tissue samples were stored at −20 °C until analysis. Inductively coupled plasma mass spectrometry (ICP-MS) was performed by SYNLAB.vet GmbH (Berlin, Germany) to determine Zn concentrations in liver and kidney samples.

RNA extraction and reverse transcription

A multiplex PCR analysis was conducted on *E. coli* isolates from affected piglets at the five farms included in this study. Total RNA from bacterial pellets was extracted using the RNAeasy Mini Kit (Qiagen, Hilden, Germany) according to the manufacturer's instructions (Protocol 4 and 7) including an on-column DNA wipeout treatment (Appendix B1–4). The RNA was eluted in 30 μl DEPC-treated water (Invitrogen) and stored at −70 °C until reverse transcription (RT). Gel electrophoresis with 1% agarose gel was used to confirm that isolated RNA was intact while the concentration and purity of the RNA extracts were analyzed by measuring the absorbances at 260 (A260) and 280 nm (A280) using a NanoDrop™ ND-1000 spectrophotometer (Thermo Scientific, Waltham, MA, USA). Only total RNA samples of high quality with A260/A280 ratios between 1.9 and 2.2 and with tight bands of 18S/28S ribosomal RNA (rRNA) were used for RT.

Reverse transcription was conducted with QuantiTect® RT kit (Qiagen) according to manufacturer's instructions for the synthesis of complementary DNA (cDNA) and included a DNase wipeout treatment. Amounts of 1 µg of RNA were used in each RT reaction conducted in a BioRad T100 (Bio-Rad, Hercules, CA, USA). In addition, to confirm the absence of any contamination with genomic DNA (gDNA) contamination, one RNA sample per round of extraction was randomly chosen and not treated with reverse transcriptase. The cDNA samples were diluted in 180 µl of DEPC-treated water and stored at −70 °C until.

Multiplex polymerase chain reaction (PCR) analysis
The E. coli strains isolated at the five case farms were characterized by applying primer sequences obtained from previous publications, targeting for the following genes/ virulence factors: (a) estB/ STb [58], (b) estA/ STa [59], (c) eltB/ LT [60], Stx2e (A subunit) [61], faeG/ F4 [62], fanA/ F5 [63], fasA/ F6 [64], fedA/ F18 [65] and fedA subunit/ F41 [66].

Statistical analyses
Data maintained on individual animal and pen-level measurements were managed in Excel (Microsoft, Windows). Data analyses were performed in STATA version 13.1 (StataCorp LP, College Station, TX) and JMP® Pro version 12.1.0 (Cary, NC, USA). Descriptive statistics and graphical plots were used to assess for any visual differences in the population starting weight, mean and range of fecal scores.

Individual piglet weight data collected at trial entry and completion was used to derive three outcome variables. The individual daily weight gain (iADG, g/ day) was calculated as overall weight gain/days in study. Then, a group-level outcome was calculated; the average daily weight gain (ADG) was calculated in gram per day (g/ day) as mean weight gain of each treatment group/ days in study. Duration variation was corrected for in statistical analyses.

To investigate whether there was a significant effect of treatment type on iADG and ADG, mixed effects linear regression models were fitted in Stata version 13.1 (Statacorp, TX). Treatment type was included as a fixed effect, and farm identity (1 to 5) as a random effect. The effect of gender (female or castrated male), pen identity and PDI were also examined as fixed effects in separate univariate models.

Mixed effects regression models were also used to examine the effect of treatment type (A to D) on fecal score, serum and tissue mineral levels in separate univariate models. Likelihood ratio tests were used to assess model significance. Model outcomes were described using coefficient β (indicating the magnitude of the effect), the 95% confidence interval (CI) and Wald p-values [67]. To assess the effect of treatment type, the baseline (β = 0) for comparison of coefficient values was set as treatment A (peat containing 2819 mg/L uncoated ZnO).

Results
Peat preparation quality
No pathogenic Mycobacteria avium were detected by applying IS901-IS902 specific primers on samples isolated from the peat preparation.

Fecal scores
Regression models found no effect of farm identity or pen identity or fecal score ($P > 0.05$). However, treatment type had a significant effect on fecal score ($P < 0.05$). Compared to pens of piglets receiving treatment A (β = 0), higher fecal scores, indicative of looser feces, were recorded in pens receiving lower levels of Zn inclusion - treatments C or D ($P < 0.05$).

Pen average daily weight gain (ADG) and individual daily weight gain (iADG)
Outbreaks of PWD and ED on Farms 4 and 5 caused mortality rates of 2.9% and 6.2%, respectively. Due to high mortality and reduced weight gain observed in affected piglets, data from Farms 4 and 5 were analyzed separately to look at the effects of different ZnO-treatments on weight gain. A summary of weight gain results are listed in Table 4.

On farm 1, no significant effect of treatment was found for iADG. Gender did not have a significant effect on iADG.

Mixed-effects models identified significantly lower iADG ($P < 0.05$) in piglets receiving treatment D, comparing with those receiving treatment A at Farms 2 and 3 (Table 4). At Farm 2, iADG in treatment groups A, B, C and D were 410 ± 90 g/ day, 390 ± 100 g/ day, 340 ± 150 g/ day and 290 ± 130 g/ day.

At Farm 3, iADG in treatment groups A, B, C and D were 410 ± 110 g/ day, 370 ± 100 kg/ day, 270 ± 80 g/ day and 230 ± 80 g/ day.

Effects on serum minerals and tissue Zn concentrations
Data from Farms 2 and 3, indicated that serum Fe, P, Cu, Ca and Mg levels were not influenced by treatment. Linear regression analysis suggested that treatment had an influence on serum Zn serum levels at Farm 2. Compared to treatments B-D, treatment A was associated

with a significantly higher Zn concentration increase in serum after 14 days of treatment ($p < 0.02$). Mean serum Zn (SD) increase was 3.43 (2.42) μmol/ L and 1.71 (2.25) μmol/ L for treatments A and B, respectively. Treatment C lead to an increase of 0.27 (2.32) μmol serum Zn/ L and treatment D lead to an increase of 1.03 (2.99) μmol serum Zn/ L. At Farm 3, no significant serum Zn increase was observed, when comparing initial and final Zn serum levels across all treatment groups.

Mean Zn concentrations (μg/ g dry weight) in liver samples of piglets at Farm 2 receiving treatments A to D for 7 days were 31.9 (4.3), 25.5 (3.1), 20.9 (2.5) and 25.7 (1.8), respectively. Mean Zn concentrations (μg/ g dry weight) in liver samples of piglets at Farm 2 receiving treatments A to D for 15 days were 57.8 (10.42), 51.37 (7.05), 29.30 (7.78) and 25.77 (3.98), respectively. Mean Zn concentrations (μg/ g dry weight) in kidneys of piglets at Farm 2 receiving treatments A to D for 7 days were 13.5 (0.9), 13.5 (0.8), 13.5 (0.2) and 12.3 (0.5), respectively. Mean Zn concentrations (μg/ g dry weight) in kidneys of piglets at Farm 2 receiving treatments A to D for 15 days were 30.23 (6.91), 27.23 (9.42), 11.95 (4.03) and 11.06 (2.48), respectively.

Clinical signs and bacteriology

Bacteriological investigations of fecal material from piglets observed with clinical signs of diarrhea revealed that pathogenic *E. coli* strains were isolated from all five farms (Table 3). At Farm 1, ETEC and the two predominant virotypes STa:F5:F41 and LT:STb:F4 were isolated. Signs of diarrhea were evident across treatment groups at initiation of the trial. Only one pen in treatment group C showed

Table 3 Pathotyping and virotyping of *E. coli* strains isolated during trials at Farms 1 to 5

Farm	Pathotype	Virotype	Fimbriae and toxin prevalence (%)
1	ETEC	STa:F5:F41	50.0
		LT:STb	12.5
		LT:STb:F4	37.5
2	ETEC	STa:STb	13.3
		STa:STb:F4	13.3
		STxA	13.3
		STb	46.7
		STb:F18	6.7
		LT:STb	6.7
3	ETEC	F18	100.0
4	ETEC	LT:STb:F4	100.0
5	STEC	Stx2e:F18	100.0

E. coli isolates from Farms 1 to 5. Pathotypes and virotypes are described. At Farms 1 to 4, the pathotype Enterotoxigenic *E. coli* (ETEC) was found. At Farm 5, Shiga-toxigenic *E. coli* (STEC) was present. At Farms 1 to 5, the predominant virotypes detected by multiplex PCR analysis were STa:F5:F41, STb, F18, LT:STb:F4 and Stx2e:F18, respectively

signs of diarrhea until eight days into the trial. ETEC STb$^+$ were the predominant pathotype and virotype at Farm 2 and clinical signs of diarrhea were seen at initiation of the trial in pens across treatment groups. The symptoms disappeared in all treatment groups except the group receiving no peat. At Farm 3, ETEC F18$^+$ was found and clinical symptoms occurred seven days into the trial in pens where piglets received treatment C and D. At Farm 4, ETEC LT:STb:F4$^+$ was associated with an outbreak of sudden death affecting 16 piglets (2.9% of the batch) within a one week period, starting 3 days prior to weaning. Postmortem examination revealed hemorrhagic enteritis in all examined piglets. At Farm 5, STEC Stx2e:F18$^+$ caused sudden death of totally 24 piglets (6.2% of the batch) within a two weeks period, the first cases occurred at weaning. Post-mortem examinations of several piglets revealed macroscopic pathological findings compatible with ED including subcutaneous edema, edema in the submucosa of the stomach and the mesocolon. One trial piglet in the control group (D) at Farm 3 died during the experimental period. Necropsy findings were consistent with a case of haemorrhagic enteritis caused by *E. coli* infection. Serotyping and multiplex PCR analysis revealed an *E. coli* 0138 F18$^+$strain.

Discussion

Therapeutic ZnO levels in diets for weaner pigs to prevent *E. coli* infections are widely used as an efficient and cost-effective preventive strategy for PWD or ED [68–70]. In Asia and the Americas, it has been standard procedure to apply up to 3000 ppm of ZnO in weaners feed [71]. However, various studies have elucidated different challenges associated with this prophylactic approach including antimicrobial resistance and environmental pollution [25, 28, 29, 72–74]. This study aimed to identify whether peat supplemented with low-level uncoated or coated ZnO preparations could offer a feasible and effective alternative to conventional therapeutic ZnO levels for the reduction of *E. coli* associated diarrhea or ED. To the authors' knowledge, there are no previous reports on the effects of coated ZnO enriched peat on weaned piglets production parameters. Data from the present study supported our hypothesis that feeding ZnO enriched coated peat to weaned piglets for 14 days can achieve the combined beneficial effects of higher weight gain and reduced fecal scores. Additionally, the usage of coated ZnO to prevent enterotoxic colibacillosis can reduce Zn emmissions from swine producing units resulting in a substantially lower environmental impact.

An effect of treatment type on fecal consistency scores was found at Farms 1 to 3. Treatment C (commercial peat without ZnO-additives) and treatment D (controls) resulted in significantly higher fecal scores than treatment A (2819 mg/L uncoated ZnO) at Farms 1 to 3.

These findings are consistent with a previously published study showing that 14 days of post weaning ZnO-inclusion in feed affected fecal consistency, and that 3125 mg/kg of uncoated ZnO led to firmer fecal consistency than the inclusion of 139 mg/kg feed of a lipid encapsulated ZnO source called Shield Zn [75]. In the present study, basal diets at Farms 1–3 contained between 16% and 19.6% crude protein. Farms feeding diets containing crude protein levels below 19% can be considered relatively low. Low-protein diets may have a diarrhea-reducing effect [76]. This, combined with a possibly suboptimal concentration of ZINCORET™ included in treatment B (321 mg/L coated ZnO), may have concealed the presumptive effect on fecal consistency. Thus, any future studies including coated ZnO in peat may require concentrations above 321 mg ZnO/ l to promote significant effects on fecal consistency and growth rates. Other reports have described beneficial effects of coated ZnO on growth rates, intestinal morphology, digestive enzyme activity and colibacillosis at rates of 100 to 200 ppm in basic feed to recently weaned piglets [28, 75, 77].

ZnO treatment had no significant effect on ADG on Farms 1, 2 and 3. Large body weight variations within each group combined with a relatively low number of pens per treatment may have contributed to these results. No treatment effect on iADG was discovered at Farm 1. These piglets entered the study at three weeks of age. A possible explanation to the lack of statistical differences in weight gain across the groups at Farm 1, may be related to the fact that the farmer did not consent to include a control or untreated group (treatment D) due to concerns regarding E. coli associated diarrhea. At Farms 2 and 3, however, treatment D was included. Ear tagged piglets receiving treatments A showed higher iADG than piglets receiving treatment D. Individual animal identification through ear tagging and individual weight measurements of a larger number of piglets across the study farms could have provided stronger evidence to support the finding of growth promoting effects of ZnO enriched peat treatment identified on Farms 2 and 3.

Serum Zn serum levels at Farm 2 were influenced by the type of Zn treatment. Compared to treatment A (2819 mg/L uncoated ZnO), treatment B (321 mg/L coated ZnO), C (commercial peat without additives) and D (controls) were associated with significantly lower increases in serum Zn concentration after 14 days of treatment. Our results are consistent with previous studies, showing that inclusion of ZnO in the feed will increase the serum Zn concentrations [78–80].

Tissue samples from only three animals per treatment group were collected at days 7 and 15 of the first trial at Farm 2 due to limited financial resources. Although no statistically significant effects of treatment were seen on

final Zn kidney and liver concentrations, the highest numerical increase of both liver and kidney Zn concentrations was observed in animals receiving treatment A, followed by animals receiving treatments B, C and D, respectively.

These results are in line with previous findings, showing greater hepatic and circulating Zn concentrations in piglets receiving therapeutic concentrations of uncoated ZnO (between 2000 ppm and 2500 ppm) than piglets fed 100 to 200 ppm of coated ZnO [28, 29, 81]. The mean Zn concentrations in liver samples from piglets receiving treatment A were 57.80 (10.42) μg/ g dry weight while Zn concentrations in liver samples from piglets receiving treatment B, C and D were 51.37 (7.05) μg/ g dry weight, 29.30 (7.78) μg/ g dry weight and 25.77 (3.98) μg/ g dry weight, respectively.

Peat B contained 321 mg/L coated ZnO while Peat A contained 2819 mg/L uncoated ZnO, equivalent with a ratio of 1:8.8. Despite the low coated versus high uncoated ZnO ratio in Peat B and Peat A, comparable Zn-levels were detected in animals receiving Peat A or Peat B. These tissue Zn concentrations suggest that the bioavailability of coated Zn added to peat is higher than uncoated Zn. Experimental studies on the pharmacological effects of Zn to reduce post-weaning scouring and improve body weight gain have shown that formulations of Zn in organic form or lipid-encapsulated Zn may be effective at relatively low concentrations, achieving comparable effect with far higher concentrations of inorganic Zn. This indicates that the bioavailability and retention of organic form or lipid-encapsulated Zn may be increased [24]. A recent study demonstrates that nanosize ZnO can increase Zn digestibility, serum growth hormone levels and carbonic anhydrase activity and enhance the immune response of weanling piglets [82]. Uncoated ZnO tend to dissociate after uptake in the low pH environment of the anterior gastrointestinal tract, allowing interaction with other nutrient and ingredient potentially leading to impaired absorption, and thus decreased bioavailability [22].

The fecal Zn concentrations were not measured in this trial due to limited financial resources, but it seems likely that fecal Zn concentrations in feces from piglets receiving treatment B would be lower than Zn concentrations in feces from piglets receiving treatment A, as shown in previous studies [83–85].

Five farms with a history of E. coli associated enteric disease were specifically included in this study. Pathogenic E. coli strains were detected at all farms. During the course of the trial, clinical signs of disease were not evident on Farms 1 and 2. At Farm 3, one piglet died due to haemorrhagic enteritis associated with E. coli whilst Farms 4 and 5 experienced outbreaks of E. coli-associated peracute-to-acute PWD and ED, respectively. The differences in clinical presentations may be explained by the fact that different pathotypes of *E. coli* were present at the different trial farms (Table 3). Possible coinfections with e.g. rotavirus [86], management, feeding and hygiene policies [87–89] may also have influenced the general enteric health and disease susceptibility among piglets at Farms 4 and 5. The detection of coinfection-causing agents was not included in this study. The passive protection of piglets against *E. coli* infections through vaccination of the dams decreases with ageing and lactogenic immunity suddenly stops at weaning [90]. It is likely that subclinical infections of the surviving weaned piglets at Farms 4 and 5 affected ADG. Reduced weight gain is indeed associated with subclinical infections in pigs [91–93]. Tables 4 shows that the ADG/ piglet in treatment groups A to C were low at Farms 4 and 5 where ETEC and STEC expressing the virulence factors LT:STb:F4 and Stx2e:F18 were found. Mortality rates of 2.9% at Farm 4 and 6.2% at Farm 5 during the first 2 weeks after weaning occurred in spite of prophylactic treatment with ZnO enriched peat. This may suggest that both uncoated or microencapsulated ZnO-concentrations in peat require optimization to achieve

broader preventive effects on piglets at farms with different infection pressure and *E. coli* variants.

The multiplex PCR results show that ETEC F4$^+$ were found at both Farms 2 and 4. There was a clear difference in strain virulence at these farms, which may be explained by differing management strategies. At Farm 2 a strict cleaning and disinfection regime between batches was maintained. This was not possible at Farm 4 due to poor growth rates and consequently a reduced duration of empty periods between batches. Additionally, a large amount of flies were present at Farm 4. Flies are known to transmit bacteria including *E. coli* [94, 95].

The actual daily consumption of peat per piglet was not feasible to measure in this study because piglets were kept in groups. Instead, an estimated daily piglet Zn consumption rate was calculated, by dividing the amount of daily added Zn in peat preparations by the number of piglets per pen [96, 97]. This field trial demonstrated that significant growth promoting and diarrhea reducing effects were maintained by adding 2819 mg uncoated ZnO/ l of peat (Treatment A). Pens of piglets receiving 2 L of peat per

Table 4 Average daily gain (ADG) results at Farms 1 to 5

Farm	Treatment	Trial duration (days)	ADG (g/ day)	SEM	n=	iADG (g/ day)	SEM	n=
1	A	21	270	12	6	270	12	57
	B		300	11	6	300	11	54
	C		280	12	6	280	12	57
2	A	15/15	400	12	9	410^a	18	12
	B		410	11	9	390	21	12
	C		340	10	9	340	31	12
	D		330	12	9	290^b	27	12
3	A	15/17	400	5	6	410^a	31	6
	B		370	10	6	370	29	6
	C		320	8	6	270	23	6
	D		370	8	6	230^b	23	6
4	A	15	220	3	18	#	#	#
	B		210	2	18	#	#	#
	C		190	4	17	#	#	#
5	A	14/15	230	8	12	#	#	#
	B		240	8	12	#	#	#
	C		210	7	12	#	#	#

The pen based and individual weight measurements are expressed as ADG/ piglet and iADG, respectively. Treatment A was peat containing 2819 mg/L uncoated ZnO (2255 mg Zn/L). Treatment B was peat containing 321 mg/L coated ZnO (257 mg Zn/L). Treatment C was commercial peat without ZnO-additives (36 mg Zn/L). Treatment D implied no feeding of peat (control groups). Individual measurements of all piglets were included at Farm 1, both group and selected individual weight registrations were included at Farms 2 and 3. Group weight registrations only were included at Farms 4 and 5. Significant differences (*P* < 0.05) between iADG at the Farms 2 and 3 are indicated by different superscripts (a or b). At Farm 3, two trials with differing duration were conducted without affecting the weight gain of piglets significantly (data not shown). Variation in trial durations were based on the need for farmers compliance to participate in the trials and the practicality at each farm. Duration variation was corrected for in statistical analyses
#Not included in the trial

day, received 5638 mg ZnO per day, which equals to 4510 mg Zn. Each piglet (10 to 12/ pen) should theoretically consume approximately between 451 mg Zn and 376 mg Zn per day. Treatments B equated to an approximate daily Zn uptake per piglet between 51 mg Zn per day and 43 mg Zn per day. Treatment C equated to an approximate daily Zn uptake per piglet between 7 mg Zn per day and 6 mg Zn per day. These levels of Zn uptake per piglet per day are much lower than the uptake levels when applying conventional pharmacological concentrations of ZnO in pelleted feed to piglets. If assuming a mean daily feed consumption of 450 g/ day during the first 14 days after weaning (32 days old piglets) [98, 99], piglets receiving conventional pharmacological levels of uncoated ZnO between 2000 and 3500 ppm (1600 and 2800 ppm Zn, respectively) added to their basal diet will consume between 720 and 1260 mg Zn per day, respectively. A comparison of feeding Peat A or Peat B with a diet added 2000 ppm uncoated ZnO (or 1600 ppm Zn) implicates a reduction of dietary Zn by 72.0% (Peat A) or even 96.8% (Peat B).

Conclusions

To the author's knowledge, this is the first field study undertaken to identify effects of supplementation with both uncoated and coated ZnO-enriched peat on fecal consistency and weight gain. This study has practical relevance for the control of enteric diseases in weaned piglets managed under European pig production systems. Since higher iADG was observed in a relatively small sample size of piglets receiving treatment A, our findings support the need for further research, conducted on a larger number of farms and under varying management conditions. The determination of optimal ZnO concentrations in peat preparations for growth-enhancing as well as PWD and ED preventive effects needs further investigation. Additionally, our promising findings support further investigation on coated ZnO in a larger randomized clinical trial, either added to peat or concentrates. Coated ZnO represents an alternative to reduce the negative impact on the environment and a way of counteracting potential co-selection for antibiotic resistance in bacteria.

In light of the current discussion regarding a possible ban on the use of ZnO in animal feed, it is important to emphasize that the usage of orally administered veterinary medicinal products containing ZnO should be reduced. Simultaneously, optimization of management strategies at pig producing units should always be strived for prior to applying ZnO as a preventive measure to avoid PWD or ED.

Abbreviations

ADG: Average daily weight gain; AR: Antibiotic resistance; Ca: Calcium; CI: Confidence interval; Cp: Ceruloplasmin; Cu: Copper; E. coli: Escherichia coli; ED: Edema disease; ETEC: Enterotoxigenic E. coli; Fe: Iron; g: Gram; HH: Hampshire/Hampshire; iADG: Individual weight gain; L: Liter; LD: Landrace/Duroc; LL: Landrace x Landrace; LT: Heat-labile enterotoxin; LY: Landrace x Yorkshire; Mg: Magnesium; P: Inorganic phosphate; PCR: Polymerase chain reaction; PWD: Post-weaning diarrhea; Stb: Heat-stable enterotoxin B; STEC: Shiga-toxigenic E. coli; Zn: Zinc

Acknowledgements

The Authors wish to acknowledge the contributions of Fossli AS and the farmers involved in this study.

Funding

This study was financed by SINTEF, Norway.

Authors' contributions

AKF and HS analyzed the bacteria isolates. MOM, CAG and TF conducted the field trials while CP analyzed the data statistically. MOM, CAG, CP, HS and TF were major contributors in writing the manuscript. All authors read and approved the final manuscript.

Competing interests

The authors declare that they have no competing interests.

Author details

[1]Department of Production Animal Clinical Sciences, Norwegian University of Life Sciences (NMBU) Faculty of Veterinary Medicine, Campus Sandnes, Sandnes, Norway. [2]Norwegian Veterinary Institute, Oslo, Norway. [3]Faculty of Veterinary Medicine, Department of Food Safety and Infection Biology, Norwegian University of Life Sciences, Oslo, Norway. [4]Department of Production Animal Clinical Sciences, Norwegian University of Life Sciences (NMBU) Faculty of Veterinary Medicine, Campus Adamstuen, Adamstuen, Norway.

References

1. Nguyen UV, Melkebeek V, Devriendt B, Goetstouwers T, Van Poucke M, Peelman L, et al. Maternal immunity enhances systemic recall immune responses upon oral immunization of piglets with F4 fimbriae. Vet Res. 2015;46:72. doi:10.1186/s13567-015-0210-3.
2. Sieverding E. Handbuch Gesunde Schweine. Germany: Kamlage Verlag; 2000.
3. Bailey M, Clarke CJ, Wilson AD, Williams NA, Stokes CR. Depressed potential for interleukin-2 production following early weaning of piglets. Vet Immunol Immunopathol. 1992;34:197–207.
4. Hessing MJC, Coenen GJ, Vaiman M, Renard C. Individual differences in cell-mediated and humoral immunity in pigs. Vet Immunol Immunopathol. 1995;45:97–113. doi:10.1016/0165-2427(94)05338-S.
5. Wattrang E, Wallgren P, Lindberg A, Fossum C. Signs of infections and reduced immune functions at weaning of conventionally reared and specific pathogen free pigs. Zentralbl Veterinärmed B. 1998;45:7–17.

6.   Melin L, Wallgren P. Aspects on Feed Related Prophylactic Measures Aiming to Prevent Post Weaning Diarrhoea in Pigs. Acta Vet Scand. 2002;43:231. doi:10.1186/1751-0147-43-231.

7.   Quiñonero J, Ramis G, Lopes E, María-Dolores E, Armero E. Effect of mixing piglets affected by Escherichia coli diarrhea on growth and welfare responses. J Swine Health Prod. 2012;20:216–22.

8.   Svensmark B, Jorsal SE, Nielsen K, Willeberg P. Epidemiological studies of piglet diarrhoea in intensively managed Danish sow herds. I. Pre-weaning diarrhoea. Acta Vet Scand. 1989;30:43–53.

9.   Svensmark B, Nielsen K, Willeberg P, Jorsal SE. Epidemiological studies of piglet diarrhoea in intensively managed Danish sow herds. II. Post-weaning diarrhoea. Acta Vet Scand. 1989;30:55–62.

10. Broes A, Fairbrother JM, Jacques M, Larivière S. Requirement for capsular antigen KX105 and fimbrial antigen CS1541 in the pathogenicity of porcine enterotoxigenic Escherichia coli O8:KX105 strains. Can J Vet Res. 1989;53:43–7.

11. Helgerson AF, Sharma V, Dow AM, Schroeder R, Post K, Cornick NA. Edema Disease Caused by a Clone of Escherichia coli O147. J Clin Microbiol. 2006; 44:3074–7. doi:10.1128/JCM.00617-06.

12. Nagy B, Fekete PZ. Enterotoxigenic Escherichia coli (ETEC) in farm animals. Vet Res. 1999;30:259–84.

13. Bertschinger HU, Gyles CL. Escherichia coli in domestic animals and humans; Oedema disease of pigs. In: Oedema Dis. Pigs. Wallingford: CAB International; 1994. p. 193–219.

14. European Commission. Ban on antibiotics as growth promoters in animal feed enters into effect. 2005. http://europa.eu/rapid/press-release_IP-05-1687_en.htm. Accessed 19 Oct 2016.

15. Food and Agriculture Organization of the United Nations (FAO). Antibiotics in Farm Animal Production Public health and animal welfare. 2011. http://www.fao.org/fileadmin/user_upload/animalwelfare/antibiotics_in_animal_farming.pdf. Accessed 15 Feb 2017.

16. Li X, Yin J, Li D, Chen X, Zang J, Zhou X. Dietary supplementation with zinc oxide increases Igf-I and Igf-I receptor gene expression in the small intestine of weanling piglets. J Nutr. 2006;136:1786–91.

17. Carlson MS, Hill GM, Link JE. Early- and traditionally weaned nursery pigs benefit from phase-feeding pharmacological concentrations of zinc oxide: effect on metallothionein and mineral concentrations. J Anim Sci. 1999;77:1199–207.

18. Zhang B, Guo Y. Supplemental zinc reduced intestinal permeability by enhancing occludin and zonula occludens protein-1 (ZO-1) expression in weaning piglets. Br J Nutr. 2009;102:687–93. doi:10.1017/S0007114509289033.

19. Jensen-Waern M, Melin L, Lindberg R, Johannisson A, Petersson L, Wallgren P. Dietary zinc oxide in weaned pigs — effects on performance, tissue concentrations, morphology, neutrophil functions and faecal microflora. Res Vet Sci. 1998;64:225–31. doi:10.1016/S0034-5288(98)90130-8.

20. Højberg O, Canibe N, Poulsen HD, Hedemann MS, Jensen BB. Influence of dietary zinc oxide and copper sulfate on the gastrointestinal ecosystem in newly weaned piglets. Appl Environ Microbiol. 2005;71:2267–77. doi:10.1128/AEM.71.5.2267-2277.2005.

21. Katouli M, Melin L, Jensen-Waern M, Wallgren P, Möllby R. The effect of zinc oxide supplementation on the stability of the intestinal flora with special reference to composition of coliforms in weaned pigs. J Appl Microbiol. 1999;87:564–73.

22. Suttle NF. Mineral Nutrition of Livestock. 4th ed. Oxfordshire: CAB International; 2010.

23. Åhman M. Zinc flow to the soil in Swedish piglet production. 2013. http://stud.epsilon.slu.se/5322/. Accessed 16 Feb 2017.

24. Norwegian Scientific Committee for Food Safety. Zinc and copper in pig and poultry production – fate and effects in the food chain and the environment. 2014. http://www.english.vkm.no/dav/3b1b6769dd.pdf. Accessed 22 Feb 2017

25. Dourmad J-Y, Jondreville C. Impact of nutrition on nitrogen, phosphorus, Cu and Zn in pig manure, and on emissions of ammonia and odours. Livest Sci. 2007;112:192–8. doi:10.1016/j.livsci.2007.09.002.

26. European Union. Commision Regulation No 1334/2003 amending the conditions for authorisation of a number of additives in feedingstuffs belonging to the group of trace elements. 2003. http://eur-lex.europa.eu/legal-content/EN/TXT/?uri=CELEX%3A32003R1334. Accessed 22 Feb 2017

27. Baker-Austin C, Wright MS, Stepanauskas R, McArthur JV. Co-selection of antibiotic and metal resistance. Trends Microbiol. 2006;14:176–82. doi:10.1016/j.tim.2006.02.006.

28. Bednorz C, Oelgeschläger K, Kinnemann B, Hartmann S, Neumann K, Pieper R, et al. The broader context of antibiotic resistance: zinc feed supplementation

29. of piglets increases the proportion of multi-resistant Escherichia coli in vivo. Int J Med Microbiol. 2013;303:396–403. doi:10.1016/j.ijmm.2013.06.004.

29. Cavaco LM, Hasman H, Aarestrup FM. Zinc resistance of Staphylococcus aureus of animal origin is strongly associated with methicillin resistance. Vet Microbiol. 2011;150:344–8. doi:10.1016/j.vetmic.2011.02.014.

30. Hölzel CS, Müller C, Harms KS, Mikolajewski S, Schäfer S, Schwaiger K, et al. Heavy metals in liquid pig manure in light of bacterial antimicrobial resistance. Environ Res. 2012;113:21–7. doi:10.1016/j.envres.2012.01.002.

31. Seiler C, Berendonk TU. Heavy metal driven co-selection of antibiotic resistance in soil and water bodies impacted by agriculture and aquaculture. Front Microbiol. 2012;3:399. doi:10.3389/fmicb.2012.00399.

32. Vahjen W, Pietruszyńska D, Starke IC, Zentek J. High dietary zinc supplementation increases the occurrence of tetracycline and sulfonamide resistance genes in the intestine of weaned pigs. Gut Pathog. 2015;7. doi:10.1186/s13099-015-0071-3.

33. Kwon C-H, Lee CY, Han S-J, Kim S-J, Park B-C, Jang I, et al. Effects of dietary supplementation of lipid-encapsulated zinc oxide on colibacillosis, growth and intestinal morphology in weaned piglets challenged with enterotoxigenic Escherichia coli. Anim Sci J Nihon Chikusan Gakkaihō. 2014; 85:805–13. doi:10.1111/asj.12215.

34. Kim SJ, Kwon CH, Park BC, Lee CY, Han JH. Effects of a lipid-encapsulated zinc oxide dietary supplement, on growth parameters and intestinal morphology in weanling pigs artificially infected with enterotoxigenic Escherichia coli. J Anim Sci Technol. 2015;57. doi:10.1186/s40781-014-0038-9.

35. Shen J, Chen Y, Wang Z, Zhou A, He M, Mao L, et al. Coated zinc oxide improves intestinal immunity function and regulates microbiota composition in weaned piglets. Br J Nutr. 2014;111:2123–34. doi:10.1017/S0007114514000300.

36. Jang I, Kwon CH, Ha DM, Jung DY, Kang SY, Park MJ, et al. Effects of a lipid-encapsulated zinc oxide supplement on growth performance and intestinal morphology and digestive enzyme activities in weanling pigs. J Anim Sci Technol. 2014;56 doi:10.1186/2055-0391-56-29.

37. Roost H, Dobberstein I, Kuntsch G, Berber H, Tardel H, Benda A, et al. Results and experience obtained from use of peat paste in industrialized piglet raising (in German). Monatsh Veterinärmed. 1990;45:239–43.

38. Trckova M, Matlova L, Hudcova H, Faldyna M, Zraly Z, Dvorska L, et al. Peat as a feed supplement for animals: a review. Vet Med. 2005;50:361–77.

39. Fuchs B, Orda J, Preś J, Muchowicz M. The effect of feeding piglets up to the 100th day of their life with peat preparation on their growth and physiological and biochemical indices. Arch Vet Pol Pol Acad Sci Comm Vet Sci. 1995;35:97–107.

40. Stackhouse RA, Benson WH. Interaction of humic acid with selected trace metals: Influence on bioaccumulation in daphnids. Environ Toxicol Chem. 1989;8:639–44. doi:10.1002/etc.5620080711.

41. Stackhouse RA, Benson WH. The effect of humic acid on the toxicity and bioavailability of trivalent chromium. Ecotoxicol Environ Saf. 1989;17:105–11.

42. Beer AM, Sagorchev P, Lukanov J. Isolation of biologically active fractions from the water soluble components of fulvic and ulmic acids from peat. Phytomed Int J Phytother Phytopharm. 2002;9:659–66. doi:10.1078/094471102321616490.

43. Kuhnert M, Fuchs V, Golbs S. Chemical characterization and pharmacologico-toxicological peculiarities of humic acid (in German). Arch Für Exp Veterinärmed. 1982;36:169–77.

44. Kuhnert M, Bartels KP, Kroll S, Lange N. Veterinary pharmaceuticals containing humic acid for therapy and prophylaxis for gastrointestinal diseases of dog and cat (in German). Monatsh Veterinärmed. 1991;46:4–8.

45. Fuchs V, Kuhnert M, Golbs S, Dedek W. The enteral absorption of iron (II) from humic acid-iron complexes in suckling piglets using radiolabeled iron (59Fe) (in German). Dtsch Tierärztl Wochenschr. 1990;97:208–9.

46. Ji F, McGlone JJ, Kim SW. Effects of dietary humic substances on pig growth performance, carcass characteristics, and ammonia emission. J Anim Sci. 2006;84:2482–90. doi:10.2527/jas.2005-206.

47. Johansen TB, Agdestein A, Lium B, Jørgensen A, Djønne B, et al. Mycobacterium avium subsp. hominissuis Infection in Swine Associated with Peat Used for Bedding, Mycobacterium avium subsp. hominissuis Infection in Swine Associated with Peat Used for Bedding. Biomed Res Int. 2014;2014:e189649. doi:10.1155/2014/189649.

48. Matlova L, Kaevska M, Moravkova M, Beran V, Shitaye VE, Pavlik I. Mycobacteria in peat used as a supplement for pigs: failure of different decontamination methods to eliminate the risk. Vet Med (Praha). 2012;57:212–7.

49. European Union. Commission Regulation (EC) No 152/2009 laying down the methods of sampling and analysis for the official control of feed. http://eur-lex.europa.eu/legal-content/EN/ALL/?uri=CELEX%3A32009R0152. 2009. Accessed 22 Feb 2017.

50. International Organization for Standardization. ISO 6869:2000 - Animal feeding stuffs - Determination of the contents of calcium, copper, iron, magnesium, manganese, potassium, sodium and zinc. Method using atomic absorption spectrometry. 2000. http://www.iso.org/iso/catalogue_detail.htm?csnumber=33707. Accessed 30 Dec 2016.

51. NordVal International. Mould and yeasts. Determination in foods and feed. 2005. http://www.nmkl.org/index.php/nb/webshop/item/nmkl-98. Accessed 30 Dec 2016.

52. NordVal International. 3MTM PetrifilmTM E.coli/ Coliform Count Plate - NordVal International Certificate. 2003. http://www.nmkl.org/dokumenter/nytt/90-no.pdf. Accessed 16 Feb 2017.

53. 3M Microbiology. 3MTM TecraTM Salmonella Visual Immunoassay (VIA). 2008. http://www.mdairysolutions.com/Brochures/other_food/3M/salmonella.pdf. Accessed 14 Feb 2017.

54. Standard Norge. Water quality - Determination of pH (ISO 10523:2008). 2008. https://www.standard.no/no/Nettbutikk/produktkatalogen/Produktpresentasjon/?ProductID=681000. Accessed 17 Feb 2017.

55. Poulsen HD. Zinc oxide for weanling piglets. Acta Agric Scand Sect A Anim Sci. 1995;45:159–67.

56. Agdestein A, Johansen TB, Polaček V, Lium B, Holstad G, Vidanović D, et al. Investigation of an outbreak of mycobacteriosis in pigs. BMC Vet Res. 2011; 7:63. doi:10.1186/1746-6148-7-63.

57. Ahrens P, Giese SB, Klausen J, Inglis NF. Two markers, IS901-IS902 and p40, identified by PCR and by using monoclonal antibodies in Mycobacterium avium strains. J Clin Microbiol. 1995;33:1049–53.

58. Lee CH, Moseley SL, Moon HW, Whipp SC, Gyles CL, So M. Characterization of the gene encoding heat-stable toxin II and preliminary molecular epidemiological studies of enterotoxigenic Escherichia coli heat-stable toxin II producers. Infect Immun. 1983;42:264–8.

59. So M, McCarthy BJ. Nucleotide sequence of the bacterial transposon Tn1618 encoding a heat-stable (ST) toxin and its identification in enterotoxigenic E. coli strains. Proc Natl Acad Sci. 1980;77:4011–2015.

60. Dallas WS, Falkow S. Amino acid sequence homology between cholera toxin and Escherichia coli heat-labile toxin. Nature. 1980;288:499–501.

61. Weinstein DL, Jackson MP, Samuel JE, Holmes RK, O'Brien AD. Cloning and sequencing of a Shiga-like toxin type II variant from Escherichia coli strain responsible for edema disease of swine. J Bacteriol. 1988;170: 4223–30.

62. Josephsen J, Hansen F, de Graaf FK, Gaastra W. The nucleotide sequence of the protein subunit of the K88ac fimbriae of porcine enterotoxigenic Escherichia coli. FEMS Microbiol Lett. 1984;25:301–6.

63. Roosendaal E, Jacobs AA, Rathman P, Sondermeyer C, Stegehuis F, Oudega B, et al. Primary structure and subcellular localization of two fimbrial subunit-like proteins involved in the biosynthesis of K99 fibrillae. Mol Microbiol. 1987;1:211–7.

64. de Graaf FK, Klaasen P. Nucleotide sequence of the gene encoding the 987P fimbrial subunit of Escherichia coli. FEMS Microbiol Lett. 1987;42:253–8. doi:10.1111/j.1574-6968.1987.tb02082.x.

65. Imberechts H, De Greve H, Schlicker C, Bouchet H, Pohl P, Charlier G, et al. Characterization of F107 fimbriae of Escherichia coli 107/86, which causes edema disease in pigs, and nucleotide sequence of the F107 major fimbrial subunit gene, fedA. Infect Immun. 1992;60:1963–71.

66. Anderson DG, Moseley SL. Escherichia coli F41 adhesin: genetic organization, nucleotide sequence, and homology with the K88 determinant. J Bacteriol. 1988;170:4890–6.

67. Long JS, Freese J. Regression Models for Categorical Dependent Variables using Stata. 2nd edn. College Station: StataCorp LP; 2006.

68. Poulsen HD, Carlson D. Zinc and copper for piglets- how do high dietary levels of these minerals function, Trace Elem Anim Prod Syst. Wageningen: Wageningen Academic Publishers; 2008. p. 151–60.

69. Pettigrew JE. Reduced Use of Antibiotic Growth Promoters in Diets Fed to Weanling Pigs: Dietary Tools, Part 1. Anim Biotechnol. 2006;17:207–15. doi:10.1080/10495390600956946.

70. Hollis GR, Carter SD, Cline TR, Crenshaw TD, Cromwell GL, Hill GM, et al. Effects of replacing pharmacological levels of dietary zinc oxide with lower dietary levels of various organic zinc sources for weanling pigs. J Anim Sci. 2005;83:2123–9.

71. Starke IC, Pieper R, Neumann K, Zentek J, Vahjen W. The impact of high dietary zinc oxide on the development of the intestinal microbiota in weaned piglets. FEMS Microbiol Ecol. 2014;87:416–27. doi:10.1111/1574-6941.12233.

72. Poulsen HD, Larsen T. Zinc excretion and retention in growing pigs fed increasing levels of zinc oxide. Livest Prod Sci. 1995;43:235–42.

73. Jondreville C, Revy PS, Dourmad JY. Dietary means to better control the environmental impact of copper and zinc by pigs from weaning to slaughter. Livest Prod Sci. 2003;84:147–56. doi:10.1016/j.livprodsci.2003.09.011.

74. Yazdankhah S, Rudi K, Bernhoft A. Zinc and copper in animal feed – development of resistance and co-resistance to antimicrobial agents in bacteria of animal origin. Microb Ecol Health Dis. 2014;25 doi:10.3402/mehd.v25.25862.

75. Park BC, Jung DY, Kang SY, Ko YH, Ha DM, Kwon CH, et al. Effects of dietary supplementation of a zinc oxide product encapsulated with lipid on growth performance, intestinal morphology, and digestive enzyme activities in weanling pigs. Anim Feed Sci Technol. 2015;200:112–7. doi:10.1016/j.anifeedsci.2014.11.016.

76. Heo JM, Kim JC, Hansen CF, Mullan BP, Hampson DJ, Pluske JR. Feeding a diet with decreased protein content reduces indices of protein fermentation and the incidence of postweaning diarrhea in weaned pigs challenged with an enterotoxigenic strain of Escherichia coli. J Anim Sci. 2009;87:2833–43. doi:10.2527/jas.2008-1274.

77. Kim JC, Hansen CF, Pluske JF, Mullan BP. Evaluating the replacement of zinc oxide with an encapsulated zinc oxide product as a means of controlling post-weaning diarrhoea in piglet. 2010. https://apri.com.au/2C-114_Final_report.pdf. Accessed 22 Feb 2017.

78. Walk CL, Srinongkote S, Wilcock P. Influence of a microbial phytase and zinc oxide on young pig growth performance and serum minerals. J Anim Sci. 2013;91:286–91. doi:10.2527/jas.2012-5430.

79. Walk CL, Wilcock P, Magowan E. Evaluation of the effects of pharmacological zinc oxide and phosphorus source on weaned piglet growth performance, plasma minerals and mineral digestibility. Anim Int J Anim Biosci. 2015;9:1145–52. doi:10.1017/S175173111500035X.

80. Schell TC, Kornegay ET. Zinc concentration in tissues and performance of weanling pigs fed pharmacological levels of zinc from ZnO, Zn-methionine, Zn-lysine, or ZnSO4. J Anim Sci. 1996;74:1584–93.

81. Jensen-Waern M, Melin L, Lindberg R, Johannisson A, Petersson L, Wallgren P. Dietary zinc oxide in weaned pigs–effects on performance, tissue concentrations, morphology, neutrophil functions and faecal microflora. Res Vet Sci. 1998;64:225–31.

82. Li M-Z, Huang J-T, Tsai Y-H, Mao S-Y, Fu C-M, Lien T-F. Nanosize of zinc oxide and the effects on zinc digestibility, growth performances, immune response and serum parameters of weanling piglets. Anim Sci J. 2016;87:1379–85. doi:10.1111/asj.12579.

83. Carlson MS, Boren CA, Wu C, Huntington CE, Bollinger DW, Veum TL. Evaluation of various inclusion rates of organic zinc either as polysaccharide or proteinate complex on the growth performance, plasma, and excretion of nursery pigs. J Anim Sci. 2004;82:1359–66.

84. Buff CE, Bollinger DW, Ellersieck MR, Brommelsiek WA, Veum TL. Comparison of growth performance and zinc absorption, retention, and excretion in weanling pigs fed diets supplemented with zinc-polysaccharide or zinc oxide. J Anim Sci. 2005;83:2380–6.

85. Wang C, Xie P, Liu LL, Lu JJ, Zou XT. Effects of Dietary Capsulated Zinc Oxide on Growth Performance, Blood Metabolism and Mineral Concentrations in Weaning Piglets. Asian J Anim Vet Adv. 2013;8:502–10.

86. Dewey C, Carman S, Pasma T, Josephson G, McEwen B. Relationship between group A porcine rotavirus and management practices in swine herds in Ontario. Can Vet J. 2003; 44:649–653.

87. Frydendahl K. Prevalence of serogroups and virulence genes in Escherichia coli associated with postweaning diarrhoea and edema disease in pigs and a comparison of diagnostic approaches. Vet Microbiol. 2002;85:169–82.

88. van Beers-Schreurs HM, Vellenga L, Wensing T, Breukink HJ. The pathogenesis of the post-weaning syndrome in weaned piglets: a review. Vet Q. 1992;14:29–34. doi:10.1080/01652176.1992.9694322.

89. Bosworth BT, Samuel JE, Moon HW, O'Brien AD, Gordon VM, Whipp SC. Vaccination with genetically modified Shiga-like toxin IIe prevents edema disease in swine. Infect Immun. 1996;64:55–60.

90. Cox E, Melkebeek V, Devriendt B, Goddeeris B, Vanrompay D. Vaccines against enteric E.coli infections in animals, Pathog Escherichia coli Mol Cell Microbiol. Caister: Academic Press; 2014. p. 255–70.

91. Rohrbach BW, Hall RF, Hitchcock JP. Effect of subclinical infection with Actinobacillus pleuropneumoniae in commingled feeder swine. J Am Vet Med Assoc. 1993;202:1095–8.
92. Kurmann, J. Subclinical porcine circovirus infection significantly decreases growth parameters of fatteningpigs. 2011. University of Zurich. http://www.zora.uzh.ch/59592/2/Diss_Kurmann_J_Titel.pdf. Accessed 18 Feb 2017.
93. Jacobs AAC. A vaccine for use against subclinical lawsonia infection in a pig. 2016. https://www.google.com/patents/WO2016124623A1?cl=en. Accessed 20 Feb 2017.
94. Usui M, Shirakawa T, Fukuda A, Tamura Y. The Role of Flies in Disseminating Plasmids with Antimicrobial-Resistance Genes Between Farms. Microb Drug Resist. 2015;21:562–9. doi:10.1089/mdr.2015.0033.
95. Literak I, Dolejska M, Rybarikova J, Cizek A, Strejckova P, Vyskocilova M, et al. Highly variable patterns of antimicrobial resistance in commensal Escherichia coli isolates from pigs, sympatric rodents, and flies. Microb Drug Resist. 2009;15:229–37. doi:10.1089/mdr.2009.0913.
96. Spreeuwenberg MA, Verdonk JM, Gaskins HR, Verstegen MW. Small intestine epithelial barrier function is compromised in pigs with low feed intake at weaning. J Nutr. 2001;131:1520–7.
97. Campbell JM, Crenshaw JD, Polo J. The biological stress of early weaned piglets. J Anim Sci Biotechnol. 2013;4:19. doi:10.1186/2049-1891-4-19.
98. Carr J. Garth Pig Stockmanship Standards. Sheffield: 5m Publishing; 1998.
99. Kjelvik O, Bøe KE. Vanntildeling til avvent smågris. 2013. http://www.umb.no/statisk/husdyrforsoksmoter/2009/13.pdf. Accessed 19 Feb 2017.

11

Modified-live PRRSV subtype 1 vaccine UNISTRAIN® PRRS provides a partial clinical and virological protection upon challenge with East European subtype 3 PRRSV strain Lena

Caroline Bonckaert[1], Karen van der Meulen[1], Isaac Rodríguez-Ballarà[2], Rafael Pedrazuela Sanz[2], Mar Fenech Martinez[2] and Hans J. Nauwynck[1*]

Abstract

Background: Western European porcine reproductive and respiratory syndrome virus (PRRSV) strains cause limited and mild clinical signs whereas more virulent strains are circulating in Eastern Europe. The emergence of such highly virulent strains in Western Europe might result in severe clinical problems and a financial disaster. In this context, the efficacy of the commercial modified-live PRRSV subtype 1 vaccine UNISTRAIN® PRRS was tested upon challenge with the East European subtype 3 PRRSV strain Lena.

Results: The mean duration of fever was shortened and the number of fever days was significantly lower in vaccinated pigs than in control pigs. Moreover, a lower number of vaccinated animals showed fever, respiratory disorders and conjunctivitis. The mean virus titers in the nasal secretions post challenge (AUC) were significantly lower in the vaccinated group than in the control group. The duration of viremia was slightly shorter (not significantly different) in the vaccinated group as compared to the control group.

Conclusions: Vaccination of pigs with the modified-live vaccine UNISTRAIN® PRRS provides a partial clinical and virological protection against the PRRSV subtype 3 strain Lena.

Keywords: Modified-live, Protection, PRRSV, subtype 1, subtype 3 Lena, UNISTRAIN® PRRS, Vaccine

Background

Porcine Reproductive and Respiratory Syndrome (PRRS), originally designated Mystery Swine Disease, was first recognized in the United States in the late 1980s and is characterized by late abortion, stillbirth, weak piglets and mummies and is associated with the porcine respiratory disease complex [1]. In 1991, an arterivirus was identified as etiological agent and was scientifically called Porcine Reproductive and Respiratory Syndrome Virus (PRRSV) [2]. During two decades, the virus and its pathogenesis have been studied in-depth, which brought many new insights. There are two main genotypes: the European genotype (genotype 1) and the North American genotype (genotype 2). Three (potentially four) subtypes were already distinguished within the European PRRSV genotype 1 [3]. Subtype 1 is only present in the EU whereas in the Russian area all three (four) subtypes are circulating. After infection with subtype 1, limited clinical signs and respiratory disorders are observed in growing pigs [4, 5]. In contrast, subtypes 2 and 3 are more virulent and infection with subtype 3 strain Lena results in rapid onset of disease with high fever, severe dyspnea and tachypnea, periorbital oedema, depression and mortality [6, 7].

To prevent PRRS, several live-attenuated and inactivated vaccines against PRRSV are commercially available.

---

* Correspondence: hans.nauwynck@ugent.be
[1]Laboratory of Virology, Department of Virology, Parasitology and Immunology, Faculty of Veterinary Medicine, Ghent University, Salisburylaan 133, B-9820 Merelbeke, Belgium
Full list of author information is available at the end of the article

Attenuated vaccines significantly shorten the viremic phase post challenge [8], but there are concerns on reversion to virulence and the low level of protection upon challenge with heterologous PRRSV strains [9]. Commercial inactivated vaccines are safe, but are not providing a sufficient level of protection [8, 10]. Despite several attempts, no vaccine is providing full protection against the currently circulating PRRSV strains [11]. This might be explained by the low antigenic degree of similarity between the vaccine and challenge strain and the immune evasive character of the virus [12–14]. The co-existence of different subtypes in Europe emphasizes the need for cross-protective vaccines.

Until recently no information was available concerning the efficacy of PRRSV subtype 1 vaccines against PRRSV subtype 3 strains, such as Lena. Surprisingly, a commercially available attenuated subtype 1 vaccine, based on the DV strain, offered partial protection upon the East European strain [15]. This positive result led to the present study, where the clinical and virological protection of another commercially available attenuated subtype 1 vaccine, based on a Spanish PRRSV isolate, was evaluated upon infection with the virulent subtype 3 PRRSV strain Lena.

Results

Clinical signs after vaccination and challenge
After vaccination - No adverse local or systemic effects were observed upon vaccination.

After challenge - The effect of vaccination on body temperature upon challenge is presented in Fig. 1. Overall, a slight beneficial effect of vaccination was observed. In brief, the mean body temperature in control pigs was higher compared to vaccinated animals between 6 and 13 days post challenge (dpc), although the difference was not statistically significant. Also, the area under the curve (AUC) value of fever (with a threshold at 40.0 °C) was higher in the non-vaccinated group (11.7 ± 2.2) than in the vaccinated group (9.7 ± 1.4). A significant beneficial effect was observed for the number of fever days, i.e. the total number of days that an animal showed fever throughout the observation period (9.2 ± 2.9 days for control animals versus 5.2 ± 1.9 days for the vaccinated animals). Also, the number of animals that showed fever per day throughout the observation period was significantly lower in the vaccinated group. Mild respiratory disorders were observed from 2 dpc in non-vaccinated animals and from 5 dpc in vaccinated animals. All animals, except for one unvaccinated pig, showed respiratory signs at least at one time point during the observation period. Respiratory disorders lasted up till 3 weeks post challenge. Scores ranged from 1 to 6 in non-vaccinated animals and from 1 to 4 in vaccinated animals. No significant differences were observed in the mean respiratory score between both groups throughout the study. The AUC value was not significantly higher in the non-vaccinated group (16.1 ± 12.6) than in the vaccinated animals (9.0 ± 9.5). A significant beneficial effect was observed for the number of animals that showed

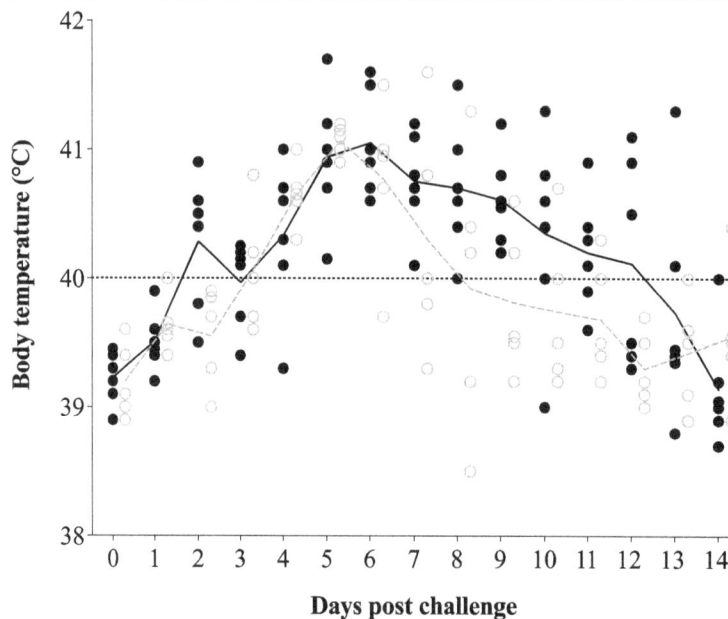

Fig. 1 Body temperature after challenge with PRRSV subtype 3 strain Lena. *Bullets* represent individual animals; *lines* represent the mean body temperature in each group. *Solid bullets* and *solid line* show the body temperature for the control group; *open bullets* and *dashed line* show the body temperature for the vaccinated group. *Dotted line* represents the threshold for fever (40.0 °C)

respiratory signs per day throughout the observation period. A slight reduction in liveliness was observed from 2 dpc in non-vaccinated animals and 5 dpc in vaccinated animals and lasted up till 3 weeks post challenge. All animals showed a reduced activity at least at two time points during the observation period and the reduction in liveliness was associated with the occurrence of fever. Discoloration of the ears was regularly observed in all control animals from 6 dpc up till the end of the experiment. In the vaccinated group, mild discoloration of the ears was observed in 4 out of 5 animals between 7 and 17 dpc. Clinical disorders of the eyes, such as conjunctivitis, were seen from 5 dpc in unvaccinated animals and from 6 dpc in vaccinated animals. All non-vaccinated animals showed mild conjunctivitis at least at two time points during the observation period. Only three out of five vaccinated animals showed mild conjunctivitis at least at one time point during the observation period. The AUC value was significantly higher in the non-vaccinated group (3.0 ± 1.7) than in vaccinated animals (0.6 ± 0.7). A significant beneficial effect was also observed for the number of days at which conjunctivitis was observed $(6.0 \pm 3.3$ days for control animals versus 1.2 ± 1.3 days for vaccinated animals). In general, all pigs showed a similar growth rate, independently of vaccination. Mean body weight in the non-vaccinated group at arrival, challenge and euthanasia was 8.1 ± 0.8 kg, 17.9 ± 3.4 kg and 28.8 ± 6.4 kg, respectively. At the same time points, body weight of the animals in the vaccinated group was 8.6 ± 1.0 kg, 15.4 ± 2.7 kg and 27.4 ± 3.9 kg, respectively. At necropsy (28 dpc), macroscopic lung lesions were found in 3/6 control pigs and in 2/5 vaccinated pigs. The total affected lung area in these pigs varied from 0.1 to 0.6 % (control group) and from 0.1 to 2.6 % (vaccinated group). The mean total affected lung area was not significantly different between the groups.

Serological response upon vaccination and challenge

At the time of arrival (-35 dpc), all pigs were serologically and virologically negative for PRRSV, as determined by immunoperoxidase monolayer assay (IPMA) and virus titration.

Figure 2 represents the evolution of the IPMA antibody titers during the course of the experiment in vaccinated and unvaccinated control pigs. All control pigs remained seronegative until challenge. The vaccinated pigs seroconverted within two weeks after vaccination with a titer of 3.2 ± 0.8 $\log_{10}$ at -7 dpc. After challenge, an increase in IPMA antibody titers was observed in all animals within two weeks. Figure 3 represents the evolution of the virus neutralizing (VN) antibody titers against PRRSV. In both vaccinated and control groups, VN antibodies against PRRSV LV were not detected before challenge. After challenge, VN antibodies against PRRSV Lena were only detected in one out of five vaccinated animals at very low titers (≤ 3 $\log_2$) at 21 dpc. A similar pattern in ELISA antibodies was observed as for IPMA antibodies.

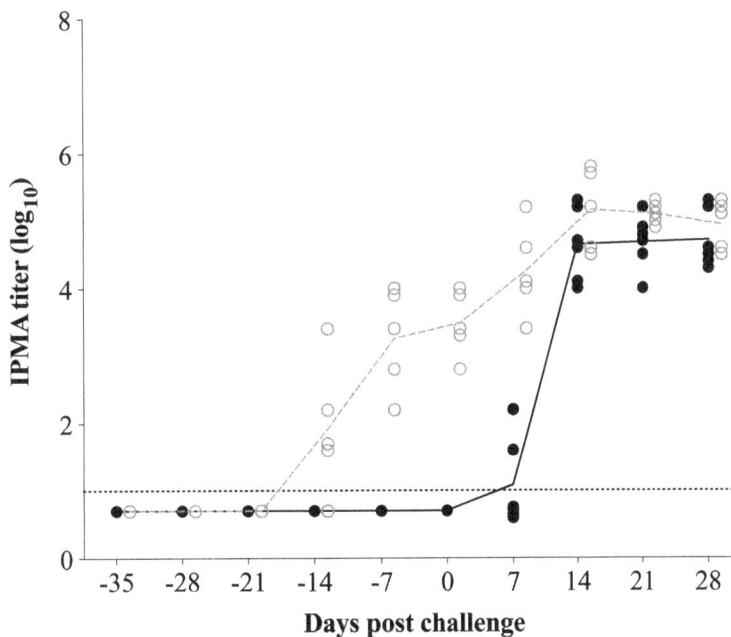

Fig. 2 IPMA antibody titers upon vaccination with PRRSV subtype 1 vaccine UNISTRAIN® PRRS and challenge with PRRSV subtype 3 strain Lena. *Bullets* represent individual animals; *lines* represent the mean titer in each group. *Solid bullets* and *solid line* show the titer for the control group; *open bullets* and *dashed line* show the titer for the vaccinated group. *Dotted line* represents the detection limit for the test

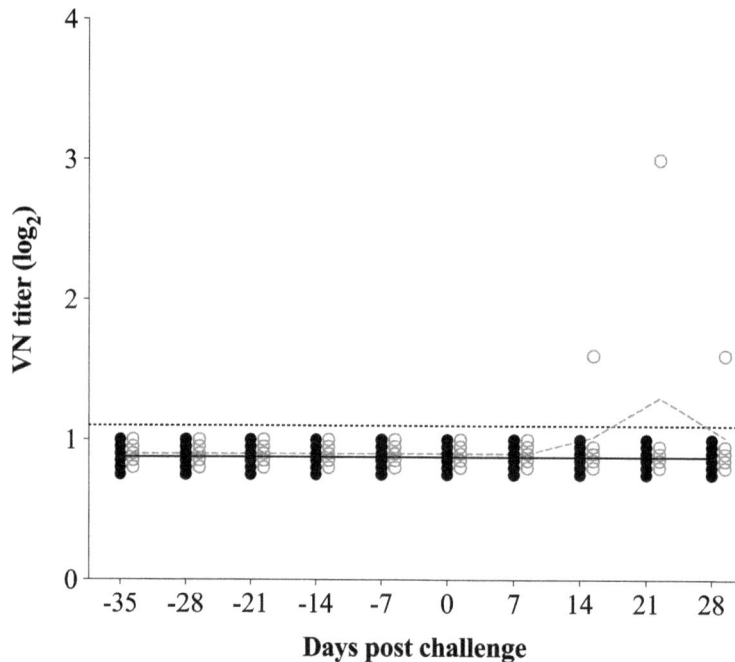

Fig. 3 VN antibody titers upon vaccination with PRRSV subtype 1 vaccine UNISTRAIN® PRRS and challenge with PRRSV subtype 3 strain Lena. *Bullets* represent individual animals; *lines* represent the mean titer in each group. *Solid bullets* and *solid line* show the titer for the control group; *open bullets* and *dashed line* show the titer for the vaccinated group. *Dotted line* represents the detection limit for the test

Protective effect of vaccination against viral shedding

Significant differences were found in viral shedding in nasal secretions. Viral shedding was observed from 3 dpc in both groups (Fig. 4). Titers peaked between 3 and 7 dpc in the control group and at 5 dpc in the vaccinated group. Peak mean titers were 5.6 ± 0.8 $\log_{10}$ tissue culture infectious dose with 50 % end point ($TCID_{50}$)/ 100 mg and 5.0 ± 0.3 $\log_{10}$ $TCID_{50}$/100 mg, respectively. In the control group, virus shedding was observed until at least 28 dpc (end of the experiment) with one out of six pigs still shedding virus (1.5 $\log_{10}$ $TCID_{50}$/100 mg). In the five vaccinated pigs, viral shedding was observed in all animals up till 10 dpc. After that, two animals shed virus up till 28 dpc. Significant differences in virus titers were found at 3, 7 and 10 dpc. Moreover, the AUC value of virus secretion was significantly lower in the vaccinated pigs (11.6 ± 3.5) than in the non-vaccinated pigs (18.4 ± 1.9).

Protective effect of vaccination against viremia

The results of virus titrations of sera (viremia) are shown in Fig. 5. Virus was present in sera of all animals from 3 dpc. A peak was observed at 10 dpc in the control group (4.2 ± 0.2 $\log_{10}$ $TCID_{50}$/ml) and at 5 dpc in the vaccinated group (4.7 ± 0.6 $\log_{10}$ $TCID_{50}$/ml). In the control group, viremia lasted until at least 28 dpc (end of the experiment) with two out of six piglets still being viremic, although at low titers (2.1 and 1.6 $\log_{10}$ $TCID_{50}$/ml). In

the vaccinated group, viremia lasted until 21 dpc. Despite the shorter duration of viremia, no significant differences were observed in the mean virus titer between control and vaccinated pigs. Also, no significant differences were seen for AUC values between both groups (15.4 ± 0.8 in control animals versus 15.9 ± 2.0 in vaccinated animals).

Discussion

Reproductive failure with early farrowing, late abortion, still- and weakborn piglets in sows and infertility in boars on the one hand and respiratory disorders in piglets on the other hand are hallmarks of PRRS. Depending on the strain genotype, host genotype and co-infections, divergent clinical signs can be observed in piglets. Pigs are well protected against a challenge or re-infection with a homologous strain after a natural infection [8, 12, 16, 17]. This can be mimicked using modified-live vaccines [18, 19]. However, after a heterologous challenge different levels of protection can be obtained [16, 18–20]. In general, animals are partially protected, both clinically and virologically. Labarque et al. found evidence that a genetic diversity within European strains of subtype 1 affects the efficacy of European vaccines and similar findings were described after natural exposure within the same subtype [12, 16]. In the present study, the efficacy of a vaccination with UNISTRAIN® PRRS (genotype 1, subtype 1) was

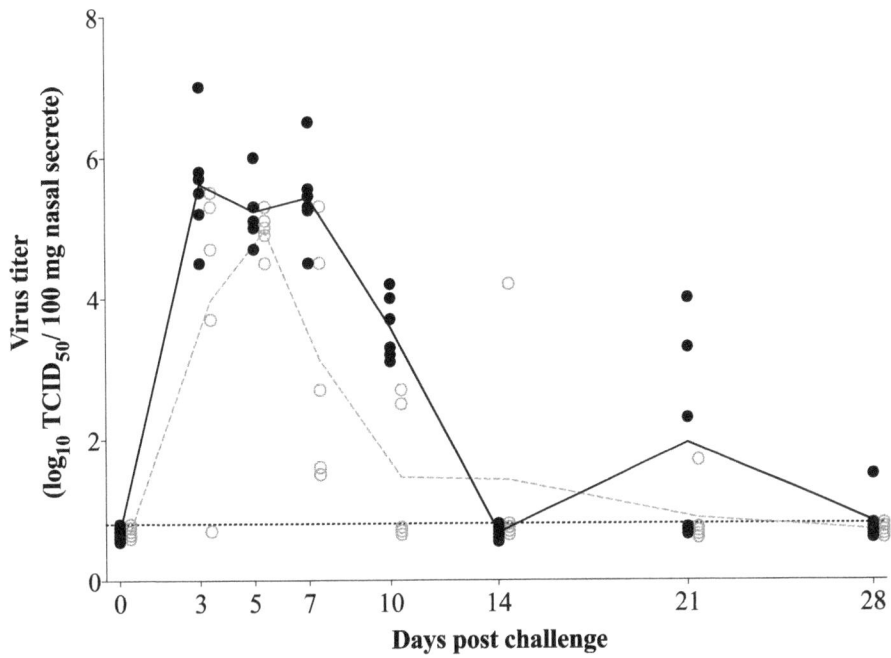

Fig. 4 Nasal viral shedding after challenge with PRRSV subtype 3 strain Lena. *Bullets* represent individual animals; *lines* represent the mean titer in each group. *Solid bullets* and *solid line* show the titer for the control group; *open bullets* and *dashed line* show the titer for the vaccinated group. *Dotted line* represents the detection limit for the test

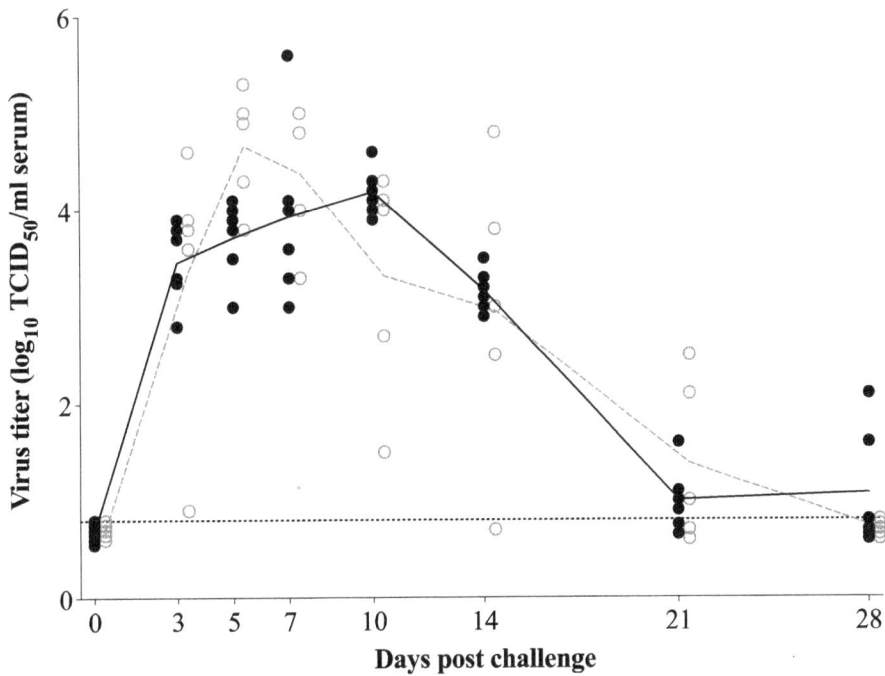

Fig. 5 Viremia after challenge with PRRSV subtype 3 strain Lena. *Bullets* represent individual animals; *lines* represent the mean titer in each group. *Solid bullets* and *solid line* show the titer for the control group; *open bullets* and *dashed line* show the titer for the vaccinated group. *Dotted line* represents the detection limit for the test

examined upon a challenge with PRRSV strain Lena (genotype 1, subtype 3). The mean duration of fever was shortened and the number of fever days was significantly reduced in vaccinated pigs compared to unvaccinated control pigs. Scores for respiratory and eye disorders were assigned to fewer vaccinated animals than to control pigs. Based on these results, the vaccine is considered to raise an immunity that gives a partial clinical protection against heterologous infection. In addition, the vaccination with UNISTRAIN° PRRS offers also a partial virological protection. Significant differences in mean nasal PRRSV titers were observed at 3, 7 and 10 dpc and titers were reduced with 1.64, 2.29 and 2.14 $\log_{10}$ TCID$_{50}$/100 mg, respectively. In addition, the total nasal viral shedding (AUC) upon challenge was significantly lowered with a factor 6.8. Similar findings concerning nasal secretion after vaccination with a commercially available live-attenuated vaccine based on the DV strain upon challenge with PRRSV Lena were recently described [15]. The high titers in nasal secretions in control animals might have influenced the process of viral shedding since transmission through viral shedding is considered to be an efficient way of re-infecting pen mates and is a measure of safety and efficacy of commercially available vaccines. In present study, a sudden drop in PRRSV-titer in nasal secretions is observed at 14 dpc in control animals, after which three control pigs secrete the virus at 21 dpc. In the vaccinated group, one piglet shed PRRSV again at 21 dpc. The ratio of 3 re-infected control pigs and 1 re-infected vaccinated piglet suggest the protective effect of vaccination, which is in agreement with previous studies [21, 22], although this experimental design did not allow us to determine the transmission ratio. Despite the positive outcome for nasal shedding, vaccination with UNISTRAIN° PRRS only slightly reduced the duration of viremia. In the study of Trus et al. [15], the viremia was significantly reduced upon challenge with PRRSV strain Lena in pigs vaccinated with a commercially available live-attenuated vaccine based on the DV strain. This difference in protection might be explained by different factors, such as age and breed of the pigs, interval between vaccination and challenge, vaccine and challenge virus titer and antigenic homology between the vaccine strain and challenge strain. Although the regions that are responsible for the induction of neutralizing antibodies and cellular immunity have been identified [23–28], there is no clear correlation between genetic homology and antigenic homology [12, 13, 15, 29]. Therefore, it is difficult to estimate the impact of slight genetic differences on the immunogenicity of the vaccine virus and the protection upon challenge (PRRSV strains DV and Lena have an identity of 88 % whereas VP-046 BIS and Lena have an 82.5 % identity (ORF5)). The different outcomes

between both studies cannot be related to the genetic background in our opinion, as the piglets came from the same farm [30, 31]. The major difference between both studies was the vaccination-challenge interval. In the studies described by Trus et al. [15], the interval was 6 and 8 weeks, which is two and four weeks longer than in the present experiment. After infection and vaccination with PRRSV, the immunity is slowly induced and it has been shown that protection six or eight weeks after vaccination is better than after four weeks [14].

The virus neutralizing (VN) antibodies have a crucial role in prevention of disease caused by Equine Arteritis Virus (EAV) in horses [32] and Lactate dehydrogenase-elevating virus (LDV) in mice [33]. Similarly, inhibition of the PRRSV replication can be achieved by VN antibodies [34]. However, neutralizing antibodies appear late after PRRSV infection [35] or vaccination with modified-live PRRSV vaccines [8, 36]. Thus, it is not surprisingly that in the present study no VN antibodies were detected during the four-week vaccination-challenge interval.

After a homologous challenge, the VN antibodies against the challenge virus are boosted [8, 15, 36, 37] in contrast with a genotypically heterologous challenge where no VN antibodies against the challenge virus are detected [38, 39]. After challenge with the subtype 3 strain Lena, VN antibodies against Lena were only detected in one UNISTRAIN° PRRS-vaccinated animal during 2 weeks. In a similar experiment using another PRRSV subtype 1 vaccine, based on the DV strain, the pigs developed VN antibodies against Lena 1-2 weeks after a PRRSV Lena challenge. In this latter study, the viremia was clearly more reduced compared to their non-vaccinated control group, which might be explained in part by the presence of the neutralizing antibodies. However, in the present study, the pig that developed VN antibodies against Lena did not show a shorter duration of viremia or nasal shedding. The role of VN antibodies in protection is therefore again disputable [40]. Certain branches of the cell-mediated immunity are most likely more important and can be assessed by measuring interferon gamma (IFN-γ) producing cells [41]. During this study, a test to determine the levels of the IFN-γ was not available in our laboratory and was therefore not assessed. We do agree that those results could have given an extra value and are implementing this technique in current studies.

Conclusions

The present study demonstrates that vaccination with the modified-live vaccine UNISTRAIN° PRRS provides a partial clinical and virological protection upon challenge with PRRSV Lena. Because only a partial clinical and virological protection has been obtained with currently commercially available subtype 1 PRRSV vaccines, there is a need to design vaccines that give a better protection against PRRSV Lena.

Methods

Experimental design

Eleven piglets were purchased from a PRRSV-negative farm immediately after weaning. Their negative PRRSV status was confirmed by serology (IPMA) and by virus titration of sera and nasal secretions that were collected upon arrival. They were acclimatized during seven days after which the animals were randomly assigned to two groups. One group ($n = 5$) was vaccinated intramuscularly with 2 ml of the commercially available live attenuated PRRSV subtype 1 vaccine (UNISTRAIN® PRRS, Laboratorios Hipra S.A.). Retitration revealed a titer of 6.8 $\log_{10}$ TCID$_{50}$ per ml. The second group was mock-vaccinated with phosphate buffered saline (PBS) ($n = 6$). At 4 weeks post vaccination, all pigs were intranasally inoculated with 2 ml of 5 $\log_{10}$ TCID$_{50}$ PRRS virus strain Lena (subtype 3) [6]. Blood was collected on a weekly base to monitor the serological status (IPMA and VN). To follow the course of viremia and nasal shedding upon challenge, blood and nasal swabs were collected on 0, 3, 5, 7, 10, 14, 21 and 28 dpc. At 4 weeks post challenge, the experiment was terminated by intravenous injection of an overdose of sodium pentobarbital (Natrium pentobarbital 20 %, Kela Laboratoria nv, Hoogstraten, Belgium).

Serology

Fixed PRRSV Lelystad virus (LV) respectively Lena infected Marc-145 cells in 96-well microtiter plates were used for the IPMA [4]. Serial twofold dilutions of the serum samples were added to the plates and incubated for 1 hour at 37 °C. After washing, secondary goat anti-swine IgG labeled with peroxidase were added for another hour at 37 °C. Plates were washed again and a substrate solution of 3-amino-9-ethylcarbazole (AEC) was added to each well, followed by incubation of the plates at room temperature for 20 minutes. The IPMA titer is the reciprocal of the highest dilution that gives a coloration of infected cells. VN antibodies were detected by SN assays in Marc-145 cells using PRRSV LV in sera collected before challenge and PRRSV Lena in sera collected after challenge. Twofold dilutions of serum samples were prepared and 100 μl of the appropriate PRRSV strain with a titer of 2 $\log_{10}$ TCID$_{50}$/50 μl was added. After mixing, the plates were incubated at 37 °C for 1 hour and 50 μl of the mixture was subsequently transferred to confluent monolayers of Marc-145 cells in 96-well microtiter plates. Cells were screened for 7 days after inoculation and the neutralization titer of the sera was recorded as the reciprocal of the highest dilution

that inhibited CPE in 50 % of the inoculated wells. Additionally, sample to positive ratios were determined using the CIVTEST SUIS PRRS E/S° ELISA (Laboratorios Hipra S.A.) with the aim to detect antibodies against European PRRSV isolates. The ELISA was performed according to the manufacturer's instructions.

Evaluation of clinical signs

Body weight was monitored for all pigs upon arrival (-35 dpc), at challenge (0 dpc) and at euthanasia (28 dpc). Local side effects as well as body temperature were recorded at 1, 2 and 3 days post vaccination (dpv). After challenge, the animals were monitored daily for the presence of clinical signs up till day 14 post challenge, with particular attention to PRRS related clinical signs. Clinical parameters included body temperature, respiratory symptoms, liveliness, discoloration of the ears, clinical symptoms at the eyes and presence of diarrhea. A score was assigned to the various parameters to allow an objective comparison between both groups. The scores were based on the methodology described by Karniychuk et al. [6] and Weesendorp et al. [7]. Lungs were collected and macroscopic lung lesions were given a score by visual observation and computer-assisted analysis. The percentage of lung surface affected by pneumonia was estimated by multiplying the lung lesion score per lobe with the relative proportion of this lobe in the entire lung [42].

Virus titrations

At 0, 3, 5, 7, 10, 14, 21 and 28 dpc, serum was tested virologically (titration) to follow the course of viremia. In addition, nasal secretions were collected with dry swabs (COPAN 160C°), 1 ml transport medium (phosphate buffered saline supplemented with antibiotics and fetal calf serum) was added and the swabs were vortexed and centrifuged. Supernatant was used for virus titration. In brief, porcine alveolar macrophages (PAM) were cultivated for 24 hours and inoculated with 10-fold dilutions of either serum or nasal secretion. After 72 hours, cells were fixed and virus-infected cells were subsequently evaluated by subsequent incubation with PRRSV-specific monoclonal antibodies against the nucleocapsid protein.

Ethics statement

The study was conducted in compliance with the provisions of Directive 86/609/EEC and KB 29/05/2013 and received approval number EC 2013/157.

Statistics

Data were analyzed with GraphPad Prism 6 software (GraphPad Software Inc., San Diego, CA, USA). All results shown represent mean ± standard deviation (S.D.)

or, for IPMA titers, geometric mean value ± S.D. Serological titers (IPMA and VN), as well as viral loads, were log-transformed prior to analysis. Gross pathology scores and area under the curve (AUC) were analyzed using the non-parametric Mann Whitney test. Duration was evaluated by the t-test. Statistical analysis of continuous data was performed using repeated-measures two-way analysis of variance (rANOVA), with Bonferroni's posttest. Results with P-values ≤ 0.05 were considered statistically significant.

Competing interests
This study was funded by Laboratorios Hipra, S.A., Spain. The authors declare that there is no conflict of interest.

Authors' contributions
BC participated in the study design, coordinated and carried out the experiment and drafted the manuscript. VDMK conceived the study and performed the statistical analysis. FMM participated actively during protocol design and publication revision. RBI and PSR reviewed the protocols and discussed the details of the agreement between the laboratory of virology and HIPRA. NHJ has been involved in discussions throughout the experiment and helped in writing this manuscript. All authors read and approved the final manuscript.

Acknowledgements
The authors wish to acknowledge Chantal Vanmaercke and Carine Boone for their excellent technical assistance and Loes Geypen for helping with the animal housing and handling.

Author details
[1]Laboratory of Virology, Department of Virology, Parasitology and Immunology, Faculty of Veterinary Medicine, Ghent University, Salisburylaan 133, B-9820 Merelbeke, Belgium. [2] Laboratorios Hipra S.A., Amer (Girona), Spain.

References
1. Tacker E.L. Porcine Respiratory Disease Complex. Proceeding, The 15th Congress of FAVA. Bangkok, Thailand: 2008.
2. Wensvoort G, Terpstra C, Pol JM, ter Laak EA, Bloemraad M, de Kluyver EP, et al. Mystery swine disease in The Netherlands: the isolation of Lelystad virus. Vet Q. 1991;13(3):121–30.
3. Stadejek T, Oleksiewicz MB, Scherbakov AV, Timina AM, Krabbe JS, Chabros K, et al. Definition of subtypes in the European genotype of porcine reproductive and respiratory syndrome virus: nucleocapsid characteristics and geographical distribution in Europe. Arch Virol. 2008;153(8):1479–88.
4. Labarque GG, Nauwynck HJ, Van Reeth K, Pensaert MB. Effect of cellular changes and onset of humoral immunity on the replication of porcine reproductive and respiratory syndrome virus in the lungs of pigs. J Gen Virol. 2000;81(Pt 5):1327–34.
5. Van Reeth K, Nauwynck H, Pensaert M. Dual infections of feeder pigs with porcine reproductive and respiratory syndrome virus followed by porcine respiratory coronavirus or swine influenza virus: a clinical and virological study. Vet Microbiol. 1996;48(3-4):325–35.
6. Karniychuk UU, Geldhof M, Vanhee M, Van Doorsselaere J, Saveleva TA, Nauwynck HJ. Pathogenesis and antigenic characterization of a new East European subtype 3 porcine reproductive and respiratory syndrome virus isolate. BMC Vet Res. 2010;6:30.
7. Weesendorp E, Morgan S, Stockhofe-Zurwieden N, Popma-De Graaf DJ, Graham SP, Rebel JM. Comparative analysis of immune responses following experimental infection of pigs with European porcine reproductive and respiratory syndrome virus strains of differing virulence. Vet Microbiol. 2013; 163(1-2):1–12.
8. Geldhof MF, Vanhee M, Van Breedam W, Van Doorsselaere J, Karniychuk UU, Nauwynck HJ. Comparison of the efficacy of autogenous inactivated

9. Porcine Reproductive and Respiratory Syndrome Virus (PRRSV) vaccines with that of commercial vaccines against homologous and heterologous challenges. BMC Vet Res. 2012;8:182.
9. Nielsen HS, Oleksiewicz MB, Forsberg R, Stadejek T, Botner A, Storgaard T. Reversion of a live porcine reproductive and respiratory syndrome virus vaccine investigated by parallel mutations. J Gen Virol. 2001;82(Pt 6):1263–72.
10. Nilubol D, Platt KB, Halbur PG, Torremorell M, Harris DL. The effect of a killed porcine reproductive and respiratory syndrome virus (PRRSV) vaccine treatment on virus shedding in previously PRRSV infected pigs. Vet Microbiol. 2004;102(1-2):11–8.
11. Diaz I, Gimeno M, Darwich L, Navarro N, Kuzemtseva L, Lopez S, et al. Characterization of homologous and heterologous adaptive immune responses in porcine reproductive and respiratory syndrome virus infection. Vet Res. 2012;43:30.
12. Labarque G, Reeth KV, Nauwynck H, Drexler C, Van Gucht S, Pensaert M. Impact of genetic diversity of European-type porcine reproductive and respiratory syndrome virus strains on vaccine efficacy. Vaccine. 2004;22(31-32):4183–90.
13. Mengeling WL, Lager KM, Vorwald AC, Clouser DF. Comparative safety and efficacy of attenuated single-strain and multi-strain vaccines for porcine reproductive and respiratory syndrome. Veterinary Microbiology. 2003;93(1):25–38.
14. Nauwynck HJ, Van Gorp H, Vanhee M, Karniychuk U, Geldhof M, Cao A, et al. Micro-dissecting the pathogenesis and immune response of PRRSV infection paves the way for more efficient PRRSV vaccines. Transbound Emerg Dis. 2012;59 Suppl 1:50–4.
15. Trus I, Bonckaert C, van der Meulen K, Nauwynck HJ. Efficacy of an attenuated European subtype 1 porcine reproductive and respiratory syndrome virus (PRRSV) vaccine in pigs upon challenge with the East European subtype 3 PRRSV strain Lena. Vaccine. 2014;32(25):2995–3003.
16. Martelli P, Gozio S, Ferrari L, Rosina S, De Angelis E, Quintavalla C, et al. Efficacy of a modified live porcine reproductive and respiratory syndrome virus (PRRSV) vaccine in pigs naturally exposed to a heterologous European (Italian cluster) field strain: Clinical protection and cell-mediated immunity. Vaccine. 2009;27(28):3788–99.
17. Lager KM, Mengeling WL, Brockmeier SL. Homologous challenge of porcine reproductive and respiratory syndrome virus immunity in pregnant swine. Vet Microbiol. 1997;58(2-4):113–25.
18. Hesse, R.A., Couture, L.P., Lau, M.L., Dimmick, B.S., Ellsworth, S.R.. Efficacy of Prime Pac PRRS in controlling PRRS reproductive disease: homologous challenge. In: Proceedings of the 27th Annual Meeting of the American Association of Swine Practitioners (1996) Nashville, TN, USA, pp. 103–105
19. Gorcyca, D.E., Schlesinger, K.J., Chladek, D.C., Morrison, R., Wensvoort, G., Dee, S., Polson, D. A summary of experimental and field studies evaluating the safety and efficacy of RespPRRS/ReproTM for the control of PRRS-induced reproductive disease. In: Proceedings of the 28th Annual Meeting of the American Association of Swine Practitioners, QueÅLbec, Canada (1997), pp. 203–214
20. Lager KM, Mengeling WL, Brockmeier SL. Evaluation of protective immunity in gilts inoculated with the NADC-8 isolate of porcine reproductive and respiratory syndrome virus (PRRSV) and challenge-exposed with an antigenically distinct PRRSV isolate. Am J Vet Res. 1999;60(8):1022–7.
21. Pileri E, Gibert E, Soldevila F, García-Saenz A, Pujols J, Diaz I, et al. Vaccination with a genotype 1 modified live vaccine against porcine reproductive and respiratory syndrome virus significantly reduces viremia, viral shedding and transmission of the virus in a quasi-natural experimental model. Vet Microbiol. 2015;175(1):7–16.
22. Rose N, Renson P, Andraud M, Paboeuf F, Le Potier MF, Bourry O. Porcine reproductive and respiratory syndrome virus (PRRSv) modified-live vaccine reduces virus transmission in experimental conditions. Vaccine. 2015;33(21): 2493–9.
23. Vanhee M, Costers S, Van Breedam W, Geldhof MF, Van Doorsselaere J, Nauwynck HJ. A variable region in GP4 of European-type porcine reproductive and respiratory syndrome virus induces neutralizing antibodies against homologous but not heterologous virus strains. Viral Immunol. 2010;23(4):403–13.
24. Oleksiewicz MB, Bøtner A, Toft P, Normann P, Storgaard T. Epitope mapping porcine reproductive and respiratory syndrome virus by phage display: the nsp2 fragment of the replicase polyprotein contains a cluster of B-cell epitopes. J Virol. 2001;75(7):3277–90.
25. Burgara-Estrella A, Díaz I, Rodríguez-Gómez IM, Essler SE, Hernández J, Mateu E. Predicted peptides from non-structural proteins of porcine

reproductive and respiratory syndrome virus are able to induce IFN-γ and IL-10. Viruses. 2013;5(2):663–77.

26. Díaz I, Pujols J, Ganges L, Gimeno M, Darwich L, Domingo M, et al. In silico prediction and ex vivo evaluation of potential T-cell epitopes in glycoproteins 4 and 5 and nucleocapsid protein of genotype-I (European) of porcine reproductive and respiratory syndrome virus. Vaccine. 2009;27(41):5603–11.

27. Parida R, Choi IS, Peterson DA, Pattnaik AK, Laegreid W, Zuckermann FA, et al. Location of T-cell epitopes in nonstructural proteins 9 and 10 of type-II porcine reproductive and respiratory syndrome virus. Virus Res. 2012;169(1):13–21.

28. Vanhee M, Van Breedam W, Costers S, Geldhof M, Noppe Y, Nauwynck H. Characterization of antigenic regions in the porcine reproductive and respiratory syndrome virus by the use of peptide-specific serum antibodies. Vaccine. 2011;29(29-30):4794–804.

29. Murtaugh M. Use and interpretation of sequencing in PRRSV control programs. In: Proceedings of the Allen D. Leman Swine Conference (2012), p. 49–55, 39.

30. Boddicker NJ, Garrick DJ, Rowland RR, Lunney JK, Reecy JM, Dekkers JC. Validation and further characterization of a major quantitative trait locus associated with host response to experimental infection with porcine reproductive and respiratory syndrome virus. Anim Genet. 2014;45(1):48–58.

31. Abella G, Pena RN, Nogareda C, Armengol R, Vidal A, Moradell L, et al. A WUR SNP is associated with European Porcine Reproductive and Respiratory Virus Syndrome resistance and growth performance in pigs. Res Vet Sci. 2016;104:117–22.

32. Hammond SA, Cook SJ, Lichtenstein DL, Issel CJ, Montelaro RC. Maturation of the cellular and humoral immune responses to persistent infection in horses by equine infectious anemia virus is a complex and lengthy process. J Virol. 1997;71(5):3840–52.

33. Chen Z, Li K, Rowland RR, Plagemann PG. Selective antibody neutralization prevents neuropathogenic lactate dehydrogenase-elevating virus from causing paralytic disease in immunocompetent mice. J Neurovirol. 1999;5(2):200–8.

34. Vanhee M, Delputte PL, Delrue I, Geldhof MF, Nauwynck HJ. Development of an experimental inactivated PRRSV vaccine that induces virus-neutralizing antibodies. Vet Res. 2009;40(6):63.

35. Yoon KJ, Zimmerman JJ, Swenson SL, Mcginley MJ, Eernisse KA, Brevik A, et al. Characterization of the Humoral Immune-Response to Porcine Reproductive and Respiratory Syndrome (Prrs) Virus-Infection. J Vet Diagn Invest. 1995;7(3):305–12.

36. Diaz I, Gimeno M, Callen A, Pujols J, Lopez S, Charreyre C, et al. Comparison of different vaccination schedules for sustaining the immune response against porcine reproductive and respiratory syndrome virus. Vet J. 2013; 197(2):438–44.

37. Osorio FA, Zuckermann F, Wills R, Meier W, Christian S, Galeota J, Doster A. PRRSV: comparison of commercial vaccines in their ability to induce protection against current PRRSV strains of high virulence. Allen D. Leman Swine Conf. Minnesota, USA: 1998;25:176-182.

38. Roca M, Gimeno M, Bruguera S, Segales J, Diaz I, Galindo-Cardiel IJ, et al. Effects of challenge with a virulent genotype II strain of porcine reproductive and respiratory syndrome virus on piglets vaccinated with an attenuated genotype I strain vaccine. Vet J. 2012;193(1):92–6.

39. Park C, Choi K, Jeong J, Chae C. Cross-protection of a new type 2 porcine reproductive and respiratory syndrome virus (PRRSV) modified live vaccine (Fostera PRRS) against heterologous type 1 PRRSV challenge in growing pigs. Vet Microbiol. 2015;177(1-2):87–94.

40. Lopez OJ, Osorio FA. Role of neutralizing antibodies in PRRSV protective immunity. Vet Immunol Immunopathol. 2004;102(3):155–63.

41. Zuckermann FA, Garcia EA, Luque ID, Christopher-Hennings J, Doster A, Brito M, et al. Assessment of the efficacy of commercial porcine reproductive and respiratory syndrome virus (PRRSV) vaccines based on measurement of serologic response, frequency of gamma-IFN-producing cells and virological parameters of protection upon challenge. Vet Microbiol. 2007;123(1-3):69–85.

42. Halbur PG, Paul PS, Frey ML, Landgraf J, Eernisse K, Meng XJ, et al. Comparison of the Pathogenicity of 2 Us Porcine Reproductive and Respiratory Syndrome Virus Isolates with That of the Lelystad Virus. Veterinary Pathology. 1995;32(6):648–60.

12

Viral and bacterial investigations on the aetiology of recurrent pig neonatal diarrhoea cases

Susana Mesonero-Escuredo[1], Katrin Strutzberg-Minder[2], Carlos Casanovas[1] and Joaquim Segalés[3,4*] (iD)

Abstract

Background: Neonatal diarrhoea represents a major disease problem in the early stages of animal production, increasing significantly pre-weaning mortality and piglets weaned below the target weight. Enteric diseases in newborn piglets are often of endemic presentation, but may also occur as outbreaks with high morbidity and mortality. The objective of this study was to assess the frequency of different pathogens involved in cases of recurrent neonatal diarrhoea in Spain.

Results: A total of 327 litters from 109 sow farms located in Spain with neonatal recurrent diarrhoea were sampled to establish a differential diagnosis against the main enteric pathogens in piglets. In total, 105 out of 109 (96.3%) case submissions were positive to one of the examined enteric organisms considered potentially pathogenic (*Escherichia coli*, *Clostridium perfringens* types A and C, *Transmissible gastroenteritis virus* [TGEV], *Porcine epidemic diarrhoea virus* [PEDV] or *Rotavirus A* [RVA]). Fifty-eight out of 109 (53.2%) submissions were positive for only one of these pathogens, 47 out of 109 (43.1%) were positive for more than one pathogen and, finally, 4 out of 109 (3.7%) were negative for all these agents. *Escherichia coli* strains were isolated from all submissions tested, but only 11 of them were classified into defined pathotypes. *Clostridium perfringens* type A was detected in 98 submissions (89.9%) and no *C. perfringens* type C was found. Regarding viruses, 47 (43.1%) submissions were positive for RVA, 4 (3.7%) for PEDV and none of them for TGEV.

Conclusion: In conclusion, *C. perfringens* type A, *E. coli* and RVA were the main pathogens found in faeces of neonatal diarrheic piglets in Spain.

Keywords: Neonatal diarrhoea, Spain, Frequency, *C. perfringens*, *E. coli*, Rotavirus, Coronavirus

Background

Neonatal diarrhoea is one of the most frequent clinical signs in young piglets, increasing significantly pre-weaning mortality and the number of piglets weaned below the target weight [1]. Enteric diseases in newborn piglets are often endemic, but may also occur as outbreaks with high morbidity and mortality [2, 3]. Although the latter ones have a major economic impact in the short-term, the economic consequences of endemic and recurrent neonatal diarrhoea can also be substantial. In studies conducted in Sweden and Denmark, diarrhoea was estimated to account for 5–24% of the overall pre-weaning mortality [4] and for a reduction in average daily gain (ADG) by 8–14 g/day in the first week of life [5, 6]. Based on these production losses, the cost of neonatal diarrhoea was recently estimated to be 134 € per sow per year in affected herds [7].

Diarrhoea can be described as faeces with excess of water in relation to faecal dry matter [8]. Clinical signs and impact of enteric diseases in newborn piglets vary depending on the infectious agent/s involved, as well as the susceptibility of piglets to infection [9]. Regardless of the cause, a rapid loss of water, electrolytes and nutrients do occur. Given the limited body reserves of the newborn piglet, this situation quickly leads to a deleterious condition of the piglet that may die in a matter of hours.

* Correspondence: joaquim.segales@irta.cat
[3]Departament de Sanitat i Anatomia Animals, Universitat Autònoma de Barcelona (UAB), 08193 Bellaterra, Barcelona, Spain
[4]UAB, Centre de Recerca en Sanitat Animal (CReSA, IRTA-UAB), Campus de la Universitat Autònoma de Barcelona, 08193 Bellaterra, Barcelona, Spain
Full list of author information is available at the end of the article

Therefore, acute diarrhoea in the newborn pig should always receive immediate attention [10].

Diarrhoea is a clinical sign and its treatment depends on the nature of the cause; therefore, a definitive diagnosis is required to take the proper control approach. Once management problems are solved, the most common causes of enteric problems are infections by one or more pathogens or changes in the microbiota [9]. The differential diagnosis includes viruses, bacteria and parasites. Among infectious causes of neonatal diarrhoea (first week of age), both bacteria and viruses may play a significant role, not only by separate but also in co-infection [9, 11].

The most widespread viral infection causing diarrhoea in neonatal swine is *Rotavirus type A* (RVA), although types B and C are also linked to enteric diseases as well [12–14]. RVA is often detected as the sole infectious agent, but the majority of studies are based on qualitative detection of RVA without histologic verification; this fact implies that the causative significance of this virus is often unknown. *Transmissible gastroenteritis* (TGE) *virus* (TGEV) and *Porcine epidemic diarrhoea* (PED) *virus* (PEDV) can also cause diarrhoea in piglets [15]. TGEV is a cause of disease in most pig-producing areas of the world [16], but the clinical impact of TGEV in Europe is low since 1980s–90s due to the extensive spread of the closely related *Porcine respiratory coronavirus* (PCRV), which resulted in immunological cross-protection [16]. PEDV was recognized for the first time in Europe during the seventies, but a major concern reappeared in the European swine production in 2014 when the virus was detected in several countries causing high piglet mortality and significant economic losses [17]. Outbreaks of PED in suckling piglets are clinically indistinguishable from outbreaks of TGE [18].

A number of bacteria are related to neonatal diarrhoea in piglets. *Escherichia coli* is probably the most important one, responsible for a range of different diseases in both man and animals [19]. The main pathotype of *E. coli* responsible for intestinal disease in pigs is enterotoxigenic *E. coli* (ETEC) [20]. However, there are other *E. coli* pathotypes also linked with piglet disease, such as enteropathogenic *E. coli* (EPEC) and those known as attaching-and-effacing (A/E) *E. coli* [21]. *Clostridium perfringens* is another important diarrhoeagenic pathogen, which is classified into five groups (A to E) based on the production of the major toxin types alpha, beta, epsilon and iota [22]. *C. perfringens* type C produces α- and β-toxin and can cause high mortality rates in newborns [23]. *C. perfringens* type A produces α-toxin and ß2-toxin; besides being considered a cause of neonatal diarrhoea, it is also considered part of the normal intestinal microbiota of piglets [24].

The objective of the present work was to investigate the presence of viral (RVA, TGEV and PEDV) and bacterial (different *E. coli* pathotypes, and *C. perfringens* types A and C) pathogens associated to cases of recurrent neonatal diarrhoea in Spain.

Methods

Case selection

A total of 327 litters from 109 sow farms located in Spain that experienced neonatal recurrent diarrhoea were sampled to establish a differential diagnosis against enteric pathogens in piglets. Therefore, a convenience sampling was designed; the inclusion criterion for all veterinarians submitting samples was the presence of diarrhoea during the first week of age in a repeated fashion through different batches.

Five piglets per litter from three litters with diarrhoea were sampled in each studied farm. Selected piglets were not treated with antibiotics and their faeces were collected individually and pooled subsequently in a plastic tube (total of 3 pools per farm, one per each litter). A swab in Amies medium was taken from each plastic tube, which was previously hand-shaken. Both samples, swab and plastic tube, were sent to IVD Innovative Veterinary Diagnostics (IVD) Laboratory (Germany) to check for several enteric pathogens causing neonatal diarrhoea. The shipment was sent by plane, with a delivery in 24 h and using a cool pack in the box during the transportation.

Bacteriological isolation

Faeces from the swab were streaked out on blood agar (Columbia agar with sheep blood; Oxoid: PB5008A) and Gassner agar (Oxoid: PO5021A) for the isolation of *Escherichia coli*. Inoculated plates were incubated aerobically at 37 °C for 24 h. Suspected *E. coli* isolated colonies were confirmed by morphological characteristics; in addition, blue colonies (lactose-positive) on Gassner agar were further confirmed by negative oxidase testing. Haemolysin presence was identified by haemolysis on blood agar.

For the isolation of *C. perfringens*, faeces from the swab were streaked out on plates containing Schaedler agar with sheep blood (Oxoid: PB5034A) and incubated anaerobically (AnaeroGen, Oxoid: AN0035A) at 37 °C for 24 to 48 h. *C. perfringens* was identified because of the double-zoned haemolysis, typical colony morphology and butyric acid smell. Suspected isolated colonies were further confirmed by PCR genotyping using the species-specific cpa-gene coding for the α-toxin.

Escherichia coli Genotyping

E. coli species were characterized by the detection of the *E. coli* species-specific glyceraldehyde phosphate dehydrogenase gene gapA [25], which was the internal amplification and positive control in the multiplex PCR used for genotyping. For genotyping purposes, a single *E. coli* colony from a pure agar culture was selected and suspended in 150 µL lysis buffer (10 mM Tris-HCl (pH 8.0), 0.05% Tween 20, 240 µg/mL Proteinase K with 0.5% Triton X-100, and then incubated for 60 min at 60 °C. Subsequently, the suspension was heated at 97 °C for 15 min and the lysate was cooled at room temperature. A total of 1.5 µL of this lysate were used as a template for genotyping PCR methods. Virulence associated genes listed in Table 1 were investigated for *E. coli* isolates by multiplex PCRs [26]. Pathotypes were defined following the combination of detected genes [21].

Clostridium perfringens Immunoblotting and genotyping
For the immunoblotting, 5 colonies were suspended in 5 mL TYCG-medium plus TYCG-supplement (liquid media for *Clostridium* spp.) and incubated 6 to 8 h at 37 °C under anaerobic conditions; 1 mL was centrifuged at 11.000 x g for 5 min. The supernatant was used to detect α-, β- and β2-toxins by immunoblotting [27]; α and β toxin presence was defined by positive or negative, and only β2 production was semi quantitatively recorded (strongly positive, positive, weakly positive and negative)

Table 1 Target genes of *Escherichia coli* virulence factors detected by multiplex PCRs

Bacterial components or products	Target genes	Virulence factors
Fimbriae	*faeG (F4)*	F4 fimbriae
	fanC (F5)	F5 fimbriae
	fasA (F6)	F6 fimbriae
	fedA (F18)	F18 fimbriae
	fim41A (F41)	F41 fimbriae
	fimH (F1)	type 1 fimbriae
	fimA (F1)	type 1 fimbriae
Adhesins	*papC*	P fimbriae
	aidA (AIDA)	AIDA-I autotransporter adhesin
	paa	porcine attaching-effacing associated protein
	eaeA (intimin)	intimin
Toxins	*eltB (LTI)*	heat-sensitive enterotoxin
	estA (STI)	heat-resistant enterotoxin
	estB (STII)	heat-resistant enterotoxin
	astA (EAST)	heat-resistant enterotoxin
	stx2e	Shiga toxin variant 2e
	cdtB	cytolethal distending toxin
	cnf1	cytotoxic necrotizing factor type 1
Others	*iucD*	aerobactin siderophore
	escV	type III secretion system
	pic	serin protease autotransporter

[28]. For genotyping purposes, a single colony from a pure agar culture was selected and suspended in 150 µL lysis buffer, incubated for 90 min at 60 °C and then heated at 97 °C for 15 min. Lysate cooled at room temperature and genotyping (cpa, cpb, and cpb2 genes) was performed following a previously published method [28].

Virological analyses
Nucleic acid was extracted from faecal samples using an RNA-DNA isolation kit (MagMAX Pathogen RNA/DNA Kit; Life Technologies GmbH, Darmstadt, Germany). Briefly, 0.5 g of faeces was suspended in 1 mL PBS and vortexed vigorously for 3 min, until the solution was fully suspended. For a separation of phases, it was centrifuged at 100 x g for 3 to 5 s. A total of 200 µL of the solution was transferred to a tube with 500 µL prepared lysis/binding solution of the RNA-DNA isolation kit. It was vortexed vigorously for 5 min and then centrifuged at 16.000 x g for 3 min to clarify the lysate. Nucleic acid isolation was performed with an automated nucleic acid isolation processor (MagMAX™ Express-96 Magnetic Particle Processor; Life Technologies GmbH) based on magnetic bead technology, according the manufacturer's protocol and instructions. Extracted nucleic acid was analysed by PCR methodologies.

RVA RNA was detected by a previously described real-time RT-PCR [29]. PEDV and TGEV were detected by a real-time multiplex RT-PCR for the simultaneously detection of both viruses, following manufacturer recommendations (virotype PEDV/TGEV RT-PCR Kit, Qiagen, Denmark).

Results
Globally, 105 out of 109 (96.3%) herds were positive to at least one of the examined enteric pathogens (pathogenic *E. coli*, *C. perfringens* types A and C, TGEV, PEDV or RVA). Fifty-eight out of 109 (53.2%) submissions were positive for only one of these pathogens, 47 out of 109 (43.1%) were positive for more than one pathogen and, finally, 4 out of 109 (3.7%) were negative for all these agents.

E. coli strains were isolated from all submissions tested. However, only 11 of them were classified into defined pathotypes (ETEC and EPEC). Specifically, 9 isolates were classified as ETEC and 2 as EPEC (Table 2). Within ETEC isolates, 7 different virulence factor profiles were found; among ETEC strains, the most frequently detected virulence factors were STII (7 isolates), STI (7 isolates) and F4 (5 isolates). Both EPEC strains showed the same combination of virulence factors, Intimin and escV.

C. perfringens type A was isolated from 98 submissions (89.9%), which were all of them cpa positive by PCR. No isolation of *C. perfringens* type C was found, and all submissions resulted negative to cpb gene detection by

Table 2 Patothypes of the 11 *E. coli* strains isolated in the present study and their combinations of virulence factors detected by PCR

Pathotype	Combination of virulence factors	Number of isolates
ETEC	F4, STI, STII	2
	AIDA, STII	2
	F4, LTI, STI, STII	1
	F5, intimin, STI	1
	F18, paa, STI, STII	1
	F4, AIDA, LTI, STI, STII	1
	F4, LTI, STI	1
EPEC	Intimin, escV	2

ETEC enterotoxigenic, *E. coli* EPEC enteropathogenic *E. coli*

PCR. The cpb2 toxin gene was found in 95 out of 98 (96.9%) *C. perfringens* type A isolates. By immunoblotting of these 95 strains, 20 isolates were β2 toxin strongly positive, 51 positive, 17 weakly positive and 7 negative. The result of production of α toxin by immunoblotting was positive in 34 isolates.

Regarding viruses, 47 out of 109 (43.1%) submissions were positive for RVA, 4 (3.7%) for PEDV and none of them for TGEV.

Table 3 summarizes all combinations of pathogens found in the studied diarrhoea cases. Noteworthy, pathogenic *E. coli* were only found in combination with other pathogens, and the maximum number of pathogens found in one submission was four (ETEC, *C. perfringens* type A, RVA and PEDV).

Discussion

The emergence of the modern pig production, with more intensified farming, has been paralleled with an increase of neonatal piglet diarrhoea prevalence [20]. Neonatal enteric problems in a herd are usually the result from the interaction of multiple factors that need to

Table 3 Combinations of different pathogens found in neonatal cases of diarrhoea in Spain

Combination of pathogens	Number of cases (percentage)
RVA and *C. perfringens* type A	34 (31.2%)
ETEC, RVA and *C. perfringens* type A	4 (3.7%)
PEDV and *C. perfringens* type A	2 (1.8%)
ETEC and *C. perfringens* type A	3 (2.7%)
ETEC, RVA, *C. perfringens* type A and PEDV	1 (0.92%)
ETEC, *C. perfringens* type A and PEDV	1 (0.92%)
EPEC, RVA and *C. perfringens* type A	1 (0.92%)
EPEC and *C. perfringens* type A	1 (0.92%)
Total	47 (43.1%)

PEDV Porcine epidemic diarrhoea virus, *RVA* Rotavirus type A, ETEC enterotoxigenic *E. coli*, EPEC enteropathogenic *E. coli*

be examined to find rational means for intervention. Major determinants for the manifestation of neonatal diarrhoea include factors such as passive immunity transferred by colostrum and milk [30], environmental temperature [31] and humidity [21], management [32] and infection pressure by specific pathogens of the herd [32]. The present study focused on different enteric pathogens able to cause neonatal diarrhoea in piglets in an important European pig producing country such as Spain, with specific focus on frequency of infections and co-infections. It was not possible, however, to address the specific role of other non-tested pathogens as well as non-infectious factors in the studied cases.

Both viral and/or bacterial pathogens were found in 96% of the submissions, which represents a fairly high number of cases with at least one infectious agent present. *C. perfringens* type A is considered rather an ubiquitous bacteria in the pig intestinal tract [24]. Therefore, it is difficult to predict if it acted as primary pathogen or its multiplication was triggered by other infectious or non-infectious factors. In consequence, it was not possible to assess in which number of submissions the primary cause was a pathogen. Noteworthy, infectious diarrhoea in newborn piglets is usually related to the presence of a single pathogen and mixed infections are considered less common [33]. However, almost half of the cases (43.1%) of the present study corresponded to mixed infections, with *C. perfringens* type A being present in all these cases.

Regarding viruses, RVA was the most frequently detected agent. Rotavirus is among the most prevalent pathogens in cases of neonatal diarrhoea, and is often detected as the sole infectious agent [34]. In fact, several recent studies have described such high prevalence in pigs in Europe and North America [13; 14]. In contrast, only 4 submissions were positive to PEDV. After the 1980s, problems with PEDV in Europe declined and disease outbreaks have been occasionally seen during the last decades [17]. In 2013, PEDV was introduced for the first time on the American continent and resulted in severe outbreaks of disease in the naïve population [17]. Recently, PEDV isolates similar to the S-INDEL variants described in America have also been detected in Europe [35, 36]. Regarding the occurrence of PED in 2014–2015 recorded by the European Food Safety Authority (EFSA) Network, countries voluntarily reported 245 cases of pig herds meeting the PED case definition and 71 pig herds with RT-PCR confirmation of PEDV-genome; such PEDV-confirmed cases were found in Austria, Belgium, Spain, France, Italy, the Netherlands and Germany (EFSA, 2015). As expected, TGEV was not found in any of the submissions. TGEV is a cause of disease in most pig-producing areas of the world [16]. However, outbreaks of TGE in Europe are rare, probably due to immunological cross-protection induced by PRCV, which is apparently ubiquitous in the continent [16].

ETEC has commonly been incriminated as the main aetiological agent of neonatal diarrhoea [37], although a recent survey conducted in Canada has suggested that the clinical importance of neonatal *E. coli* enteric problems have decreased during recent years [34]. Pathogenic pathotypes of *E. coli* were found only in 10% of the submissions in the present study which may reflect such a decrease in prevalence. Anyway, it is known that the major pathotype of *E. coli* responsible for intestinal disease in pigs is ETEC [20] and these data fit with the results of the current work, since 9 out of 11 *E. coli* pathotypes were ETEC (with major virulence factors being STII and STI toxins and F4 fimbriae). Curiously, two of the *E. coli* isolates consisted of EPEC strains, which are usually related with post-weaning diarrhoea [21]. However, EPEC isolates from neonatal diarrhoea have been already described [38, 39]. In contrast, all tested submissions yielded non-pathogenic *E. coli* strains, which is in line with other published works. In a Danish study on neonatal diarrhoea in four commercial swine herds, non-haemolytic *E. coli* were the most predominant isolate obtained after aerobic culturing of both diarrhoeic and non-diarrhoeic piglets [40]. This was also the case in a similar Swedish study on neonatal diarrhoea, where non-haemolytic *E. coli* was found in all piglets [41]. The prevalence of classical porcine ETEC in both Scandinavian studies was very low in diarrhoeic piglets (less than 3%). This fact can be associated to modern swine production, in which pre-farrowing vaccination of sows against *E. coli* fimbriae antigens (F4, F5 and F6) is common.

C. perfringens type A was found in most of the submissions (89.9%), with detection of the cpb2 gene by PCR in the majority of cases. Moreover, in 88 cases such results were reinforced with the production in vitro of the β2 toxin by immunoblotting. This result fits well with a recent report from Poland [42], who found a 91.4% prevalence of *C. perfringens* type A at herd level. Such a high rate of detection raises the question of this bacterium as a true cause of diarrhoea or part of the microbiota, which may be up-regulated in enteric disease scenarios. In fact, the impact of α and β2 toxins on disease pathogenesis has not been conclusively answered [43]. In contrast, *C. perfringens* type C was not detected in any of the samples. This bacterium causes disease in piglets in many areas of the world, but in a global perspective, it is considered much less important than other enteric pathogens [22]. In the same Polish survey, for example, they found a 1.4% herd prevalence of this bacterium [42]. Probably, during recent years, *C. perfringens* type C infections are rare in cases of neonatal diarrhoea due to sow vaccination [34]. Indeed, in Spain, routine vaccination of sows pre-farrowing with beta toxoid vaccines is usual.

Conclusions

In summary, the present study shows that RVA, ETEC and *C. perfringens* type A are the main pathogens involved in persistent neonatal diarrhoea in Spain. In almost half of the cases, more than one enteric pathogen was found. Noteworthy, pathogenic *E. coli* was only found in combination with other pathogens, and the maximum number of pathogens found in one submission, occurring once, was four.

Acknowledgements
The authors wish to thank all swine veterinarians who submitted samples for the study. Susana Mesonero-Escuredo is a resident of the European College of Porcine Health Management (ECPHM). The funding from CERCA Programme (*Generalitat de Catalunya*) to IRTA is also acknowledged.

Funding
Not applicable.

Authors' contributions
SME and CC designed the study protocol. KSM performed the laboratory analyses. SME and JS analysed the results and drafted the manuscript; CC and KSM critically revised the manuscript. All authors read and approved the final manuscript.

Competing interests
The authors declare that they have no competing interest. This study did not use or evaluate any commercial product.

Author details
[1]IDT Biologika SL, Gran Vía Carles III, 84, 3°, 08028 Barcelona, Spain. [2]IVD Innovative Veterinary Diagnostics (IVD GmbH) Albert-Einstein-Str. 5, 30926 Seelze, Germany. [3]Departament de Sanitat i Anatomia Animals, Universitat Autònoma de Barcelona (UAB), 08193 Bellaterra, Barcelona, Spain. [4]UAB, Centre de Recerca en Sanitat Animal (CReSA, IRTA-UAB), Campus de la Universitat Autònoma de Barcelona, 08193 Bellaterra, Barcelona, Spain.

References
1. Holland RE. Some infectious causes of diarrhea in young farm animals. Clin Microbiol Rev. 1990 Oct;3(4):345–75.
2. Morin M, Turgeon D, Jolette J, Robinson Y, Phaneuf JB, Sauvageau R, Beauregard M, Teuscher E, Higgins R, Lariviere S. Neonatal diarrhea of pigs in Quebec: infectious causes of significant outbreaks. Can J Comp Med. 1983;47(1):11–7.
3. Svensmark B, Jorsal S, Nielsen K, Willeberg P. Epidemiological studies of piglet diarrhoea in intensively managed Danish sow herds. I Pre-weaning diarrhoea Acta Vet Scand. 1988;30(1):43–53.
4. Svendsen J, Bille N, Nielsen N, Larsen J, Riising H. Preweaning mortality in pigs. Diseases of the gastrointestinal tract in pigs. Nordisk Veterinär. 1975; 27(2):85–101.

5. Kongsted H, Stege H, Toft N, Nielsen JP. The effect of new neonatal porcine Diarrhoea syndrome (NNPDS) on average daily gain and mortality in 4 Danish pig herds. BMC Vet Res. 2014;10(1):90.

6. Johansen M, Alban L, Kjærsgård HD, Bækbo P. Factors associated with suckling piglet average daily gain. Prev Vet Med. 2004;63(1):91–102.

7. Sjölund M, Zoric M, Wallgren P. Financial impact of disease on pig production. Part III. Gastrointestinal disorders. In: Proceedings of 6th European symposium of porcine health management. Italy: Sorrento; 2014. p. 189.

8. Brown CC, Baker DC, Barker IK. Alimentary system. In: Grant Maxie M, editor. Jubb, Kennedy, and Palmer's pathology of domestic animals, vol. 2. 5th ed. Philadelphia: Elsevier Saunders; 2007. p. 81–2.

9. Thomson JR, Friendship RM. Digestive system. In: Zimmerman J, Karriker LA, Ramirez A, Schwartz KJ, Stevenson GW, editors. Diseases of swine. 10th. ed: Chichester: Wiley-Blackwell; 2012. p. 216–8.

10. Muirhead Michael R, Alexander Thomas JL. Managing Pig Health. In: Chapter 8: managing health in the farrowing and sucking period. second ed; 2013. p. 269–327.

11. Wang X, Ren W, Nie Y, Cheng L, Tan W, Wang C, Wei L, Zhang R, Yan G. A novel watery diarrhoea caused by the co-infection of neonatal piglets with *Clostridium perfringens* type a and *Escherichia coli* (K88, 987P). Vet J. 2013; 197(3):812–6.

12. Vlasova AN, Amimo JO, Saif LJ. Porcine rotaviruses: epidemiology, immune responses and control strategies. Viruses. 2017;9(3):48.

13. Theuns S, Vyt P, Desmarets LMB, Roukaerts IDM, Heylen E, Zeller M, Matthijnssens J, Nauwynck HJ. Presence and characterization of pig group a and C rotaviruses in feces of Belgian diarrheic suckling piglets. Virus Res. 2016;213:172–83.

14. Marthaler D, Homwong N, Rossow K, Culhane M, Goyal S, Collins J, Matthijnssens J, Ciarlet M. Rapid detection and high occurrence of porcine rotavirus a, b, and C by RT-qPCR in diagnostic samples. J Virol Methods. 2014;209:30–4.

15. Kim O, Chae C. In situ hybridization for the detection and localization of porcine epidemic diarrhea virus in the intestinal tissues from naturally infected piglets. Vet Pathol. 2000;37(1):62–7.

16. Saif LJ, Pansaert MB, Sestak K, Yeo SG, Jung K. Coronaviruses. In: Zimmerman J, Karriker LA, Ramirez A, Schwartz KJ, Stevenson GW, editors. Diseases of swine. 10th ed: Chichester: Wiley-Blackwell; 2012. p. 501–24.

17. Carvajal A, Argüello H, Martínez-Lobo FJ, Costillas S, Miranda R, de Nova PJ G, Rubio P. Porcine epidemic diarrhoea: new insights into an old disease. Porcine Health Manag. 2015;1:12.

18. Stevenson GW, Hoang H, Schwartz KJ, Burrough EB, Sun D, Madson D, Cooper VL, Pillatzki A, Gauger P, Schmitt BJ. Emergence of porcine epidemic diarrhea virus in the United States: clinical signs, lesions, and viral genomic sequences. J Vet Diagn Investig. 2013;25(5):649–54.

19. Kaper JB, Nataro JP, Mobley HL. Pathogenic *Escherichia coli*. Nature Reviews Microbiol. 2004;2(2):123–40.

20. Alexander TJL. Neonatal diarrhoea in pigs. In: Gyles CL, editor. *Escherichia coli* In domestic animals and humans. Wallingford: CAB International; 1994. p. 151–70.

21. Fairbrother JM, Gyles CL. Colibacillosis. In: Zimmerman J, Karriker LA, Ramirez A, Schwartz KJ, Stevenson GW, editors. Diseases of Swine. 10th ed. Chichester: Wiley-Blackwell; 2012. p. 723–49.

22. Songer GJ. Clostridiosis. In: Zimmerman J, Karriker LA, Ramirez A, Schwartz KJ, Stevenson GW, editors. Diseases of swine. 10th ed. Chichester: Wiley-Blackwell; 2012. p. 709–22.

23. Morin M, Phaneuf JB, Malo R. *Clostridium perfringens* type C enteritis in a Quebec swine herd. Can Vet J. 1981;22(3):58.

24. Petri D, Hill J, Van Kessel A. Microbial succession in the gastrointestinal tract (GIT) of the preweaned pig. Livest Sci. 2010;133(1):107–9.

25. Jandu N, Ho NKL, Donato KA, Karmali MA, Mascarenhas M, Duffy SP, Tailor C, Sherman P. Enterohemorrhagic *Escherichia coli* O157:H7 gene expression profiling in response to growth in the presence of host epithelia. 2009; 4(3):e4889.

26. Lee SI, Kang SG, Kang ML, Yoo HS. Development of multiplex polymerase chain reaction assys for detecting enterotoxigenic *Escherichia coli* and their application to field isolates from piglets with diarrhea. J Vet Diagn Investig. 2008;20:492–6.

27. Unterweger C, Kahler A, Gerlach GF, Viehmann M, von AA, Hennig-Pauka I. Administration of non-pathogenic isolates of *Escherichia coli* and *Clostridium perfringens* type a to piglets in a herd affected with a high incidence of neonatal diarrhoea. Animal. 2016 August;30:1–7.

28. Baums CG, Schotte U, Amtsberg G, Goethe R. Diagnostic multiplex PCR for toxin genotyping of Clostridium Perfringens isolates. Vet Microbiol. 2004; 100(1–2):11–6.

29. Pang Xiaoli L. Bonita lee, Nasim Boroumand, Barbara Leblanc, Jutta K. Preiksaitis, Charlotte C, Yu Ip. Increased detection of rotavirus using a real time reverse transcription-polymerase chain reaction (RT-PCR) assay in stool specimens from children with diarrhea. J Med Virol. 2004;72:496–501.

30. Le Dividich J, Noblet J. Colostrum intake and thermoregulation in the neonatal pig in relation to environmental temperature. Biol Neonate. 1981; 40(3–4):167–74.

31. Pedersen LJ, Malmkvist J, Kammersgaard T, Jorgensen E. Avoiding hypothermia in neonatal pigs: effect of duration of floor heating at different room temperatures. J Anim Sci. 2013;91(1):425–32.

32. Martineau GP, Vaillancourt JP, Broes A. Principal neonatal diseases. In: Varley MA, editor. The neonatal pig- development and survival. Wallingford: CAB International; 1995. p. 239–64.

33. Katsuda K, Kohmoto M, Kawashima K, Tsunemitsu H. Frequency of enteropathogen detection in suckling and weaned pigs with diarrhea in Japan. J Vet Diagn Investig. 2006;18(4):350–4.

34. Chan G, Farzan A, DeLay J, McEwen B, Prescott JF, Friendship RM. A retrospective study on the etiological diagnoses of diarrhea in neonatal piglets in Ontario, Canada, between 2001 and 2010. Can J Vet Res. 2013; 77(4):254–60. (7)

35. Boniotti MB, Papetti A, Lavazza A, Alborali G, Sozzi E, Chiapponi C, Faccini S, Bonilauri P, Cordioli P, Marthaler D. Porcine epidemic diarrhea virus and discovery of a recombinant swine enteric Coronavirus. Italy Emerg Infect Dis. 2016;22(1):83–7.

36. Pensaert MB, Martelli P. Porcine epidemic diarrhea: a retrospect from Europe and matters of debate. Virus Res. 2016;226:1–6.

37. Ngeleka M, Pritchard J, Appleyard G, Middleton D, Fairbrother JM. Isolation and association of *Escherichia coli* AIDA-I/STb, rather than EAST1 pathotype, with diarrhea in piglets and antibiotic sensitivity of isolates. J Vet Diagn Investig. 2003;15(3):242–52.

38. Alustiza FE, Picco NY, Bellingeri RV, Terzolo HR, Vivas AB. Frequency of virulence genes of *Escherichia coli* among newborn piglets from an intensive pig farm in Argentina. Rev Argent Microbiol. 2012;44(4):250–4.

39. Wada Y, Kato M, Yamamoto S, Shibahara T, Ishikawa Y, Kadota K. Invasive ability of *Escherichia coli* O18 isolated from swine neonatal diarrhea. Vet Pathol. 2004;41(4):433–7.

40. Kongsted H, Jonach B, Haugegaard S, Angen Ø, Jorsal SE, Kokotovic B, Larsen LE, Jensen TK, Nielsen JP. Microbiological, pathological and histological findings in four Danish pig herds affected by a new neonatal diarrhoea syndrome. BMC Vet Res. 2013;9:206.

41. Larsson J, Aspán A, Lindberg R, Grandon R, Båverud V, Fall N, Jacobson M. Pathological and bacteriological characterization of neonatal porcine diarrhoea of uncertain aetiology. J Med Microbiol. 2015;64(8):916–26.

42. Dors A, Czyżewska-Dors E, Wasyl D, Pomorska-Mól M. Prevalence and factors associated with the occurrence of bacterial enteropathogens in suckling piglets in farrow-to-finish herds. Vet Rec. 2016;179(23):598.

43. Springer S, Finzel J, Florian V, Schoepe H, Woitow G, Selbitz HJ. Vorkommen und Bekämpfung des *Clostridium-perfringens*-Typ-A-assoziierten Durchfalls der Saugferkel unter besonderer Berücksichtigung der Immunprophylaxe. Tierärztl Prax. 2012;40(G):375—82.

13

Swine enteric colibacillosis: diagnosis, therapy and antimicrobial resistance

Andrea Luppi

Abstract

Intestinal infection with enterotoxigenic *Escherichia coli* (ETEC) is an important disease in swine resulting in significant economic losses. Knowledge about the epidemiology, the diagnostic approach and methods of control are of fundamental importance to tackle the disease. The ETEC causing neonatal colibacillosis mostly carry the fimbriae F4 (k88), F5 (k99), F6 (987P) or F41, while the ETEC of post-weaning diarrhoea carry the fimbriae F4 (k88) and F18. These fimbriae adhere to specific receptors on porcine intestinal brush border epithelial cells (enterocytes), starting the process of enteric infection. After this colonization, the bacteria produce one or more enterotoxins inducing diarrhoea, such as the heat stable toxin a (STa), the heat stable toxin b (STb), and the heat labile toxin (LT). A role in the pathogenesis of the disease was demonstrated for these toxins. The diagnosis of enteric colibacillosis is based on the isolation and quantification of the pathogenic *E.coli* coupled with the demonstration by PCR of the genes encoding for virulence factors (fimbriae and toxins). The diagnostic approach to enteric colibacillosis must consider the differential diagnosis and the potential different causes that can be involved in the outbreak.
Among the different methods of control of colibacillosis, the use of antimicrobials is widely practiced and antibiotics are used in two main ways: as prophylactic or metaphylactic treatment to prevent disease and for therapeutic purposes to treat diseased pigs.
An accurate diagnosis of enteric colibacillosis needs an appropriate sampling for the isolation and quantification of the ETEC responsible for the outbreak by using semi-quantitative bacteriology. Definitive diagnosis is based on the presence of characteristic lesions and results of bacteriology along with confirmation of appropriate virulence factors to identify the isolated *E.coli*. It is important to confirm the diagnosis and to perform antimicrobial sensitivity tests because antimicrobial sensitivity varies greatly among *E. coli* isolates. Growing concern on the increase of antimicrobial resistance force a more rational use of antibiotics and this can be achieved through a correct understanding of the issues related to antibiotic therapy and to the use of antibiotics by both practitioners and farmers.

Keywords: Colibacillosis, ETEC, Pig, Diarrhoea, Diagnosis, Control

Background

Escherichia coli is a gram negative peritrichously flagellated bacteria belonging to the family Enterobatteriaceae and is the causative agent of a wide range of diseases in pigs, including neonatal diarrhoea and post-weaning diarrhoea (PWD), which are important causes of death occurring worldwide in suckling and weaned pigs respectively [1].

Two main pathotypes are involved in enteric colibacillosis: enterotoxigenic *E.coli* (ETEC) and enteropathogenic *E.coli* (EPEC). ETEC is the most important pathotype in swine and include different virotypes (this term is used to describe strains characterized by different combinations of toxins and fimbriae). Outbreaks of neonatal and post-weaning diarrhoea due to ETEC infection, generally affecting a high proportion of pigs, are often recurrent in the same herds and require expensive control measures. Enteric colibacillosis may result in significant economic losses due to mortality, decreased weight gain, cost for treatments, vaccinations and feed supplements [1]. Depending on the severity of the disease, the cost of PWD was estimated to range from €40 to €314 per sow [2]. ETEC possess fimbriae which adhere to enterocytes and elaborate one or several enterotoxins (Fig. 1) that induce secretory diarrhoea, causing some of the most

Correspondence: andrea.luppi@izsler.it
Istituto Zooprofilattico Sperimentale della Lombardia e dell'Emilia Romagna (IZSLER), Brescia, Italy

Pathotype	Adhesins	Toxins	Disease
ETEC	F5 (K99), F6, F41	Sta	Neonatal diarrhoea
	F4 (K88)	STa, STb, LT, EAST-1, α-hemolysin	
	F4 (K88) AIDA	STa, STb, LT, EAST-1, α-hemolysin	PWD
	F18 AIDA	STa, STb, LT, EAST-1, Stx2e, α-hemolysin	
EPEC	Eae	-	PWD

Fig. 1 Pathotypes, adhesins and toxins of porcine pathogenic *E.coli* responsible for neonatal and post-weaning colibacillosis (AIDA: Adhesin involved in diffuse adherence; EAST-1: Enteroaggregative heat stable enterotoxin)

significant diseases in the pig industry worldwide, such as neonatal colibacillosis and PWD.

Strategies commonly used to prevent and control neonatal colibacillosis should be aimed to reduce the number of pathogenic *E.coli* in the environment, implementing hygienic measures and internal and external biosecurity. The maintenance of suitable environmental conditions and piglets' high level of immunity, guaranteed by lactogenic immunity and by vaccinations of sows against ETEC F4 (k88), F5 (k99), F6 (987P) and F41, reduce the risk of the disease's development.

Various approaches have been used to prevent ETEC PWD, including passive administration with specific antibodies, dietary supplementation such as prebiotics and probiotics and dietary preventive measures, genetic breeding for ETEC-resistant herds and live oral nontoxigenic *E.coli* vaccines [3].

Even if some of the preventive approaches reported above for both neonatal and post-weaning colibacillosis have shown some promise and efficacy, antibiotics are still frequently used to treat enteric colibacillosis, administered by the parenteral and oral routes. Under-dosing is frequent with oral administration in pigs and this condition can favour the selection of resistant bacteria [4]. Antimicrobials commonly used to treat enteric colibacillosis must be chosen for their ability to achieve therapeutic concentrations in the intestinal content. The most frequently used are enrofloxacin, apramycin, ceftiofur, neomycin, gentamicin, amoxicillin/clavulanic acid, trimethoprim/sulphonamide and colistin [1]. Antimicrobial resistance to apramycin, neomycin, trimethoprim-sulfonimide and colistin has been increasingly observed, in particular in ETEC strains causing PWD [3].

Managing enteric colibacillosis in pigs requires an understanding of the pathotypes and the virotypes of *E.coli* involved and the conditions under which they are capable of causing disease, in order to implement appropriate diagnostics and strategies for prevention and control. The key element for approaching an outbreak of colibacillosis in order to reach a reliable and accurate diagnosis, is the knowledge of the diagnostic process and the interpretative criteria of diagnostic methods.

This paper is aimed at addressing some of the major questions that are frequently asked when faced with ETEC enteric neonatal and post-weaning colibacillosis in the field, which are the main subjects of this review, concerning the diagnostic approach and the interpretation of the specific investigations, the measures of control based on antibiotic therapy and the impact of antimicrobial resistance in the control of these diseases.

Pathogenesis of pig enteric colibacillosis
Neonatal enteric colibacillosis
ETEC causing neonatal enteric colibacillosis enter the animal by ingestion and in the presence of predisposing environmental conditions and host factors, proliferate in the intestine and cause disease by means of specific virulence factors. The degree of colonization and proliferation determine whether or not disease results from infection. ETEC responsible for neonatal diarrhoea possess adhesins, surface proteins called fimbriae, identified as F4 (k88), F5 (k99), F6 (987P) and F41 (Fig. 1). The fimbriae allow the microorganism to adhere to specific receptors on the brush borders of the small intestine's enterocytes. ETEC with the fimbriae F4 colonize the length of jejunum and ileum, while ETEC with fimbriae F5, F6, F41 mostly colonize the posterior jejunum and ileum [1]. Susceptibility to ETEC F5, F6 and F41 decreases with age and has been related to a reduction in the number of active receptors present on the intestinal epithelial cells with age. Most ETEC strains of neonatal colibacillosis produce heat stable enterotoxin STa, which binds guanylyl cyclase C glycoprotein receptor on the brush border of villous and crypt intestinal epithelial cells, stimulating the production of cyclic guanosine monophosphate (cGMP) leading to electrolyte end fluid secretion [1]. Excessive secretion leads to dehydration and eventual death [1]. Metabolic acidosis, defined as a state of decreased systemic pH, is a severe complication of neonatal colibacillosis and is due to lactate production. Most of the clinical signs that were formerly attributed to acidosis were in fact due to elevated blood levels of D-lactate. The source of D-lactataemia is bacterial fermentation of undigested substrate that reaches the large intestine due to the damage to the small intestinal mucosal epithelium. Respiratory compensation of acidosis occurs by hyperventilation, but this mechanism falls short due to an inadequate bicarbonate buffer [5].

Based on the concentration and affinity of the STa receptors, the posterior jejunum appears to be the major site of hypersecretion in response to STa. In the development of neonatal enteric colibacillosis, passive immunity plays a very important role. In particular, most neonatal infections can be prevented by passive colostral and lactogenic immunity [6]. Because ETEC infections are non-invasive gastrointestinal infections, mucosal i.e. lactogenic immunity rather than colostral i.e. systemic immunity is important to fight the disease [6]. For this reason, the presence of high levels of IgA in the milk of sows vaccinated or exposed to the pathogenic *E.coli* present in the environment of the piglets are able to prevent the small intestine colonization by ETEC. Because maternal vaccines are applied parenterally, the vaccination success, in particular of gilts, depends largely on these animals' previous mucosal exposure to ETEC. Piglets are more prone to disease if specific antibodies are absent from the sow's milk or they do not have access to a sufficient amount of milk.

Post-weaning enteric colibacillosis

As described for neonatal colibacillosis, *E.coli* causing PWD enter the animal by ingestion and in the presence of appropriate predisposing environmental conditions and host factors, proliferate in the intestine and cause disease by means of specific virulence factors [1].

Post-weaning ETEC strains mostly possess fimbriae F4 and F18, with some rare exceptions. Both fimbrial types (F4 and F18) have several variant subtypes based on antigenic differences. F4 variants ab, ac and ad have been described, even if almost all strains isolated from cases of PWD belong to the F4 ac subtype. F18 has two known variants, ab and ac. F18 ab is commonly associated with oedema disease (OD) strains, while F18 ac with PWD strains [7].

A non-fimbrial adhesin identified as adhesin involved in diffuse adherence (AIDA) has been associated with ETEC strains recovered from weaned pigs with PWD and there is evidence that it is causatively involved in diarrhoea experimentally induced in colostrum-deprived new-born piglets with STb encoding *E. coli* [8]. However, the role of EAST1 and AIDA in colibacillosis in pigs remains to be elucidated [9]. Post-weaning ETEC strains produce one or more of the known following enterotoxins: heat stable enterotoxins STa, STb, the heat-labile enterotoxin LT and the Enteroaggregative *E.coli* heat-stable enterotoxin (EAST1) [1]. The mechanism of action of STa has been described for neonatal colibacillosis. STb does not alter cGMP as described for STa, showing a different mechanism of action. Binding of STb to its receptor leads to an uptake of Ca^{2+} into the cells inducing the duodenal and jejunal secretion of water and electrolytes. In vivo significant accumulation of Na + and Cl – occur intraluminally following STb intoxication. In addition, STb stimulates bicarbonate (HCO3–) secretion [10].

LT is part of an important group of toxins - the AB5 toxin family. Two subtypes of LT, LTI and LTII have been described. Differences between LTI and LTII are largely due to dissimilarity in their B subunit. LTI can be divided in LTIh and LTIp, produced respectively by human and porcine ETEC. Strains expressing LT have also been shown to have an advantage in colonization promoting the adherence of ETEC in vitro and in vivo [10, 11]. LT permanently activates adenyl cyclase in the cell's basolateral border and leads to hypersecretion of electrolytes and water [10] causing to dehydration. Metabolic acidosis is a complication of post-weaning colibacillosis, but is limited until circulatory collapse occurs.

EAST1 was reported in ETEC isolated from pigs with diarrhoea, however its role in the development of diarrhoea has not been elucidated [9].

Intestinal microbiota and etec

Environmental and maternal bacteria quickly colonize offspring gut after birth and shape theonset of a healthy intestinal immune system and its future development [12]. Intestinal microbiota is characterised by its high population density, extensive diversity, and complexity of interactions throughout the gastrointestinal tract [13]. Studies on the characterisation of the intestinal microbiota show that the major bacterial groups isolated from the pig intestine are *Streptococcus, Lactobacillus, Prevotella, Selenomona, Mitsuokella, Megasphera, Clostridia, Eubacteria, Bacteroides, Fusobacteria, Acidodaminococci,* and *Enterobacteria* [13]. Interestingly, it was reported that there is clear evidence that gut microbiota play an important role in driving host metabolism and that the diversity of the faecal bacterial community and their changes over time were different in pigs depending on their subsequent susceptibility to post-weaning diarrhoea [12]. The stomach and proximal small intestine (duodenum) contain relatively low numbers of bacteria (10^3–10^5 bacteria/g or ml of contents) due to low pH and/or rapid digesta flow. In contrast, the distal small intestine harbours a more diverse and numerically greater (10^8 bacteria/g or ml of contents) bacterial population [13].

The mean number of *E.coli* biochemical phenotypes in piglets increased as animals aged [14] and *E. coli* populations in the pig faecal microbiota and in the farm environment are dynamic and show high levels of diversity [15].

Clinical manifestations of enteric colibacillosis obviously require the presence of pathogenic *E.coli* but also environmental changes and recognized risk factors [16]. Moredo et al. [17] demonstrated that the percentage of ETEC positive non-diarrhoeic pigs was 16.6% during the lactation period, 66% in the nursery phase and 17.3% in the finisher population. These data demonstrated that these pathogens can also be shed in faeces from healthy animals as already reported by Osek, in 1999 [18].

The barrier functions of the gastrointestinal tract in the neonatal piglet is not as developed as in mature animals due to the higher pH in the stomach, the lower proteolytic capacity, and the dependence on passive immune protection due to immunological immaturity [19]. The regeneration time of the small intestinal epithelium in day-old piglets is reported to be 7–10 days, as compared to 2–4 days in 3-week-old pigs. This difference is probably contributing to the susceptibility of infectious enteritis in new-born piglets, as a rapid turnover of enterocytes is considered a defence mechanism by the expulsion of infected cells [20]. Taken together, all of these conditions combined with predisposing factors, contribute to the neonatal piglet's vulnerability to ETEC enteric infections.

After weaning, the change in the intestinal environment of piglets, mainly due to dietary changes, results in an alteration of the composition of the indigenous flora. The diversity of E.coli strains of intestinal flora is usually high in healthy pigs [15], while in enteric colibacillosis we observe an alteration of the balance between the bacteria present in the normal intestinal flora [14]. This condition leads to the proliferation of a dominating pathogenic strain, which colonizes the small intestine [21], rapidly reaching massive numbers to the order of 10^9/g of contents. This is the reason why frequently, if not always, samples collected in diarrhoeic pigs affected by colibacillosis allow the isolation of a pure culture of pathogenic E.coli.

This information must be considered for a correct interpretation of diagnostic results. In particular, the evaluation of diagnostic findings should be made only in consideration of both clinical signs and pathological lesions, while also taking into account the number of isolated pathogenic E.coli strains belonging to the identified pathotype and virotype.

The diagnostic approach
The diagnosis of neonatal and post-weaning enteric colibacillosis includes the combination of different diagnostic procedures, starting from the observation of clinical signs and gross lesions, followed by appropriate bacteriological investigations and typing of the isolated bacterial strains.

Clinical signs, gross lesions and sampling
Neonatal diarrhoea due to enterotoxigenic E.coli is observed most commonly in piglets aged from 0 to 4 days of life, and in general, in an endemic condition, litters from first-parity sows could be more involved due to a lack of protection by passive immunity.

PWD due to E.coli is commonly observed 2–3 weeks after weaning and although not exceptionally, it can be recorded at 6–8 weeks after weaning.

When ETEC sustains neonatal diarrhoea, large quantities of watery to a creamy consistency scour are observed, with a distinctive smell and often white to yellow in colour.

The cases of post-weaning colibacillosis due to ETEC are usually characterized by yellowish, grey or slightly pink watery diarrhoea with a characteristic smell, generally lasting one week (Fig. 2).

Affected pigs are usually depressed with a reduced appetite and a rough sticky wet haircoat. Sudden deaths can occur, particularly at the start of the outbreak and dead pigs are usually dehydrated with sunken eyes. The small intestine is usually dilated, slightly oedematous and hyperaemic (Fig. 3). The stomach, usually dilated and full of clotted milk or dried feed, in neonatal or post weaning colibacillosis respectively, shows hyperaemia of the fundus (Fig. 4). The mesenteric lymph-nodes are enlarged and commonly hyperaemic. These lesions, even if not pathognomonic, are suggestive of enteric colibacillosis. For this reason the necropsy, both in the cases of neonatal and post-weaning colibacillosis, helps the pathologist in the choice of subsequent laboratory examination.

The most effective approach is to select a number of untreated pigs (3–5) suffering from diarrhoea for less than 12–24 h, and to humanely euthanize them and perform an accurate necropsy in order to evaluate gross lesions (evaluating the small intestine, colon, ileo-caecal valve, mesenteric lymph-nodes) and collect samples. Unopened segments of small intestine (in particular ileum and jejunum) and large intestine with the ends tied off

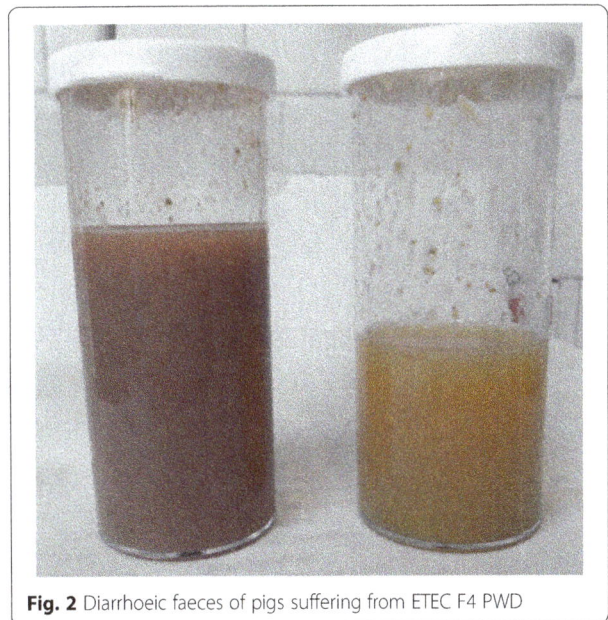

Fig. 2 Diarrhoeic faeces of pigs suffering from ETEC F4 PWD

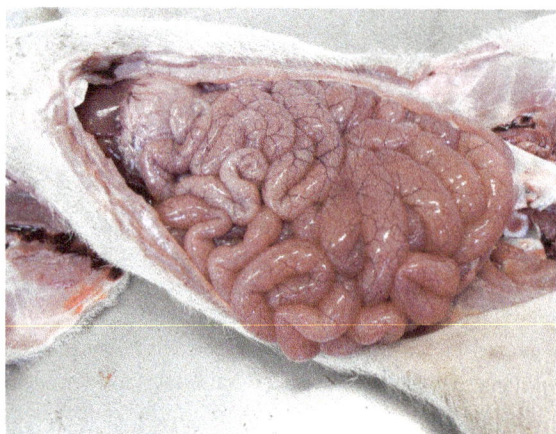

Fig. 3 Intestine of a pig suffering from ETEC F4 PWD appears dilated, oedematous and hyperemic

should be taken and sent to the laboratory (fresh samples for bacteriological investigations and fixed in 10% buffered formalin for histology), with a bacteriological examination request for the isolation of the pathogenic *E. coli* strain involved in the outbreak, its quantification (pure culture or not), its typing and evaluation of the sensitivity to antibiotics (Fig. 5). Fresh samples should be stored at +4 °C and should arrive at the laboratory in less than 24 h.

Recent spontaneously dead animals can also be used for microbiological analysis. Since autolysis of the gut after death occurs promptly, tissues obtained from animals 4–6 h after death are usually not suitable for histopathological analyses. If there are no pigs showing characteristic clinical signs of enteric colibacillosis to euthanize or recently dead pigs available, it is advisable

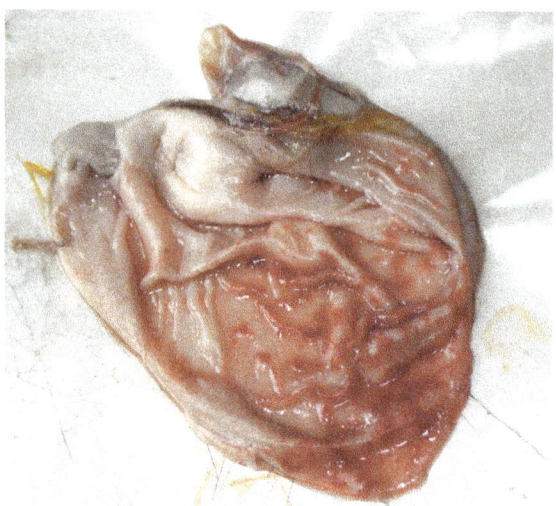

Fig. 4 Stomach of a pig suffering from ETEC F4 PWD. The gastric fundus shows a severe hyperemia

to collect faeces (directly from the animals and not from the soil) or rectal swabs from 3 to 5 pigs (Fig. 5).

The definitive diagnosis requires the combination of several investigations including quantitative bacteriology, the identification of virulence factors, usually by PCR, and histopathology as a complementary analysis, in order to have an integrated interpretation of the microscopic lesions observed with the pathogen detected. A diagnostic tree and diagnostic criteria that should be followed in the diagnosis of enteric colibacillosis is reported in Fig. 6.

Bacteriology and characterization of bacterial isolates
The diagnosis of enteric colibacillosis is based on the bacteriological examination of samples of luminal content (first choice) or rectal swabs. The samples should be inoculated onto blood agar and McConckey agar or other media which are selective for Enterobatteriaceae such as Hektoen agar. These selective media allow differentiation of lactose fermenting (such as *E.coli*) from lactose non-fermenting Gram negative enteric bacilli. Colonies on solid media reach their full size within 1 day of incubation and vary from smooth to rough or mucoid. The characteristics of the colonies grown on blood agar and lactose fermentation on selective media give a first diagnostic indication. In particular, the presence of haemolytic colonies, both in neonatal diarrhoea and PWD, is often used as a rapid tool for the diagnosis of ETEC diarrhoea (Fig. 7). In general terms, ETEC isolated from cases of neonatal colibacillosis can appear as haemolytic (ETEC F4 positive) or non-haemolytic (ETEC F5, F6, F41) colonies on blood agar plates [1, 22]. ETEC isolated from cases of PWD are mostly haemolytic (ETEC F4 or F18) even if non-haemolytic strains can be observed. In a recent study, the authors reported that *E.coli* strains isolated from cases of PWD, and characterized as ETEC, were haemolytic in 97.6% of the cases. The remaining 2.4% non-haemolytic ETEC isolates, for which haemolytic activity was consistently tested, were recovered in France, Italy and Germany, and sharing the same virotype: F4, STa, STb [23].

The detection of pathogenic strains does not justify the disease in every case and it is important to consider that *E. coli* pathotypes can, of course, also be isolated from the gut habitat of healthy hosts as reported above.

Evaluation of diagnostic findings can therefore be made only in consideration of both the clinical and pathological observations, coupled with the quantification of the isolated pathogenic *E.coli*. For this reason, the high concentration of pathogenic *E.coli* in pure or nearly pure culture isolated from the small intestine (ileum and jejunum) are indicative of enteric colibacillosis. Since almost all ETEC F4 or F18 are haemolytic, the presence of a pure culture of haemolytic colonies can be used as a presumptive diagnosis of neonatal colibacillosis

Are there pigs showing **characteristic clinical signs of enteric colibacillosis** to euthanize?

yes   no

Select **3-5 pigs** for necropsy

Are there **recently, untreated dead** pigs?

Select a **significant number of them (3-5)** for necropsy   yes   no

Perform **necropsy and gross lesions evaluation**

Collect **feaces or rectal swabs** from a significant number of pigs (3-5)

Collect **fresh samples**

Bacteriology (and possible other investigations)

Collect formalin-fixed samples for histology

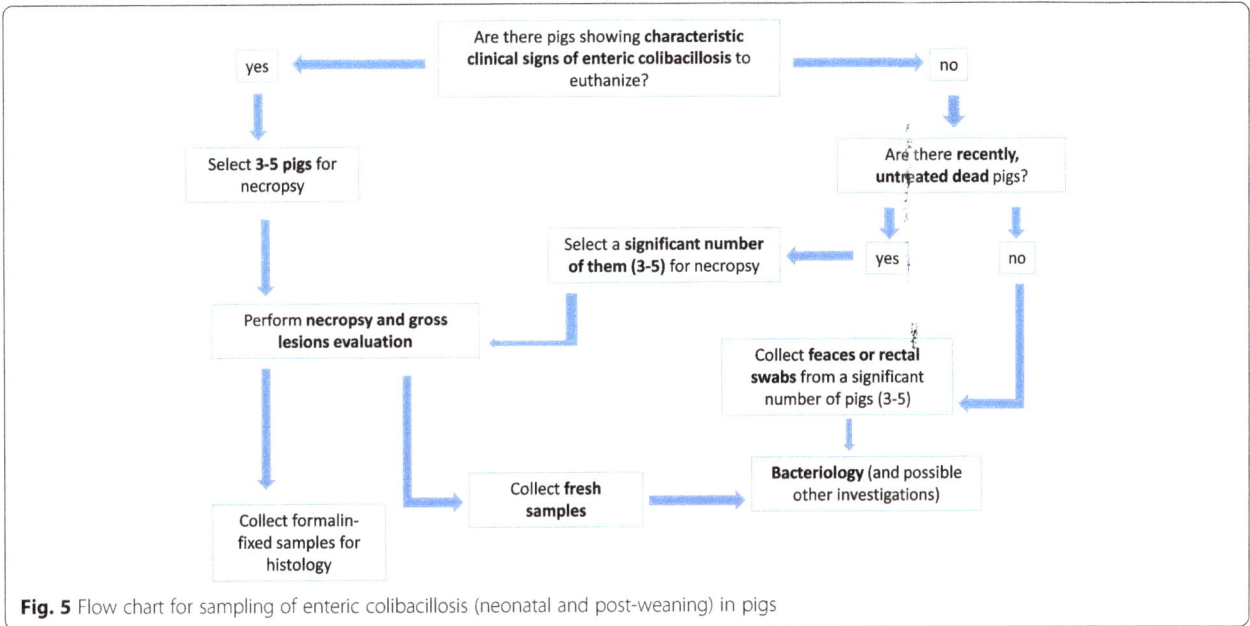

Fig. 5 Flow chart for sampling of enteric colibacillosis (neonatal and post-weaning) in pigs

(ETEC F4) or post-weaning colibacillosis (ETEC F4 or F18) [1].

The interpretation of bacteriological negative results in animals treated with antibiotics is unreliable and requires repeating the examination with untreated pigs.

The identification of virulence genes encoding for the fimbriae and toxins of the isolated strain is crucial to ascertain its role in the clinical problem observed.

Currently, in the diagnostic routine, genotypic analysis such as the polymerase chain reaction (PCR) for the detection of genes encoding for virulence factors is performed in many laboratories to characterize the isolated strains. Primers recognising genes encoding for toxins (STa, STb, LT and EAST1) and fimbriae (F4, F5, F6, F18, F41) of ETEC, for the outer membrane protein Eae or intimin in enteropathogenic *E.coli* (EPEC) and for Stx2e

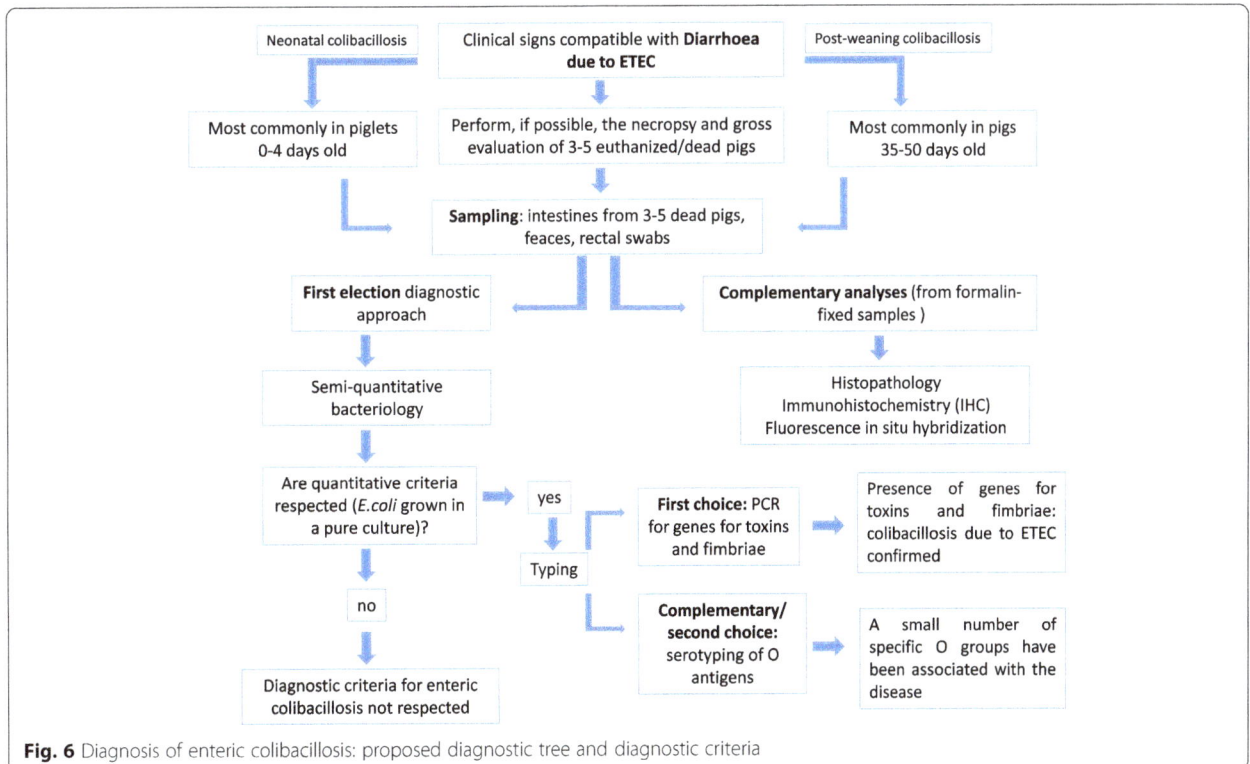

Neonatal colibacillosis

Clinical signs compatible with **Diarrhoea due to ETEC**

Post-weaning colibacillosis

Most commonly in piglets 0-4 days old

Perform, if possible, the necropsy and gross evaluation of 3-5 euthanized/dead pigs

Most commonly in pigs 35-50 days old

Sampling: intestines from 3-5 dead pigs, feaces, rectal swabs

First election diagnostic approach

Complementary analyses (from formalin-fixed samples)

Semi-quantitative bacteriology

Histopathology
Immunohistochemistry (IHC)
Fluorescence in situ hybridization

Are quantitative criteria respected (*E.coli* grown in a pure culture)?   yes

First choice: PCR for genes for toxins and fimbriae

Presence of genes for toxins and fimbriae: colibacillosis due to ETEC confirmed

Typing

no

Complementary/ second choice: serotyping of O antigens

A small number of specific O groups have been associated with the disease

Diagnostic criteria for enteric colibacillosis not respected

Fig. 6 Diagnosis of enteric colibacillosis: proposed diagnostic tree and diagnostic criteria

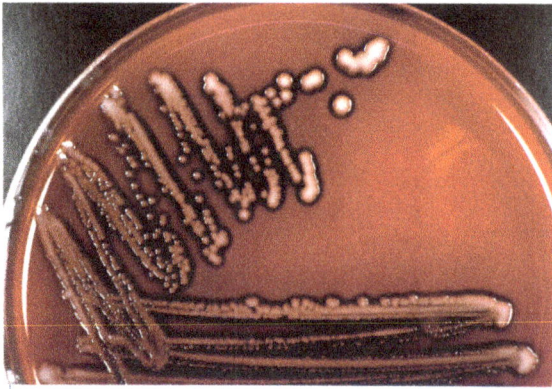

Fig. 7 ETEC F4 isolated from the intestinal content of a pig suffering from PWD. The picture shows a pure culture of haemolytic *E.coli* on blood agar

toxin in STEC (*E.coli* strains involved in oedema disease) strains, are available and can be used to perform PCR assays for daily routine diagnostics [24]. Interestingly, certain F18 strains produce both enterotoxins and the Stx2e toxin. These strains are classified ETEC rather than STEC, since they produce clinical PWD more than oedema disease [1].

The use of end point PCR for the direct identification of virulence factors in samples from diseased pigs, without performing a semi-quantitative bacteriology and typing of individual isolates, can make the interpretation difficult and unreliable. This diagnostic approach does not allow the quantification of the pathogen, and can give a mix of all the detectable virulence factors belonging to different *E.coli* strains present in the sample and, as a result, false combinations of these factors. In addition, it cannot be excluded that similar genes of virulence factors of other intestinal Enterobacteriaceae might be detected. As an example, a study performed on bacteria isolated from cases of diarrhoea in Children in Mexico showed the ST toxin gene of one strain identified as *M. morganii* being 100% identical to an ST toxin gene of *E. coli* [25]. The presence of genes encoding the LT toxin was previously reported in *M. morganii* obtained from stool samples of travelers with diarrhoea [26].

Development of quantitative PCR assays (qPCR) has become a feasible option for diagnosis [27] alone or combined with bacteriology. Ståhl and colleagues reported that the sensitivity of the qPCR was higher when compared to cultivation of *E. coli* F4 and *E. coli* F18 from faecal specimens from pigs with diarrhoea. In 34% of the samples that were positive in F4-qPCR and/or F18-qPCR, pathogenic *E. coli* were not detected by cultivation. When more than 10^7 CFU/g of *E. coli* F4 and/or *E. coli* F18 were detected, this was correlated with the cultivation of a high number of potentially pathogenic *E.*

coli [27]. Even if the quantification of the pathogenic *E.coli* using qPCR represents a promising diagnostic method for enteric colibacillosis, semi-quantitative bacteriology is of fundamental importance to perform the isolation and antimicrobial susceptibility testing of the *E.coli* strain responsible for the outbreak.

Usually, outbreaks of F4 positive *E.coli* tend to involve only one strain at any one time, even if mixed infections with the isolation of different virotypes in the same outbreak were observed. In these cases, one virotype probably predominates in any given outbreak [1]. For these reasons, it would be appropriate to type more isolates obtained from different pigs involved in the outbreak, after the quantitative bacteriological examination and compatibly with the costs for the examinations, in order to determine if more than one virotype is involved in an outbreak of enteric colibacillosis. As an example, it might be advisable to test samples from 5 representative pigs with diarrhoea and typing 3 isolates previously chosen for their cultural and biochemical characteristics. Although this approach does not give absolute results, it certainly increases the reliability of the results obtained.

A study performed on 160 European herds during PWD outbreaks, following the protocol of sampling reported above, showed that mixed infections (ETEC F4 and F18) were observed in 13% of the cases (data not published) (Fig. 8).

Pathogenic *E.coli* may be also identified by the serotyping of O antigens (cell wall LPS), since a small number of specific O groups have been associated with the disease (Table 1).

A complete serotyping of H (flagellar protein antigen) and O antigens, with the additional identification of K antigens (capsular polysaccharide), is the standard method

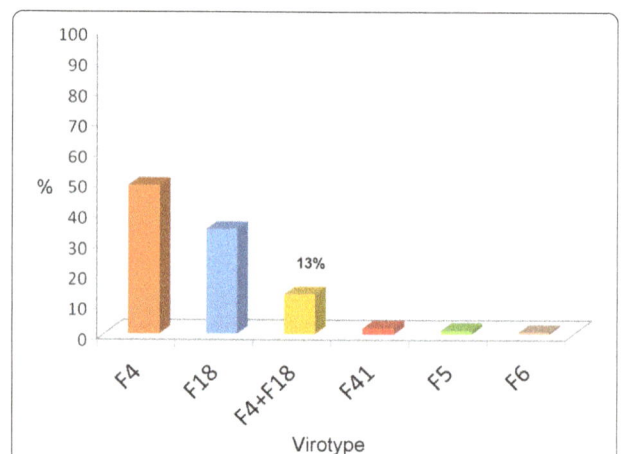

Fig. 8 Different virotypes isolated from 160 cases of PWD in different European countries, sampling 5 pigs with diarrhoea and typing 3 isolates previously chosen for their cultural and biochemical characteristics for each outbreak (data not published)

Table 1 O serogroups most frequently implicated as enterotoxigenic *E.coli* that cause neonatal diarrhoea in pigs

ETEC Adhesins	O serogroups	Disease
F5, F6, F41	O8, O9, O20, O64, O101	Neonatal diarrhoea
F4	O8, O138, O141, O145, O147, O149, O157	

for the definition of all serotypes, but in general is carried out in few reference laboratories.

Different clones within a serogroup may have evolved acquiring different virulence genes, resulting in clonal variation associated with a particular region or country. As an example, ETEC of serogroup O139, associated worldwide with the F18ab fimbriae, typically cause PWD in Australia and OD in Europe, while the predominant serogroup associated with PWD in pigs worldwide is O149 [1] (Table 2).

Histopathology

Histopathology in formalin-fixed, paraffin embedded tissues (ileum, jejunum and large intestine should be included) can be used as an additional investigation for a definitive diagnosis of colibacillosis. In piglets suffering from neonatal enteric colibacillosis, F4 positive ETEC are observed adhering to most of the jejunum and ileum's enterocyte brush border membrane of intestinal mucosa, while other ETEC mainly colonize the distal jejunum or the ileum [1]. Other changes include vascular congestion, haemorrhages and an increased number of inflammatory cells (neutrophils and macrophages in the *lamina propria*) [1]. Microscopic lesions in ETEC PWD are characterized by bacterial layers observed in patches on the apical surface of villous epithelial cells in the ileum and less consistently in the jejunum. Mild villous atrophy and an increased number of neutrophils may be observed in the superficial *lamina propria* [1]. Immuno-histochemistry and fluorescence in situ hybridization can be used as tools for the confirmation of the aetiology of the miscroscopic lesions observed.

Table 2 Common serovirotypes of pathogenic *E.coli* from pigs with PWD (modified from Fairbrother and Gyles [1])

Fimbrial adhesins	Serovirotypes
F4	O149:LT:STb:EAST-1
	O149:LT:STa:STb:EAST-1
	O149:LT:STb
F18	O149:LT:STb:EAST-1
	O138:STa:STb
	O138:LT:STb:EAST-1:Stx2e
	O139:Stx2e:(AIDA)
	O147: STa:STb:AIDA

Criteria and methods used for the identification of *E.coli* strains isolated from cases of neonatal and post-weaning colibacillosis have been reported in Table 3.

Differential diagnosis

Enteric disease outbreaks in pigs are frequently multifactorial. Focusing on the diagnosis and subsequent control strategies without take into account all the possible differential diagnoses or multiple agents involved can misguide practitioners. The diagnostic evaluation of neonatal and post-weaning colibacillosis requires similar standard diagnostic procedures. The diagnostic pathway is kept easy if the lesions observed during necropsy are strongly suggestive. This is the case in enteric colibacillosis, where bacteriology can usually easily confirm the suspect given by the recorded pathological lesions. Diarrhoea in the pre-weaned piglet is probably more straightforward to identify, treat, and prevent than post-weaning diarrhoea. In particular, ETEC neonatal diarrhoea must be differentiated from other causes of diarrhoea, such as *Clostridium difficile*, *Clostridium perfrigens* type A and C, enteric coronavirus (TGEV, PEDV) and rotavirus groups A, B and C. In piglets older than 7 days, coccidiosis due to *Isospora suis* should also be considered [28] (Table 4).

ETEC PWD should be differentiated from other causes of diarrhoea already described in piglets such as EPEC, enteric coronavirus (TGEV, PEDV), rotavirus groups A, B and C, salmonellosis, proliferative enteropathy due to *Lawsonia intracellularis* and *Brachyspira spp.* [28] (Table 5).

Treatments of enteric colibacillosis
Symptomatic treatment

The effect of diarrhoea in pigs affected by enteric colibacillosis is a loss of liquids that leads to the dehydration of the animals. The administration of saline solution and rehydration is essential in many cases [1]. Pigs represent a particular problem in rehydration, since the intravenous route is impractical, as is subcutaneous administration. Intraperitoneal injection can be used, but the volume which can be infused is limited, and uptake is uncertain [29]. Fluid therapy consisting in electrolyte replacement solutions containing glucose given orally, is used for the treatment of dehydration and metabolic acidosis in pigs affected by colibacillosis [1]. Studies in rats and clinical studies in children have shown that oral rehydration solutions with low osmolality promoted intestinal fluid absorption, with beneficial effects on the course of diarrhoea [30].

Zinc oxide

Feed containing between 2400 and 3000 ppm of zinc reduce diarrhoea, mortality and improve growth. For a

Table 3 Interpretative criteria used for the diagnosis of *E.coli* neonatal and post-weaning diarrhoea (modified from Fairbrother and Gyles, 2012) [1]

Criteria	ETEC		ETEC			EPEC
	F4	F18	F5	F6	F41	
Haemolytic colonies	Nearly all		None			None
Genotypic analysis	Fimbriae and toxins					Eae (intimin)
Serogroups (most prevalent)	O8, O138, O139, O141, O147, O149, O157		O8, O9, O20, O64, O101			O45, O103
Slide agglutination (F adhesin serotyping)	All	Not reliable	Not reliable			Not reliable
Histology	Bacterial layers are observed in patches on the apical surface of villous epithelial cells in the ileum and to a lesser extent in the jejunum					Multifocal "attaching and effacing" (AE) lesions involving the small intestine (duodenum, ileum, cecum)

long while, it was thought that zinc oxide must have an antibacterial effect, especially against *E. coli.* Several antimicrobial mechanisms of zinc oxide were proposed based on studies performed in vitro: 1) hydrogen peroxide, which is generated from the surface of zinc oxide, can penetrate through the cell membrane, produce some type of injury, and inhibit the growth of the cells; 2) the affinity between zinc oxide and bacterial cells is an important factor for antibacterial activity. Other investigators showed that zinc oxide reduced

bacterial adherence of ETEC F4 and blocked bacterial invasion by preventing increased tight junction permeability and modulating cytokine gene expression [31].

Zinc is poorly absorbed, so it becomes highly concentrated in manure with implications in terms of environmental pollution. The therapeutic use of zinc is currently debated. In general terms, bacteria in animals may develop resistance to Zn as well as to other heavy metals such as Cu. Resistance genes to Zn are often located on plasmids, which may be transferable to other

Table 4 Differential diagnosis of the main agents of neonatal diarrhoea (modified from Martelli et al. 2013) [28]

Disease/Etiological Agent	Age	Diarrhoea	Gross Lesions	Lethality	Laboratory diagnostic methods
Colibacillosis *E.coli* (ETEC)	Most commonly from 0 to 4 days	Yellowish, grey or slightly pink alkaline pH	Distension, congestion of small intestine. Stomach full of curdled milk	Can reach 70%	Culture/isolation. Typing of isolates usually by PCR Histopathology
Clostridiosis *C.perfrigens* type C	PA: 1 days A: 3 days SA: 7 days C: 10–14 days	PA: watery yellowish bloody A: brown bloody SA: watery grey/yellow C: yellow/grey	Jejunum and ileum mostly involved. Haemorrhagic enteritis Bloody ascitis	100% in PA and A forms	Culture/isolation. Typing/toxin identification. Histopathology
Clostridiosis *C.perfrigens* type A	Generally diarrhoea is observed within 48 h of birth	Mucoid, pink without blood	Jejunum and ileum mostly involved Pasty content Presence of necrotic membrane	Generally low if not complicated	Culture/isolation. Typing/toxin identification. Histopathology
Clostridiosis *Clostridium difficile*	In the first week of life	Pasty and yellow	Mesocolon oedema. Typhlocolitis with focal erosions	Variable. Up to 50%	Culture/isolation. Toxin identification
Coronavirus PEDV TGEV	All	Watery yellow/white/grey Watery yellow, white, grey, greenish; acid pH	Empty stomach. Small intestine was thinned and congested	Differs between strains and between naïve and endemic infected herds. Very high (80–100%) in suckling piglets belonging to naïve infected herds	PCR Histopathology Viral isolation
Rotaviral enteritis Rotavirus	From 1 to 5 weeks	Watery, sometime pasty. Acid pH	Small intestine was thinned. Milk in the stomach	Low (in endemic infected herds) <20%	PCR Histopathology Viral isolation
Coccidiosis *Isospora suis*	Not before 5 days. More frequent around 14 days	Yellow and pasty. Alkaline pH	Small intestine. Enteritis with fibrino-necrotic membrane	Very low or not observed	Microscopic evaluation after flotation

PA per-acute, *A* acute, *SA* sub-acute, *C* chronic

Table 5 Differential diagnosis of the main agents of post-weaning diarrhoea (modified from Martelli et al. 2013) [28]

Disease/Etiological Agent	Age	Diarrhoea	Gross Lesions	Lethality	Laboratory diagnostic methods
Colibacillosis E.coli (ETEC, EPEC)	Most commonly post-weaning until 45–50 days	Yellowish, grey or slightly pink alkaline pH	Distension, congestion of small intestine. Gastritis and stomach full of feed	Can reach 25%	Culture/isolation. Typing of isolates usually by PCR. Histopathology
Swine dysentery Brachyspira hyodysenteriae	Frequent in the growing-fattening periods	Muco-haemorrhagic	Muco-haemorrhagic and fibrino-necrotic typhlocolitis	Variable, usually low	Culture/isolation. Typing by PCR. Histopathology
Salmonellosis (Salmonella typhimurium)	Mostly in the growing-fattening periods	Yellowish, greenish, muco-haemorrhagic	Necrotic lesions yellowish membrane (small and large intestine); Prominent Payer patches	Low	Culture/isolation
PED and TGE Coronavirus PEDV TGEV	All	Watery yellow/white/grey Watery yellow, white, grey, greenish; acid pH	Empty stomach. Small intestine was thinned and congested	Can be high; less severe than in neonates	PCR Histopathology Viral isolation
Rotaviral enteritis Rotavirus	From 1 to 5 weeks	Watery, sometime pasty. Acid pH	Small intestine was thinned.	Low, <20%	PCR Histopathology Viral isolation
Proliferative enteropathy Lawsonia intracellularis	Post-weaning	A: haemorrhagic C: greenish	Ileitis	Low	PCR Histopathology

A acute, *C* chronic

bacteria, intra- and inter-species. Exposure to trace metals may also contribute to antibiotic resistance, even in the absence of antibiotics themselves. Zn supplementation to animal feed may increase the proportion of multi-resistant *E. coli* in gut microbiota [32]. Several studies have focused attention on heavy metals used in animal farming and possible mechanisms that could promote the spread of antibiotic resistance via co-selection. One report associated zinc with methicillin-resistant *Staphylococcus aureus* (MRSA) CC398 in Denmark [33], concluding that zinc compounds may be partly implicated in the emergence of MRSA clones. The co-selection mechanisms include co-resistance and cross-resistance. Co-resistance is defined as the close proximity of two or more genetic elements encoding for resistances. Sulphonamide resistance, for example, would follow the co-resistance path. The cross-resistance evolves when an antibacterial agent attacks the same target, for instance efflux systems that simultaneously transport two or more types of antibacterial agents. An example of cross resistance could be done with tetracycline, as zinc resistant strains would also expel tetracycline using the same efflux system [34].

Recently, the Committee for Medicinal Products for Veterinary Use (CVMP) of the European Medicines Agency (EMA) concluded the referral procedure for veterinary medicinal products containing zinc oxide to be administered orally to food-producing species. The Committee adopted an opinion by consensus concluding that the benefits of zinc oxide for the prevention of diarrhoea in pigs do not outweigh the risks for the environment. The CVMP highlighted that there is a risk of co-selection for resistance associated with the

use of zinc oxide, but at the present time, that risk is not quantifiable. The Committee therefore recommended the refusal of the granting of marketing authorisations and the withdrawal of existing marketing authorisations for veterinary medicinal products containing zinc oxide [35].

Antimicrobials

The treatment of enteric colibacillosis: general principles of antimicrobial therapy Antimicrobial therapy is required in many cases of enteric colibacillosis, besides using approaches to avoid infectious agents and clinical diseases. Antimicrobial therapy must be selected which reaches therapeutic concentrations in the intestinal lumen, as observed for different classes of antibiotics: β-lactam antibiotics (amoxicillin and the combination containing amoxicillin/clavulanic acid), cephalosporins (ceftiofur, cefquinome), aminoglucosides (apramycin, neomycin, gentamycin), aminocyclitols (spectinomycin) sulphonamide combined with trimethoprim (such as trimethoprim/sulphametoxazole), fluorochinolones (enrofloxacin, marbofloxacin and danofloxacin), quinolones (flumequine) and polymyxins (colistin sulphate) [1, 36].

The therapeutic approach and, consequently, the choice of the antibiotic for the treatment must consider several aspects:

1. The infection is located mainly in the small intestine. The antibiotic selected for the therapy must reach sufficient concentrations in the small intestine.

2. Empiric treatments are performed on the basis of knowledge on the individual herd and local data on the resistance pattern.
3. In many cases the evaluation of the isolated strain's antimicrobial susceptibility is fundamental for a correct therapy.

An outbreak of colibacillosis frequently requires quick actions and therefore the use of antibiotics almost always precedes the results of the resistance pattern. As a result, in most cases the right choice of antibiotics remains the practitioner's responsibility, for which the laboratory gives a retrospective result. The most basic information that the laboratory can provide is qualitative susceptibility results (the bacterial strain is susceptible, intermediate, or resistant to a specific antibiotic). Quantitative results obtained by the minimal inhibitory concentration (MIC) may be more useful than the traditional qualitative results, because MIC data define the degree of the pathogen's susceptibility more precisely.

Figure 9 reports, as an example, the steps in the initiation, management and reassessment of antibiotic therapy in an outbreak of enteric colibacillosis.

Some European Countries, such as the Netherlands, introduced a classification of all antibiotics into first,

second and third choice (last resort). This kind of approach was described by Burch et al. [37]. These classifications are continuously under revision. In general terms, first choice antibiotics can be used after a clinical diagnosis (empirical treatment), while second-choice antibiotics should be reserved for cases where sensitivity testing or clinical results has proven first-choice antibiotics are not effective, and third-choice antibiotics (such as third and fourth generation cephalosporins, fluorochinolones and macrolides) being reserved as last-resort antimicrobials, if no other options are available.

The antibiotic should be administered to all animals showing clinical signs referable to colibacillosis and sick pigs must be treated parenterally, since they eat and drink very little. In practice when mortality occurs, a metaphylactic approach is applied wherein all animals in the pens are treated where mortality has been observed. Guidelines for the prudent use of antimicrobials in veterinary medicine (2015/C 299/04) published on the official journal of the European Union considered the use of metaphylaxis and stated that antimicrobial metaphylaxis should be prescribed only when there is a real need for treatment and that the veterinarian should justify and document the treatment on the basis of clinical findings on the development of a disease in a herd or flock [38].

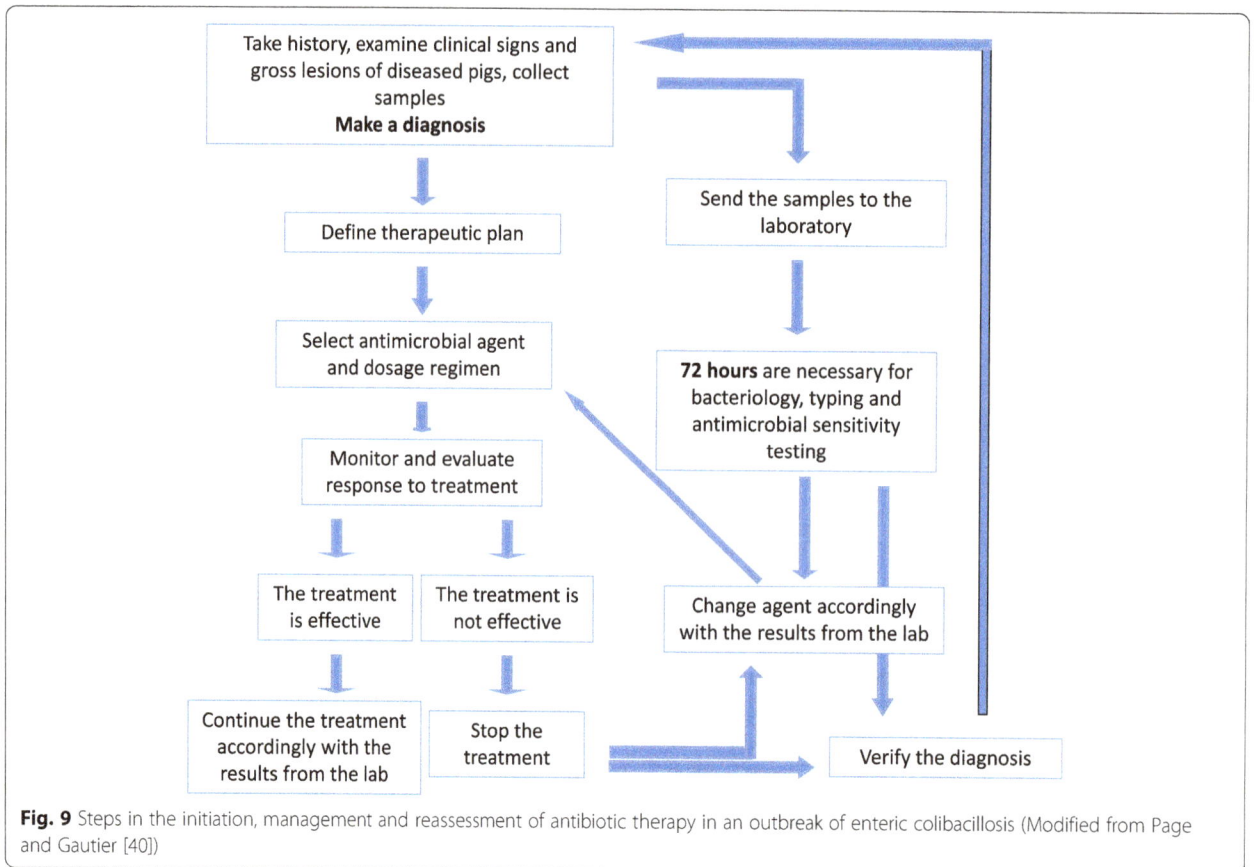

Fig. 9 Steps in the initiation, management and reassessment of antibiotic therapy in an outbreak of enteric colibacillosis (Modified from Page and Gautier [40])

Pharmacokinetic/pharmacodynamic indices: general information on antimicrobial drugs used in the treatment of enteric colibacillosis The efficacy of antimicrobial therapy is dependent upon the pathogen's ability to respond to antimicrobial therapy, the drug exposure characteristics necessary to elicit the targeted microbiological response, and the ability to achieve the necessary active drug concentrations at the site of infection [39]. The relationship between systemic drug exposure and its corresponding clinical and microbiological effects is termed pharmacokinetics/pharmacodynamics (PK/PD) (Table 6). This PK/PD relationship, in turn, dictates the dose, dosing frequency, and duration of drug administration necessary to achieve the desired clinical and microbiological outcome. The PK component describes the handling of the drug by the host (absorption, distribution, metabolism, and elimination) (Table 7). The PD component describes the effect of the drug over time on the bacteria at the site of infection. Thus, the interplay between PK and PD reflects the relationship between the fluctuating concentrations of biologically active drug at the site of infection, as reflected by its serum or plasma drug concentrations, versus its effects on the targeted microbial pathogen [39].

Three PK/PD indices have been proposed to allow predictions of antimicrobial efficacy: the ratio of the maximum unbound (free) concentration and the MIC (Cmax/MIC), the ratio of the free area under the concentration-time curve and the MIC (AUC/MIC), and the percentage of time thatthe concentration of free drug is above the MIC (T > MIC) [40].

Proper use of the PK/PD indices can optimize the dosage which, in turn, increase the possibility of therapeutic success, reduce toxicity and the emergence of resistance. To achieve a high probability of microbiological and clinical cure requires an adequate exposure of the bacteria to the antimicrobial agent. The exposure depends on the dose applied and is a function of different pharmacokinetic parameters such as drug bioavailability and clearance, as well as of the pathogen's susceptibility (e.g. MIC). Interestingly, clinical breakpoints used for the MIC evaluation are calculated taking into account different criteria and are mainly influenced by PK/PD parameters [41].

For different antimicrobials, the approach based on pharmacokinetic parameters and MIC distribution are used to assess the potential of dose to treat a systemic infection by a pathogen. The distributions of MIC values for a pathogen are used to estimate the range of doses necessary to obtain a probability of therapeutic success according to the population pharmacokinetics data. Appropriate dosing of antibiotic is the key to control or clear bacteria on the site of infection but also to limit antimicrobial resistance. The PK/PD indices are mostly used as targets for efficacy in the process of dose selection, but it is also necessary to work on the dosage regimen optimization (frequency, length of the treatment) to reach the best clinical outcome and the lowest resistant bacteria selection [41].

Main characteristics of antimicrobials used in the treatment of enteric colibacillosis ß-lactam antibiotics (such as penicillins, amoxicillin, cephalosporins, monobactams and carbapenem) prevent the bacterial cell wall from forming by interfering with the final stage of peptidoglycan synthesis. ß-lactam antibiotics act by binding to cell wall synthesis enzymes known as penicillin-binding proteins (PBPs), thereby inhibiting peptidoglycan synthesis. The drugs exert a bactericidal action, but cause lysis only of growing cells, that is, cells that are undergoing active cell-wall synthesis [42].

Amoxicillin achieves high tissue concentrations because it is well absorbed by the intestine. Amoxicillin, as most ß-lactams, is eliminated almost entirely by the kidneys, resulting in very high levels in the urine. Resistance to ß-lactams is mediated by efflux mechanisms and modification of porins in Gram negative bacteria that prevent the entry of the antibiotic [42].

Clavulanic acid is combined with amoxicillin in the ratio of 2:1 and the combinations are usually bactericidal. The combination has potential application in the treatment of a variety of infections in swine caused by plasmid-mediated ß-lactamase-producing bacteria, including

Table 6 Classification of antibacterial drugs frequently used in the treatment of enteric colibacillosis according to pharmacokinetics and pharmacodynamics indices (modified from Ahmad et al. [41])

Drugs	Bacterial effect	PK/PD parameters
Fluoroquinolones (enrofloxacin)	Concentration dependent	Cmax/MIC and AUC/MIC
Cephalosporins (ceftiofur)	Time dependent	T > MIC
Sulphonamides + Diaminopyrimidines (trimethoprim + sulfamethoxazole)	Time dependent	T > MIC
Aminoglycosides (neomycin)	Concentration dependent	Cmax/MIC or AUC/MIC
Aminocyclitols (spectinomycin)		T > MIC
Polymyxins (colistin)	Concentration dependent	AUC/MIC

Table 7 Main antimicrobials used in swine for the treatment of enteric colibacillosis: routes of administration, dosages and main pharmacokinetic properties (modified from Burch [37])

Antimicrobial class/ compounds	Administration and dosage (mg/kg body weight)			Pharmacokinetic Properties	Administration in enteric colibacillosis
	Injection	In water	In feed		
Trimethoprim/sulfonamide	15 (2.5 + 12.5)	30 (5 + 25)	15 (2.5 + 12.5)	Rapidly absorbed from intestine, well distributed in tissues;crosses uninflamed blood–brain barrier	IM and orally
Amoxicillin	7	20	15–20		IM and orally
Amoxicillin + Clavulanic acid	7 + 1,75				IM
Ceftiofur	3			Poorly absorbed from intestine,relatively poorly distributed intissues; crosses only inflamedblood–brain barrier	IM
Cefquinome	1–2				IM
Enrofloxacin	2.5			Well absorbed and distributed intissues	IM
Neomycin		11	11	Poorly absorbed from intestine,relatively poorly distributed intissues	Orally
Apramycin		7.5–12.5	4–8	Poorly absorbed from intestine,relatively poorly distributed intissues	Orally
Spectinomycin		10–50	1.1–2.2	Poorly absorbed from intestine,relatively poorly distributed intissues	Orally
Colistin sulphate		100,000 IU/Kg body weight	100,000 IU/Kg body weight	Not absorbed from intestine.	Orally

neonatal diarrhoeal *E. coli*. Clavulanic acid is well absorbed after oral administration and has pharmacokinetic properties similar to amoxicillin [43].

Cephalosporins have the advantages of ß-lactamase stability, good activity against target proteins (PBPs), and good ability to penetrate bacterial cell walls. Fourth-generation cephalosporins are effective against Enterobacteriaecae and other Gram-negative bacteria resistant to earlier generations of cephalosporins because of acquired ß-lactamase-based resistance. Cephalosporins are among the safest antimicrobial drugs. The broad spectrum of antibacterial activity of second to fourth generation drugs may cause overgrowth of resistant bacteria including *Clostridium difficile*, which no longer have to compete with susceptible members of the microbial flora [44]. Ceftiofur sodium is available for use on swine in the treatment of neonatal colibacillosis. Fourth and third-generation cephalosporins are not first choice antimicrobial agents and should be reserved for use where susceptibility testing indicates that alternatives are not available. Narrower-spectrum drugs are often effective and should be preferred [44].

In general, the 3 mechanisms of ß-lactam resistance are: reduced access to the PBPs, reduced PBP binding affinity, and destruction of the antibiotic through the expression of ß-lactamase (enzymes that bind and hydrolyze ß-lactams) [45].

Antibacterial diaminopyrimidines are combined with a variety of sulfonamides (sulfadiazine, sulfamethoxazole, and sulfadoxine) in a fixed (1:5) ratio. The combination

of a diaminopyrimidine with a sulfonamide inhibits sequential steps in the synthesis of folic acid and thus of the purines required for DNA bacterial synthesis. The interference by the diaminopyrimidine with recycling of tetrahydrofolic or dihydrofolic acid is probably responsible for the combination's synergistic interaction. The combination has a wide margin of safety, and adverse effects can mainly be attributed to the sulfonamide. The diaminopyrimidine component is concentrated in tissues whereas the sulfonamide component moves only slowly from plasma into tissues. Trimethoprim-sulfonamide combinations have been used successfully in controlling a wide variety of conditions in pigs, including neonatal and post-weaning colibacillosis [46].

The aminoglycoside antibiotics kanamycin, gentamicin, amikacin, and neomycin are large molecules with numerous amino acid groups, making them basic polycations that are highly ionized at physiological pHs. The antibacterial action of the aminoglycosides is directed primarily against aerobic, Gram-negative bacteria. The bactericidal action of the aminoglycosides on aerobic Gram-negative bacteria is markedly influenced by pH, being most active in an alkaline environment. Increased local acidity secondary to tissue damage or bacterial destruction may explain the failure of aminoglycosides to kill usually susceptible pathogens. Aminoglycosides are poorly absorbed from the normal gastrointestinal tract, but are well absorbed after IM or SC injection. Elimination is entirely by renal excretion (glomerular filtration), and unchanged drug is rapidly excreted in the urine. Nephrotoxicity (acute tubular necrosis) is the most common adverse effect of aminoglycoside therapy. Most clinically important resistance to aminoglycosides is caused by plasmid-mediated enzymes, broadly classified as phosphotransferases, acetyltransferases, and adenyltransferases [47]. Gentamicin is used to treat neonatal colibacillosis in piglets from day 1 to day 3 of age, with either a single IM injection or an oral dose of 5 mg. [47].

Spectinomycin is an aminocyclitol antibiotic that lacks most of the toxic effects of the aminoglycoside antibiotics but, is limited in application by the ready development of resistance. Spectinomycin is a usually bacteriostatic, relatively broad-spectrum drug that can be bactericidal at concentrations 4 times the MIC. Chromosomal one-step mutation to high-level resistance develops readily in vivo and in vitro. Chromosomally resistant strains do not show cross-resistance with aminoglycosides. Pharmacokinetic properties are similar to those of the aminoglycosides. In pigs, spectinomycin is available as an oral solution for the treatment of colibacillosis [47].

After administration, fluoroquinolones exhibit rapid and extensive tissue distribution because of their hydrophilic nature and low (<50%) protein binding. High concentrations are found in the bile and organs of excretion (liver, intestine, and urinary tract). The fluoroquinolones are predominantly excreted as unchanged drug in the urine by glomerular filtration and active tubular secretion. Fluoroquinolones are relatively safe antimicrobial drugs. Administered at therapeutic doses, toxic effects are mild and generally limited to gastrointestinal disturbances such as nausea, vomiting, and diarrhoea. Resistance to fluoroquinolones occurs by target modification, decreased permeability, efflux and/or target protection. Each of these fluoroquinolone resistance mechanisms can occur simultaneously within the same cell, thereby leading to very high resistance levels [48]. Fourth and third generation cephalosporins and fluoroquinolones are not first choice antimicrobial agents and should be reserved for use where susceptibility testing indicates that alternatives are not available.

Colistin (polymyxin E) is a cationic, multicomponent, lipopeptide antibacterial agent discovered soon after the end of the Second World War (1949). Colistin is a bactericidal drug that binds to lipopolysaccharide (LPS) and phospholipids in the outer membrane of Gram negative bacteria. This process results in an increase in the permeability of the cell envelope, leakage of cell contents, and subsequent cell death. Colistin sulphate is the only approved product in some countries for oral use in pig production, to control intestinal infections caused by Enterobacteriaceae [49]. Polymyxins are well tolerated after oral or local administration, but systemic use causes nephrotoxic, neurotoxic, and neuromuscular blocking effects.

The use of colistin in Europe varies widely between countries. Countries with intensive livestock production can have a level of usage below 1 mg/PCU (e.g. Denmark and the UK) or much higher, up to 20 to 25 mg/PCU (Italy and Spain) [50]. Due to its importance in human medicine, the public health impact of current or future use of colistin products in animals has been under discussion for long time [49]. The usually recommended dose for therapy is 100,000 IU/kg BW (100,000 IU/kg body weight per day or 50,000 IU/kg administered at 12-h intervals), but in some non-European countries the use of colistin is authorised at lower dosage, as feed additive for growth promotion [51].

***E.coli* and antimicrobial resistance** Antimicrobial resistance to several antibiotics such as apramycin, neomycin, trimethoprim-sulphametoxazole and colistin has been increasingly observed in ETEC strains causing PWD [3]. The development of resistance to a wide range of antimicrobial drugs, as well as the demonstrated trend of resistance in ETEC strains to the antibiotics used for the treatment of colibacillosis in pigs, is nowadays a reason for concern [52]. Multidrug resistance among ETEC isolates has been described and recently there has been an increasing tendency for porcine ETEC to express a multidrug-resistant phenotype [33].

It is difficult, if not impossible, to provide general data on resistance, because the situation is variable in different countries and pig populations, and mainly depends on the antimicrobials preferentially used. Table 8 reports the data of resistance of *E.coli* strains to different antibiotics commonly used in the treatment of colibacilloisis.

In a study performed in Italy, aiming to evaluate the trend of resistance of ETEC isolated in a 10-year period (2002–2011), 442 strains of F4-positive *E.coli* isolated from cases of porst-weaning colibacillosis were tested against several antibiotics using the disc diffusion method [52]. In the study, intermediate strains were grouped with the resistant one. Isolates showed a statistically significant increasing trend of resistance over the whole period of study to: enrofloxacin (from 14.5% to 89.3%), flumequine (from 49.1% to 92.9%) and cefquinome (from 3.8% to 44%). An increasing resistance (not statistically significant) was also observed to gentamicin (from 63.6% to 85.7%), apramycin (from 61.8% to 82.1%), and trimethoprim-sulphametoxazole (from 75% to 89.3%).

Resistance to enrofloxacin was described in *E. coli* strains isolated in Brazil, where nearly 30% of the isolates from cases of neonatal colibacillosis were resistant to this antibiotic [53]. Fluorochinolones resistance has been strongly correlated with the quantity of the drug used to treat pigs and plasmid-borne transfer of fluorochinolones resistance has been demonstrated in pig *E. coli* strains [54].

Table 8 Examples of resistance rates to different antibiotics of *E.coli* strains isolated from healthy and diseased pigs in different countries (Modified from Aarestrup et al. 2008) [33]

ANTIBIOTIC	USA[a]	Brazil[b]	Korea[c]	China[d]	Spain[e]	Belgium[e]	Germany[e]	France[e]	Poland[f]
Fluoroquinolones	0%	30%	64.9%	64%	14%	39%	8%	6%	30%
Ceftiofur	22%	-	-	-	4%	1%	1%	1%	-
SXT	23%	62%	75.7%	90%	-	71%	51%	66%	78.8%
Neomycin	66%	32.8%	-	9.4%	20%	2%	-	11%	-
Apramycin	30%	-	-	-	13%	13%	10%	3%	-
Gentamicin	48%	39%	77%	57%	20%	46%	12%	6%	45%
REFERENCE	[59]	[53]	[57]	[60]	[33]	[33]	[33]	[33]	[61]

[a](*E.coli* isolated form pigs with diarrhoea and septicemia); [b](E.coli isolated from cases of neonatal colabacillosis; [c](*E.coli* isolated from pigs with diarrhoea); [d](pathogenic and commensal *E.coli* isolated from pigs); [e](*E.coli* isolated from diseased pigs); [f](commensal *E.coli*)

High levels of resistance to gentamicin were reported in *E. coli* isolated form diseased pigs in Belgium (46%), Poland (45%) and Spain (20%) [33]. Resistance to gentamicin and other aminoglycosides is usually transmissible and cross-resistance between gentamicin and apramycin was described [55].

The *E. coli* isolates from cases of PWD in Australia resulted resistant to streptomycin spectinomycin, ampicillin and trimethoprim-sulphametoxazole. In the same study, a smaller number of isolates were resistant to neomycin and apramycin, and a proportion of these showed resistance to gentamicin. None of the isolates were resistant to enrofloxacin or ceftiofur [56].

A study performed in Korea showed how *E. coli* strains isolated from diarrhoeic pigs were multi-resistant (resistant to more than 4 antibiotics) with high levels of resistance to several antibiotics: gentamicin (77%), trimethoprim-sulphametoxazole (75.7%), amoxicillin (75.7%), ampicillin (73%) and enrofloxacin (64.9%) [57].

In the last few years, *E. coli* strains resistant to colistin has become more common. Strains of *E. coli* with acquired resistance are encountered among pathogenic isolates, commonly in pigs suffering from diarrhoea [51] (Table 9).

Resistance to colistin is based on mutations responsible for modification of the LPS charge. Until now, polymyxin resistance has involved chromosomal mutations making the resistance mechanism unstable and incapable of spreading to other bacteria but has never been reported via horizontal gene transfer. A study performed in China on antimicrobial resistance in commensal *E. coli* from food animals has shown an increase of colistin resistance and has described the emergence of the first transmissible, plasmid-mediated polymyxin resistance in the form of *mcr*-1 [58]. The gene can be easily transferred between different types of bacteria, potentially leading to rapid development of resistance. While the gene was first detected in *E.coli* in China, it has subsequently also been found in the EU. In terms of antibiotic resistance, plasmids play a

central role as vehicles for resistance gene capture and subsequent dissemination.

The European Commission, following the recent discovery of this new mechanism of resistance in bacteria to colistin (caused by the *mcr*-1 gene), requested an update from the EMA's Antimicrobial Advice Ad Hoc Expert Group (AMEG) on its 2013 advice on the "use of colistin products in animals within the European Union". In its advice published in July 2016, the Expert Group describes several measures that should be considered to tackle the problem. These are summarised as follow:

- Over the course of the next 3–4 years, all Member States should reduce the use of colistin in animals at least to a target level of 5 mg colistin/PCU.
- Member States are also encouraged to set stricter national targets, ideally below 1 mg colistin/PCU as a desirable level.
- The reduction of colistin sales should not be compensated for by an increase in the use of other types of antimicrobials, but should be achieved through other measures such as improved farming

Table 9 Examples of colistin resistance in *E.coli* strains isolated from healthy and diseased pigs in different countries (Modified from Kempf et al. [51])

Country	Origin of the isolates	% of resistance/ non-wild type strains	Reference
France	faeces, healthy pigs	0.5%	[62]
Sweden	healthy pigs	0%	[63]
Denmark	healthy pigs	0%	[64]
Belgium	pigs with diarrhoea	9.6%	[65]
Croatia	pigs with diarrhoea	3%	[66]
Brazil	pigs with diarrhoea	28.1%	[53]
UK	Slaughterhouse, healthy pigs	34,1%	[67]
China	pigs with diarrhoea	33.3%	[68]

conditions, biosecurity between production cycles, and vaccination of livestock.
– Colistin should be reclassified and added to Category 2 of the AMEG classification system, which includes medicines reserved for treating infections in animals for which no effective alternative treatments exist [50].

Conclusion

The control of a disease begins with a correct diagnostic approach. The diagnosis of colibacillosis require an appropriate sampling for isolation of the pathogen and standardized diagnostic criteria, including the evaluation of antimicrobial susceptibility.

The therapeutic use of antimicrobials is widely practiced to control both neonatal and post-weaning colibacillosis, even if in many countries the prophylactic and metaphylactic use of the antibiotics is still common. Growing concern on the increase of antimicrobial resistance among pathogenic *E. coli* strains with an increased prevalence of multi-resistant *E. coli* strains from diarrhoeic pigs is leading to more attention on the alternatives to antibiotics such as vaccines, probiotics, prebiotics, additives, and management practices. Even if some preventive approaches have shown some promise and efficacy, in many cases the use of antibiotics is preferred to treat and control enteric colibacillosis.

Nowadays, there is concern over the increased phenomenon of antimicrobial resistance among bacteria isolated from production animals. The risk linked to this phenomenon increases if antimicrobials are used inappropriately, for example, in an untargeted manner (e.g. mass medication or use on non-susceptible microorganisms), at sub-therapeutic doses, repeatedly, or for inappropriate periods of time. These conditions force a more rational and judicious use of antibiotics.

Abbreviations

AIDA: Adhesin involved in diffuse adherence; AMEG: Antimicrobial Advice Ad Hoc Expert Group; AUC: Area under the plasma concentration time curve; BW: Body weight; cGMP: Cyclic guanosine monophosphate; Cmax: Maximum plasma concentration; EAST1: Enteroaggregative *E. coli* heat stable enterotoxin; ED: Oedema disease; EMA: European Medicines Agency; EPEC: Enteropathogenic *E.coli*; ETEC: Enterotoxigenic *Escherichia coli*; IM: Intramuscular; LPS: Lipopolysaccharide; LT: Heat labile toxin; MIC: Minimum inhibitory concentration; PBPs: Penicillin-binding protein; PCR: Polymerase chain reaction; PCU: Population correction unit; PD: Pharmacodynamics; PEDV: Porcine epidemic diarrhoea virus; PK: Pharmacokinetics; PWD: Post-weaning diarrhoea; qPCR: Quantitative PCR; SC: Subcutaneous; STa: Heat stable toxin a; STb: Heat stable toxin b; STEC: Shiga toxin *E.coli*; Stx2e: Shiga toxin; T: Time; TGEV: Transmissible gastro enteritis virus

Acknowledgements
The author wish to thank Prof. Paolo Martelli.

Funding
Not applicable.

Authors' Contributions
Not applicable.

Authors' information
AL, DVM, PhD and Diplomate ECPHM is in charge of the Diagnostic Laboratory of Reggio Emilia (IZSLER).

Competing interests
The author declare that they have no competing interests.

References
1. Fairbrother JM, Gyles CL. Colibacillosis. In: Zimmerman JJ, Karriker LA, Ramirez A, Schwartz KJ, Stevenson GW, editors. Disease of Swine. 10th ed; 2012. p. 723–47.
2. Sjölund M, Zoric M, Wallgren P. Financial impact on pig production: III. Gastrointestinal disorders: Proceedings of the 6th European Symposium of Porcine Health Management, Sorrento; 2014. p. 189–Italy.
3. Zhang W. Progress and Challenges in Vaccine development against enterotoxigenic *Escherichia coli* (ETEC) – Associated porcine Post-weaning Diarrhea (PWD). J Vet Med Res. 2014;1(2):1006.
4. Burrow E, Simoneit C, Tenhaggen BA, Käsbohrer A. Oral antimicrobial resistance in porcine *E. coli* – A systematic review. Prev Vet Med. 2014; 113:364–75.
5. Lorenz I. D-Lactic acidosis in calves. Vet J. 2009;179(2):197–203.
6. Melkebeek V, Goddeeris BM, Cox E. ETEC vaccination in pigs. Vet Immunol Immunopathol. 2013;152(1–2):37–42.
7. Francis DH. Enterotoxigenic *Escherichia coli* infection in pigs and its diagnosis. J Swine Health Prod. 2002;10(4):171–5.
8. Ravi M, Ngeleka M, Kim SH, Gyles C, Berthiaume F, Mourez M, et al. Contribution of AIDA-I to the pathogenicity of a porcine diarrheagenic *Escherichia coli* and to intestinal colonization through biofilm formation in pigs. Vet Microbiol. 2007;120:308–19.
9. Zajacova ZS, Faldyna M, Kulich P, Kummer V, Maskova J, Alexa P. Experimental infection of gnotobiotic piglets with *Escherichia coli* strains positive for EAST1and AIDA. Vet Immunol Immunopathol. 2013;152:176–82.
10. Dubreuil JD, Isaacson RE, Schifferli DM. Animal Enterotoxigenic *Escherichia coli*. EcoSal Plus. 2016; doi:10.1128/ecosalplus.ESP-0006-2016.
11. Johnson AM, Kaushik RS, Francis DH, Fleckenstein JM, Hardwidge PR. Heat-Labile Enterotoxin Promotes *Escherichia coli* Adherence to Intestinal Epithelial Cells. J Bacteriol. 2009;191(1):178–86.
12. Dou S, Gadonna-Widehem P, Rome V, Dounia Hamoudi D, Thibaut Larcher T, Bahi-Jaber N, Pinon-Quintana A, Guyonvarch A, Huërou-Luron ILE, Abdennebi-Najar L. Characterisation of Early-Life Fecal Microbiota in Susceptible and Healthy Pigs to Post-Weaning Diarrhoea. PLoS One. 2017; doi: 10.1371/journal.pone.0169851.
13. Pluske JR, Pethick DW, Hopwood DE, Hampson DJ. Nutritional influences on some major enteric bacterial diseases of pigs. Nutr Res Rev. 2002;15:333–71.
14. Katouli M, Lund A, Wallgren P, Kühn I, Söderlind O, Möllby R. Phenotypic characterization of intestinal *Escherichia coli* of pigs during suckling, postweaning, and fattening periods. Appl Environ Microbiol. 1995;61(2):778–83.
15. Marchant M, Moreno MA. Dynamics and Diversity of *Escherichia coli* in Animals and System Management of the Manure on a Commercial Farrow-to-Finish Pig Farm. Appl Environ Microbiol. 2013;79(3):853–9.
16. Laine TM, Lyytikäinen T, Yliaho M, Anttila M. Risk factors for post-weaning diarrhoea on piglet producing farms in Finland. Acta Vet Scand. 2008;50:21.

17. Moredo FA, Piñeyro PE, Márquez GC, Sanz M, Colello R, Etcheverría A, et al. Enterotoxigenic *Escherichia coli* Subclinical Infection in Pigs: Bacteriological and Genotypic Characterization and Antimicrobial Resistance Profiles. Foodborne Pathog Dis. 2015;12(8):704–11.

18. Osek J. Prevalence of virulence factors of *Escherichia coli* strains isolated from diarrheic and healthy piglets after weaning. Vet Microbiol. 1999;68(3–4):209–17.

19. Lawley TD, Walker AW. Intestinal colonization resistance. Immunology. 2013;138(1):1–11.

20. Kim M, Ashida H, Ogawa M, Yoshikawa Y, Mimuro H, Sasakawa C. Bacterial interactions with the host epithelium. Cell Host Microbe. 2010;8(1):20–35.

21. Hampson DJ, Fu ZF, Bettleheim KA, Wilson MW. Managemental influences on the selective proliferation of two strains of haemolytic *Escherichia coli* in weaned pigs. Epidemiol Infect. 1988;100(2):213–20.

22. Fairbrother JM, Nadeau É, Gyles CL. *Escherichia coli* in postweaning diarrhea in pigs: an update on bacterial types, pathogenesis, and prevention strategies. Anim Health Res Rev. 2005;6:17–39.

23. Luppi A, Gibellini MV, Gin T, Vangroenweghe F, Vandenbroucke V, Bauerfeind R, et al. Prevalence of virulence factors in enterotoxigenic *Escherichia coli* isolated from pigs with post-weaning diarrhoea in Europe. Porcine Health Manag. 2016;2:20. doi:10.1186/s40813-016-0039-9.

24. Casey TA, Bosworth BT. Design and evaluation of a multiplex polymerase chain reaction assay for the simultaneous identification of genes for nine different virulence factors associated with *Escherichia coli* that cause diarrhea and edema disease in swine. J Vet Diagn Investig. 2009;21:25–30.

25. Vazquez-Marrufo G, Rosales-Castillo JA, Robinson-Fuentes VA, Tafolla-Munoz I, Carreras-Villase N, Vazquez-Garcidue MS. Multi-Typing of Enterobacteria Harboring LT and ST Enterotoxin Genes Isolated from Mexican Children. Jpn J Infect Dis. 2017;70:50–60.

26. Ouyang-Latimer J, Ajami NJ, Jiang ZD, Okhuysen PC, Paredes M, Flores J, et al. Biochemical and genetic diversity of enterotoxigenic *Escherichia coli* associated with diarrhea in United States students in Cuernavaca and Guadalajara, Mexico, 2004–2007. J Infect Dis. 2010;201:1831–8.

27. Ståhl M, Kokotovic B, Hjulsager CK, Breum SØ, Angen Ø. The use of quantitative PCR for identification and quantification of *Brachyspira pilosicoli*, *Lawsonia intracellularis* and *Escherichia coli* fimbrial types F4 and F18 in pig feces. Vet Microbiol. 2011;151:307–14.

28. Martelli P. Tabelle diagnosi differenziale. In: Martelli P, editor. "Le patologie del maiale". Point Veterinaire Italie Editor; 2013. p. 2–5.

29. Biwater RJ. Diarrhoea treatments, fluid replacement and alternatives. Ann Rech Vet. 1983;14(4):556–60.

30. Thomson J, Friendship RM. Digestive System. In: Zimmerman JJ, Karriker LA, Ramirez A, Schwartz KJ, Stevenson GW, editors. Disease of Swine. 10th ed; 2012. p. 199–226.

31. Roselli M, Finamore A, Garaguso I, Britti MS, Mengheri E. Zinc oxide protects cultured enterocytes from the damage induced by *Escherichia coli*. J Nutr. 2003;133(12):4077–82.

32. Yazdankhah S, Rudi K, Bernhoft A Zinc and copper in animal feed - development of resistance and co-resistance to antimicrobial agents in bacteria of animal origin. Microb Ecol Health Dis. 2014. doi: 10.3402/mehd.v25.25862.

33. Aarestrup FM, Oliver Duran C, Burch DG. Antimicrobial resistance in swine production. Anim Health Res Rev. 2008;9(2):135–48.

34. Vahjen W, Pietruszyńska D, Starke IC, Zentek J. High dietary zinc supplementation increases the occurrence of tetracycline and sulfonamide resistance genes in the intestine of weaned pigs. Gut Pathog. 2015;7:23.

35. CVMP opinions on veterinary medicinal products. Committee for Medicinal Products for Veterinary Use (CVMP) Meeting of 14–16 March 2017 EMA/CVMP/147249/2017. European Medicines Agency. Press release. http://www.ema.europa.eu/.

36. DGS B. Antimicrobial Drug use in swine. In: Giguère S, Prescott JF, Dowling PM, editors. Antimicrobial Therapy in Veterinary Medicine. Fifth ed; 2013. p. 553–68.

37. Burch DGS, Duran OC, Aarestrup FM. Guidlines for antimicrobial use of in swine. In: Guardabassi L, Jensen LB, Kruse H, editors. Guide to Antimicrobial Use in Animals. Oxford: Blackwell; 2008. p. 102–24.

38. COMMISSION NOTICE. Guidelines for the prudent use of antimicrobials in veterinary medicine (2015/C 299/04). Off J Eur Union. Available at http://www.ema.europa.eu/docs/en_GB/document_library/Report/2009/11/WC500008770.pdf

39. Martinez MN, Toutain PL, Turnidge J. The Pharmacodynamics of Antimicrobial Agents. In: Giguère S, Prescott JF, Dowling PM, editors. Antimicrobial Therapy in Veterinary Medicine. Fifth ed; 2013. p. 79–104.

40. Page SW, Gautier P. Use of antimicrobial agents in livestock. Rev Sci Tech Off Int Epiz. 2012;31(1):145–88.

41. Ahmad I, Huang L, Hao H, Sanders P, Yuan Z. Application of PK/PD Modeling in Veterinary Field: Dose Optimization and Drug Resistance Prediction. BioMed Res Int. 2016. http://dx.doi.org/10.1155/2016/5465678

42. Prescott JF. Beta-lactam Antibiotics: Penam Penicillins. In: Giguère S, Prescott JF, Dowling PM, editors. Antimicrobial Therapy in Veterinary Medicine. Fifth ed; 2013. p. 135–52.

43. Prescott JF. Beta-lactam Antibiotics: Beta-lactamase Inhibitors, Carbapenems, and Monobactams. In: Giguère S, Prescott JF, Dowling PM, editors. Antimicrobial Therapy in Veterinary Medicine. Fifth ed; 2013. p. 175–88.

44. Prescott JF. Beta-lactam Antibiotics: Cephalosporins. In: Giguère S, Prescott JF, Dowling PM, editors. Antimicrobial Therapy in Veterinary Medicine. Fifth ed; 2013. p. 153–74.

45. Rice LB. Mechanisms of Resistance and Clinical Relevance of Resistance to ß-Lactams, Glycopeptides, and Fluoroquinolones. Mayo Clin Proc. 2012;87(2):198–208.

46. Prescott JF. Sulfonamides, Diaminopyrimidines, and Their Combinations. In: Giguère S, Prescott JF, Dowling PM, editors. Antimicrobial Therapy in Veterinary Medicine. Fifth ed; 2013. p. 279–94.

47. Dowling PM. Aminoglycosides and Aminocyclitols. In: Giguère S, Prescott JF, Dowling PM, editors. Antimicrobial Therapy in Veterinary Medicine. Fifth ed; 2013. p. 233–56.

48. Giguère S, Dowling PM. Fluoroquinolones. In: Giguère S, Prescott JF, Dowling PM, editors. Antimicrobial Therapy in Veterinary Medicine. Fifth ed; 2013. p. 295–314.

49. Rhouma M, Beaudry F, Letellier A. Resistance to colistin: what is the fate for this antibiotic in pig production? Int J Antimicrb Agents. 2016;48(2):119–26.

50. European Medicines Agency: Updated advice on the use of colistin products in animals within the European Union: development of resistance and possible impact on human and animal health. 2016. http://www.ema.europa.eu/docs/en_GB/document_library/Scientific_guideline/2016/07/WC500211080.pdf

51. Kempf I, Fleury MA, Drider D, Bruneau M, Sanders P, Chauvin C, et al. What do we know about resistance to colistin in Enterobacteriaceae in avian and pig production in Europe? Int J Antimicrob Agents. 2013;42(5):379–83.

52. Luppi A, Bonilauri P, Dottori M, Gherpelli Y, Biasi G, Merialdi G, et al. Antimicrobial resistance of F4+ *Escherichia coli* isolated from Swine in Italy. Transbound Emerg Dis. 2015;62(1):67–71.

53. Costa MM, Drescher G, Maboni F, Weber SS, Schrank A, Vainstein MH, et al. Virulence factors, antimicrobial resi stance, and plasmid content of *Escherichia coli* isolated in swine commercial farms. Arg Bras Med Vet Zootec. 2010;62(1):30–6.

54. Barton MD. Impact of antibiotic use in the swine industry. Curr Opin Microbiol. 2014;19:9–15.

55. Jensen VF, Jakobsen L, Emborg HD, et al. Correlation between apramycin and gentamicin use in pigs and an increasing reservoir of gentamicin-resistant *Escherichia coli*. J Antimicrob Chemother. 2006;58:101–7.

56. Smith MG, Jordan D, Chapman TA, Chin JJ, Barton MD, Do TN, et al. Antimicrobial resistance and virulence gene profiles in multi-drug resistant enterotoxigenic *Escherichia coli* isolated from pigs with post-weaning diarrhoea. Vet Microbiol. 2010;145(3–4):299–307.

57. Lee SI, Rayamahji N, Lee WJ, Cha SB, Shin MK, Roh YM, et al. Genotypes, antibiogram, and pulsed-field gel electrophoresis profiles of *Escherichia coli* strains from piglets in Korea. J Vet Diagn Investig. 2009;21(4):510–6.

58. Liu YY, Wang Y, Walsh TR, Yi LX, Zhang R, Spencer J, et al. Emergence of plasmid-mediated colistin resistance mechanism MCR-1 in animals and human beings in China: a microbiological and molecular biological study. Lancet Infect Dis. 2016;16(2):161–8.

59. Malik YS, Chander Y, Olsen K, Goyal SM. Antimicrobial resistance in enteric pathogens isolated from Minnesota pigs from 1995 to 2004. Can J Vet Res. 2011;75(2):117–21.

60. Jiang HX, Lü DH, Chen ZL, Wang XM, Chen JR, Liu YH, et al. High prevalence and widespread distribution of multi-resistant *Escherichia coli* isolates in pigs and poultry in China. Vet J. 2011;187(1):99–103.

61. Mazurek J, Bok E, Stosik M, Baldy-Chudzik K. Antimicrobial resistance in commensal *Escherichia coli* from pigs during metaphylactic trimethoprim and sulfamethoxazole treatment and in the post-exposure period. Int J Environ Res Public Health. 2015;12(2):2150–63.

62. Belloc C, Nam Lam D, Laval A. Low occurrence of colistin-resistant *Escherichia coli* in faecal content of pigs in French commercial herds. Revuede Med Vet. 2008;159:634–7.

63. Statens Veterinärmedicinska Anstalt (SVA). SVARM 2010. Swedish veterinary antimicrobial resistance monitoring. SVA. 2011. http://www.sva.se/globalassets/redesign2011/pdf/om_sva/publikationer/trycksaker/svarm2010.pdf.

64. Statens Serum Institut; Danish Veterinary and Food Administration; DanishMedicines Agency; National Veterinary Institute; Technical University of Denmark; National Food Institute. DANMAP 2009—Use of antimicrobial agents and occurrence of antimicrobial resistance in bacteria from food animals, foods and humans in Denmark. 2010. http://orbit.dtu.dk/files/6329669/Danmap+2010.pdf.

65. Boyen F, Vangroenweghe F, Butaye P, De Graef E, Castryck F, Heylen P, et al. Disk prediffusion is a reliable method for testing colistin susceptibility in porcine E. coli strains. Vet Microbiol. 2010;144(3–4):359–62.

66. Habrun B, Dragica S, Kompes G, Benic M. Antimicrobial susceptibility of entero-toxigenic strains of Escherichia coli isolated from weaned pigs in Croatia. Acta Vet. 2011;61:585–90.

67. Enne VI, Cassar C, Sprigings K, Woodward MJ, Bennett PM. A high prevalence of antimicrobial resistant Escherichia coli isolated from pigs and a low preva-lence of antimicrobial resistant E. coli from cattle and sheep in Great Britain at slaughter. FEMS Microbiol Lett. 2008;278:193–9.

68. Lu L, Dai L, Wang Y, Wu C, Chen X, Li L, et al. Characterization of antimicrobial resistance and integrons among Escherichia coli isolated from animal farms in Eastern China. Acta Trop. 2010;113:20–5.

14

Comparison of the antimicrobial consumption in weaning pigs in Danish sow herds with different vaccine purchase patterns during 2013

Carolina Temtem[1], Amanda Brinch Kruse[2], Liza Rosenbaum Nielsen[2], Ken Steen Pedersen[3] and Lis Alban[3*]

Abstract

Background: There is growing concern about development of antimicrobial resistance due to use of antimicrobials (AMs) in livestock production. Identifying efficient alternatives, including vaccination, is a priority. The objective of this study was to compare the herd-level amount of AMs prescribed for weaner pigs, between Danish sow herds using varying combinations of vaccines against Porcine Circovirus Type 2 (PCV2), *Mycoplasma hyopneumoniae* (MYC) and *Lawsonia intracellularis* (LAW). It was hypothesised that herds purchasing vaccines, use these to prevent disease, and hence reduce their AM consumption, compared to herds purchasing fewer or no vaccines against these pathogens.

Data summarised over year 2013 were obtained from the Danish Central Husbandry Register and the Danish VetStat database, in which prescriptions of medication are recorded. All one-site indoor pig herds with >50 sows and >200 weaners were selected. AMs prescribed for weaners was measured in animal daily doses (ADD) and divided according to three indication groups (gastro-intestinal, respiratory indication or total use). The analysis was based on three multivariable linear regression models of the herd-level ADD for each indication group. The eight vaccination combinations (2x2x2) were included as one explanatory variable, and herd size, measured as the number of weaner pen places was included in the models as a potential confounder.

Results: Out of the 1513 herds in the study, 1415 had AMs prescribed for gastro-intestinal disorders, and 836 for respiratory disorders. PCV2 vaccines were purchased in 880 herds, MYC vaccines in 787 and LAW vaccines in 115 herds. Herds purchasing PCV2 and MYC vaccines had significantly more AMs prescribed than herds not purchasing vaccines or only purchasing LAW vaccines.

Conclusion: In the present study, using register data covering 1 year, we found an association between use of vaccination and increased amount of AMs prescribed for weaners. This does not exclude that the vaccines work, just that we were unable to detect this. The findings might be explained by some herds experiencing clinical problems associated with MYC or PCV2 despite use of vaccination. In other herds, it might reflect that vaccines applied to weaners are used for disease prevention in finishers rather than in the weaners. Information about vaccination protocols and herd health status was not available at the time of the study. Hence, further studies are required to investigate causality of the associations between use of AMs, vaccination practices and other confounding on-farm factors.

Keywords: Antimicrobial consumption, Alternatives, Vaccination, Pigs, VetStat, Denmark

* Correspondence: lia@lf.dk
[3]Danish Agriculture & Food Council, Axeltorv 3, Copenhagen V DK-1609, Denmark
Full list of author information is available at the end of the article

Background

In Denmark, there has been political and public focus on the use of antimicrobials (AMs) in livestock and the risk of development of AM resistance since the 1990s. Focus is in particularly on the Danish pig industry, because it is the largest livestock industry in Denmark; around 28 million pigs are produced annually, and around 10 million of these are exported as weaners [1]. As a result, a series of events emerged in and around the pig industry: (a) in 1995, the veterinary profit from sales of AMs was officially limited to 5-10 % [2]; (b) in 1998, an industry initiative leading to the phasing out of growth promoters was introduced for finishing pigs, and this was expanded to weaners in 1999 (effective from January 1, 2000) [3] (c) increased surveillance and regulation of veterinary practice and prescriptions was undertaken [4], as well as (d) recommendations and guidelines for prudent use of AMs were developed. Moreover, in 2010, an industry-driven ban was implemented to stop the use of cephalosporins in pigs produced in Denmark [1].

To support the Danish policy, data regarding medical consumption for production animals are collected in a national database called VetStat established mid-2000 [5]. VetStat collects prescription records from pharmacies, feed mills and veterinary practitioners [5]. A prescription record includes information about the type, concentration and amount of AMs, the treatment indication, the age group, the individual herd number, the date of issue, the name of the veterinarian prescribing, and the name of the producer [5].

Between 2008 and the first half of 2010, the AM consumption in pigs increased, leading to a public debate [1]. Consequently, in 2010 the Danish veterinary authorities adopted the "Yellow Card" initiative, a scheme that sets permit limits to AM use in swine herds [1]. Until June 2013, the Yellow Card permit limit for weaners was 28 ADD per 100 weaners per day. Thereafter, the permit limit was reduced to 25 ADD per 100 animal days [1] and www.foedevarestyrelsen.dk. By November 2014, the permit limits were further reduced to 22.9 ADD per 100 weaners per day (Please see www.foedevarestyrelsen.dk for further updates).

The introduction of the Yellow Card scheme reflected the political pressure that is forcing Danish pig producers to reduce the usage of AMs on their farms. Therefore, efficient alternatives to routinely applied AMs have become crucial.

Vaccines are being considered a potential tool to decrease the burden of animal diseases and also to reduce the need for AMs with therapeutic purposes [6, 7].

According to data from VetStat, the three most commonly used vaccines in Danish pig production is against *Mycoplasma hyopneumoniae* (MYC) (36 %),

Porcine Circovirus Type 2 (PCV2) (26 %), and *Actinobacillus pleuropneumoniae* (APP) (8 %), whereas only 3 % of the vaccine doses were prescribed for *Lawsonia intracellularis* (LAW) and only 2 % for Porcine Reproductive and Respiratory Syndrome (PRRS). These endemic disease agents are representing common production-related diseases in weaners and finishers in modern pig production. We decided to focus on the effect of MYC, PCV2 and LAW. We included MYC and PCV2 because they are the most commonly used vaccines, and we included LAW to have a vaccine with an effect on gastro-intestinal lesions. We excluded PRRS for two reasons: 1) low use and 2) apparently, in Denmark PRRS vaccines are used more commonly in breeding animals than in weaners.

PCV2 has a causal role in a large number of clinical syndromes, which are collectively named as Porcine Circovirus Diseases (PCVDs) and is highly prevalent worldwide [8]. The most economically significant condition within PCVDs is post-weaning multi-systemic wasting syndrome (PMWS) [8]. However, PCV2 can also play a role in the occurrence of reproductive failure, enteritis, porcine dermatitis and nephropathy syndrome and proliferative necrotizing pneumonia [9]. Furthermore, when there is an interaction between bacterial and viral agents, the syndrome is called porcine respiratory disease complex (PRDC) [10].

MYC is the primary agent responsible for swine enzootic pneumonia, which is a chronic respiratory disease that causes significant economic losses worldwide and is highly prevalent in most areas of pig production (present in between 38 to 100 % of the pig farms world-wide) [9]. MYC predisposes the infected animals to secondary infections, which can increase the severity of the disease for example seen as PRDC [9].

LAW is the causative bacterium of proliferative enteropathy, and it is a common high prevalence intestinal infection worldwide including Denmark [11]. This has a direct impact on pig production and herd economics as it affects growing pig performance due to the decrease in growth rates and feed conversion in some herds [12, 13].

PCV2, MYC and LAW can be controlled and prevented by different interventions. In Denmark, these include all in/all out production, multisite production, increased hygiene, antibiotic medication and use of vaccination. In Denmark, these vaccines have been used as an alternative to antibiotic medication and to increase productivity in weaners and finishers. The use of these vaccines has increased substantially since 2010. This was observed in particular right after the introduction of the Yellow Card, e.g. the use of vaccines against PCV2 infections increased by 31 % [1].

To explore the potential of using vaccination as an alternative to AMs, the present study was carried out using data from VetStat and the Danish Central Husbandry Register (CHR) from all one-site pig herds with >50 sows and >200 weaners in the year 2013. The objective was to compare the total amount of AMs prescribed for weaning pigs between Danish sow herds using varying combinations of vaccines against PCV2, MYC and LAW that year. It was assumed that year 2013 represented a steady-state in the use of vaccines and AMs. Hence, bias caused by confounding factors related to dynamics in overall health and production conditions including changes in legislation and market forces could be avoided. It was also assumed that the AMs and vaccines prescribed were used in the herd.

Results
Basic statistics
The median number of sows in the 1513 herds was 435 and the maximum was 3100 sows. For weaners, the median number of pen places was 1500 whereas the maximum was 21,000. Around half (52 %) of the herds also had production of finishing pigs on the same premises.

Out of the 1513 herds selected for the study, 1415 herds had AMs prescribed for gastrointestinal disorders in weaners, and 836 herds had AMs prescribed for respiratory disorders, corresponding to 94 and 55 % of the herds, respectively. There were no herds with no AMs prescribed.

With respect to total AM consumption (AC-TOTAL), the median use was 10.0 ADD per 100 weaners per day (Min: 0.004; Max: 79.33). The herd-level distribution of the total AM consumption was not normal but positively skewed with 58 herds corresponding to 4 % having AM consumption above 28 ADD per 100 weaners per day, which was the initial Yellow Card threshold.

The main part (67 %) of the AM consumption for weaners was prescribed for gastro-intestinal disorders. The overall median was 6.9 ADD per 100 weaners per day (Min: 0.02; Max: 67.16). The herd-level distribution of AM consumption with gastro-intestinal indication (AC-GI) was not normal, but positively skewed with 20 herds having AM consumption above 28 ADD per 100 weaners per day.

The median AM consumption with respiratory indication (AC-RESP) was 2.5 ADD per 100 weaners per day (Min: 0.01; Max: 56.20). The herd-level distribution of AM consumption with respiratory indication was not normal; and 17 of the herds had AM consumption above 28 ADD per 100 weaners per day.

Concerning the vaccines, 58 % ($n = 880$) of the herds purchased PCV2 vaccines in 2013. MYC vaccination was purchased in 52 % ($n = 787$) of the herds, and LAW vaccination was the least used vaccine, with just 8 % ($n = 115$) of the herds having at least one registered purchase of Enterisol®Ileitis. A total of 380 herds did

not have any of these three vaccines prescribed in 2013 (Table 1).

Results of multivariable analyses
With respect to total AM consumption (Table 1), the variable herd size and the variable representing vaccine use were both statistically significant ($P < 0.0001$). Some degree of confounding between herd size and the vaccine use variable was observed but only for the parameter describing use of PCV2 and LAW ($n = 35$ herds). The interaction between herd size and vaccine use was non-significant ($P = 0.48$). A model with vaccine use and herd size only explained 7 % of the variance in the total AM consumption ($R^2 = 0.07$, $F = 12.2$, $P < 0.001$). The highest use was observed in Group 4 (10.3 ADD/100 weaners/day), representing use of MYC and PCV2 vaccination, whereas the lowest consumption was observed in Group 6 (6.0 ADD/100 weaners/day), representing use of MYC and LAW vaccination. Group 1, 2, and 4, representing three different combinations of use of MYC and PCV2 vaccination, were all associated with a statistically higher AM consumption than the use of no vaccine at all (group 0); between 1.8 and 3.7 higher ADD per 100 weaners per day compared with group 0. The remaining vaccine combination groups were not associated with statistically different levels of AM consumption compared to the group not using any of the three vaccines ($P > 0.05$). Smaller herds had a significantly lower total AM consumption than medium-sized herds (6.6 versus 8.0 ADD/100 weaners/day), which again had a significantly lower consumption than large herds where the mean AM consumption was 9.2 ADD/100 weaners/day (Table 1).

Regarding AM consumption for gastro-intestinal indication (Table 2), only herd size was statistically significant ($P = 0.02$). Some degree of confounding between herd size and the vaccine use variable was observed but only for the parameter related to the group using LAW vaccine alone ($n = 21$ herds). The variable describing the vaccine use had a P-value of 0.2, and the interaction term between herd size and vaccine use had a P-value of 0.37. A model including vaccine use and production size only explained 0.6 % of the variance in the AM consumption ($R^2 = 0.006$, $F = 2.0$, $P = 0.03$) (Table 2). Large herds had significantly higher AM consumption than small herds (6.8 versus 5.7 ADD/100 weaners/day), whereas the AM consumption in medium-sized herds were in between. A detailed look into Table 2 shows that the lowest AM consumption was observed in Group 0, 2, 3 and 6 (5.7–6.0 ADD/100 weaners/day) and the highest use in Group 5 (7.0 ADD/100 weaners/day).

In relation to the AC with respiratory indication (Table 3), herd size was non-significant ($P = 0.06$) but some confounding between herd size and vaccine use

Table 1 Final multivariable model* of the associations between the use of vaccines and total consumption of antimicrobials (AC-TOTAL) measured as Animal Daily Doses (ADD) per 100 weaners per day in 1513 Danish sow herds after controlling for production size, 2013. Group 0 (no vaccination) and small herd size were used as reference classes

Variables and classes	AC-TOTAL (ADD/100 weaners/day)			Converted AC-TOTAL (ADD/100 weaners/day)		
	Estimate of square root-transformed outcome	Standard error	P-value	Mean estimate	Lower 95 % CI	Upper 95 % CI
Intercept	2.573	0.0732	<0.0001	6.6	5.9	7.4
Combinations of vaccines			<0.0001			
Group 0: PCV2 = 0 & MYC = 0 & LAW = 0 (n = 380)[a]	0.000	n.a.		6.6	n.a.	n.a.
Group 1: PCV2 = 1 & MYC = 0 & LAW = 0 (n = 290)[b,d]	0.324	0.096		8.4	7.3	9.5
Group 2: PCV2 = 0 & MYC = 1 & LAW = 0 (n = 221)[b,c,d]	0.433	0.103		9.0	7.9	10.3
Group 3: PCV2 = 0 & MYC = 0 & LAW = 1 (n = 21)[a,b,c,d]	0.192	0.274		7.6	5.0	10.9
Group 4: PCV2 = 1 & MYC = 1 & LAW = 0 (n = 507)[c,d]	0.635	0.084		10.3	9.3	11.4
Group 5: PCV2 = 1 & MYC = 0 & LAW = 1 n = 35)[a,d]	0.083	0.216		7.1	5.0	9.5
Group 6: PCV2 = 0 & MYC = 1 & LAW = 1 (n = 11)[a,b,c,d]	−0.118	0.374		6.0	3.0	10.2
Group 7: PCV2 = 1 & MYC = 1 & LAW = 1 (n = 48)[a,b,c,d]	0.202	0.188		7.7	5.8	9.9
Herd size (number of weaner pen places)			<0.0001			
Small (n = 528)[a]	0.000	n.a.		6.6	n.a.	n.a.
Medium (n = 607)[b]	0.264	0.073		8.0	7.3	8.9
Large (n = 378)[c]	0.459	0.083		9.2	8.2	10.2

n.a. not applicable, *PCV2* Porcine Circovirus Type 2, *MYC* Mycoplasma hyopneumoniae, *LAW* Lawsonia intracellularis
[a, b, c, d] – different letters indicate variable classes with significantly different parameter estimates of antimicrobial consumption according to an F-test
*Model statistics: $R^2 = 0.07$, $F = 12.2$, $P < 0.001$

Table 2 Final multivariable model* of the associations between use of vaccines and consumption of antimicrobials with gastro-intestinal indications (AC-GI) in 1415 Danish sow herds after controlling for production size, 2013. Group 0 (no vaccination) and small herd size were used as reference classes

Variables and classes	AC-GI (ADD/100 weaners/day)			Converted AC-GI (ADD/100 weaners/day)		
	Estimate of square root-transformed outcome	Standard error	P-value	Mean estimate	Lower 95 % CI	Upper 95 % CI
Intercept	2.384	0.076	<0.0001	5.7	5.0	6.4
Combinations of vaccines			0.2			
Group 0: PCV2 = 0 & MYC = 0 & LAW = 0 (n = 351)	0.000	n.a.		5.7	n.a.	n.a.
Group 1: PCV2 = 1 & MYC = 0 & LAW = 0 (n = 277)	0.145	0.097		6.4	5.5	7.4
Group 2: PCV2 = 0 & MYC = 1 & LAW = 0 (n = 204)	−0.004	0.106		5.7	4.7	6.7
Group 3: PCV2 = 0 & MYC = 0 & LAW = 1 (n = 21)	0.021	0.270		5.8	3.5	8.6
Group 4: PCV2 = 1 & MYC = 1 & LAW = 0 (n = 476)	0.183	0.085		6.6	5.8	7.5
Group 5: PCV2 = 1 & MYC = 0 & LAW = 1 (n = 32)	0.258	0.222		7.0	4.9	9.5
Group 6: PCV2 = 0 & MYC = 1 & LAW = 1 (n = 9)	0.058	0.405		6.0	2.7	10.5
Group 7: PCV2 = 1 & MYC = 1 & LAW = 1 (n = 45)	−0.026	0.190		5.6	3.9	7.5
Herd size (number of weaners pen places)			0.02			
Small (n = 468)[a]	0.000	n.a.		5.7	n.a.	n.a.
Medium (n = 585)[a,b]	0.151	0.075		6.4	5.7	7.2
Large (n = 362)[b]	0.227	0.085		6.8	6.0	7.7

n.a. not applicable, *PCV2* Porcine Circovirus Type 2, *MYC* Mycoplasma hyopneumoniae, *LAW* Lawsonia intracellularis
[a, b] – different letters indicate variable classes with significantly different parameter estimates of antimicrobial consumption according to an F-test
*Model statistics: $R^2 = 0.006$, $F = 2.0$, $P = 0.03$

Table 3 Final multivariable model* of the associations between use of vaccines and consumption of antimicrobials with respiratory indications (AC-RESP) in 836 Danish sow herds after controlling for production size, 2013. Group 0 (no vaccination) and small herd size were used as reference classes

Variables and classes	AC-RESP (ADD/100 weaners/day)			Converted AC-RESP (ADD/100 weaners/day)		
	Estimate of log-transformed outcome	Standard error	P-value	Mean estimate	Lower 95 % CI	Upper 95 % CI
Intercept	0.497	0.145	<0.0001	1.6	1.2	2.2
Combinations of vaccines			<0.0001			
Group 0: PCV2 = 0 & MYC = 0 & LAW = 0 (n = 155)[a,c]	0.000	n.a.		1.6	n.a.	n.a.
Group 1: PCV2 = 1 & MYC = 0 & LAW = 0 (n = 136)[a]	0.404	0.177		2.5	1.7	3.5
Group 2: PCV2 = 0 & MYC = 1 & LAW = 0 (n = 134)[b]	0.648	0.177		3.1	2.2	4.4
Group 3: PCV2 = 0 & MYC = 0 & LAW = 1 (n = 10)[a,c]	0.160	0.490		1.9	0.7	5.0
Group 4: PCV2 = 1 & MYC = 1 & LAW = 0 (n = 349)[b]	0.672	0.146		3.2	2.4	4.3
Group 5: PCV2 = 1 & MYC = 0 & LAW = 1 (n = 13)[c]	−0.994	0.434		0.6	0.3	1.4
Group 6: PCV2 = 0 & MYC = 1 & LAW = 1 (n = 6)[a,b,c]	−0.166	0.626		1.4	0.4	4.7
Group 7: PCV2 = 1 & MYC = 1 & LAW = 1 (n = 33)[a,b,c]	0.220	0.289		2.0	1.2	3.6
Herd size (number of weaners pen places)			0.06			
Small (n = 235)	0.000	n.a.		1.6	n.a.	n.a.
Medium (n = 331)	−0.261	0.129		1.3	1.0	1.6
Large (n = 270)	−0.295	0.136		1.2	0.9	1.6

n.a. not applicable, PCV2 Porcine Circovirus Type 2, MYC Mycoplasma hyopneumoniae, LAW Lawsonia intracellularis
a, b, c – different letters indicate variable classes with significantly different parameter estimates of antimicrobial consumption according to an F-test
*Model statistics: $R^2 = 0.04$, $F = 4.8$, $P = 0.001$

was observed for two of the parameter estimates of the vaccine variable (use of LAW vaccine alone: 10 herds; use of MYC and LAW vaccines: 6 herds). The interaction term between herd size and vaccine use was non-significant ($P = 0.80$), whereas the variable describing vaccine use was statistical significant ($P < 0.0001$), but it only explained 4 % of the variance in the AM consumption ($R^2 = 0.04$, $F = 4.8$, $P = 0.001$). The lowest AM consumption was observed in Group 5, representing the use of PCV2 and LAW vaccination (0.6 ADD/100 weaners/day). However, this was not significantly different from Group 0, statistically speaking (1.6 ADD/100 weaners/day). Group 2 and 4 representing use of MYC vaccination with and without concurrent use of PCV2 vaccination were associated with a statistically higher AM consumption than the use of no vaccines (Group 0) – 3.1 and 3.2 versus 1.6 ADD/100 weaners/day. The changes in AM consumption associated with the rest of the combinations were not statistically significant ($P > 0.05$).

Discussion

General discussion

Almost all herds (96 %) had a total AM consumption lower than 28 ADD per 100 weaners per day This implies that the majority of the producers were able to raise weaners while fulfilling the requirements regarding AM consumption set by the Danish veterinary authorities.

The statistical analyses showed that in general the pig herds using vaccines against MYC, PCV2 and LAW had a higher – and not as hypothesised a lower AM consumption – in the weaning stage compared to not using vaccination at all. This is in line with results presented by Potsma et al. (2016) [14]. This may be explained by some herds experiencing clinical problems associated in particular with MYC or PCV2 despite use of vaccination. The herds not applying vaccination are probably herds with a high health status, where these three infections are not present – or at least not causing clinical problems. In other herds, the lack of impact of vaccination on the AM consumption in weaners might reflect that vaccines are used for disease prevention in finishers rather than in the weaners as pointed out by Raidt et al. [15]. Alternatively, other infections may be present which we could not adjust for in the statistical analyses. Moreover, in Denmark much has already been done to lower the antimicrobial consumption; latest with the Yellow Card scheme setting limitations to the consumption in an age group such as the weaners as described above. Finally, the lack of effect of the vaccine combinations on the AM with gastro-intestinal indication may be explained by the fact that only the LAW vaccine has a direct impact on gastro-intestinal infections.

Effect of PCV2 vaccination

Control of PCV2-related diseases has traditionally been based on preventive measures such as: (1) improved management practices in order to control risks or triggering factors, (2) control of concurrent infections and (3) changes of the boar genetic background [8]. Currently, disease control is mainly based on vaccination, which has been shown to be very effective in reducing viraemia, improving production parameters (e.g. reducing mortality and increasing average daily weight gain) and the probability of co-infection by other pathogens [16–18].

In the present study, herds using PCV2 vaccination had a statistically significantly higher total AM consumption and AM consumption with respiratory indication compared to herds not using the vaccines – except from the case when LAW vaccination was applied as well (Table 1). This is contrary to results presented by Raidt et al. [15] who followed the consumption of antimicrobials in 65 Austrian swine herds after the first licensing of the PCV2 in Austria. The Danish results can probably be explained by reverse causality hereby pointing to PCV2's presence in the herds and its ability to cause disease. Moreover, as explained above, there may be an effect of vaccination on the finishers as shown by [15].

As described above, PCV2 has been linked with various clinical syndromes in different organs. This might justify the application of a major amount of AMs [19, 20]. PCV2 can be considered a necessary but not sufficient factor to develop clinical disease [17]. Therefore, farmers and practitioners could very well have decided to routinely use PCV2 vaccination in these herds to avoid this predisposing factor and consequently, the occurrence of PCVDs.

Effect of MYC vaccination

Use of vaccination against MYC has been shown to be associated with reduced clinical signs, fewer treatment costs and with increased average daily weight gain [21, 22]. Vaccination is therefore considered the most adequate measure for controlling MYC infection in practice [23]. Vaccination is performed in piglets, weaners and to a smaller extent in grower-finishing pigs. Vaccination of piglets during lactation is the most common. Vaccination of replacement gilts and sows is also performed in some herds.

According to the results of the multivariable analysis, on average herds using MYC vaccination had a higher total AM consumption and AM consumption with respiratory indication than herds not using the vaccines. This finding may be explained by reverse causality: herds using the vaccines were likely infected with this pathogen – some with clinical problems. Subsequently, these herds were using AMs with respiratory indication to control MYC and, simultaneously using the vaccines to avoid the predisposition of the infected animals to secondary invaders, especially other pulmonary pathogens [9]. Other herds neither vaccinated nor treated, presumably because they were not infected with MYC.

Effect of LAW vaccination

In 2013, only one vaccine was available in Denmark against proliferative enteropathy caused by LAW. It is used for piglets in the last part of lactation or (more commonly) in the first week post weaning. The positive effect of the LAW vaccine has been shown by Bak & Rathkjen, who undertook a study in a Danish Specific Pathogen Free herd [12]. Here, proliferative enteropathy was prevented by use of the vaccination and improved growth rate and a reduction in the use of AMs was observed after initiation of vaccination. However, the positive effect may be more limited in non-SPF herds due to presence of other infections. But Thaker & Bilkei (2006) also concluded that vaccination reduced LAW-associated losses as well as improved health and the immune state of pigs in highly infected herd [24].

As LAW vaccination is used to prevent proliferative enteropathy [12], it would be expected that herds using the vaccination would have been associated with a lower AM consumption with gastrointestinal indication – or lower total AM consumption. However, there was no statistically significant effect of the vaccine on AM consumption in the weaner section (neither the total AM consumption, nor the consumption with a gastrointestinal indication or respiratory indication). There were some indications that use of LAW vaccination was associated with a lower AM consumption with respiratory indication – but the findings were not statistical significant (Table 3). This may be because LAW vaccine has no effect on respiratory disease. However, to some extent AMs are being used for other disease categories than those officially prescribed for. Certain AMs, as for example some doxycyclines, are not officially registered for treating infections with gastro-intestinal indication in Denmark, although they are known to be effective in everyday practice. This may result in recordings indicating that these AM were used for respiratory indication although the aim was to treat gastro-intestinal infections.

Considerations, limitations and further work for the study

We assumed that the AM and vaccines prescribed in a herd were also used in the same herd. For some countries there may be a difference between prescription and use. However, for Denmark it is the general belief that VetStat data (consisting of prescription data) approximate AM use closely over a longer period of time. One reason is that it is the only legal way to get AM for livestock in Denmark. This was underpinned by a recent report from the Danish veterinary authorities stating that there are no indications of a systematic illegal import of AMs [25].

On average, 36 % of the total amount of AMs used for the production of a pig until slaughter is used during the weaning period [26] although weaners only cover the production from 7 to 30 kg, which corresponds to around

4 weeks. This reflects that the treatment incidence is much higher in weaners compared with finishers and sows [24]. This is one of the reasons why the present study focused on the AM consumption for weaners. However, it would also be of interest to study the effect of vaccination in the sow herd on the consumption of AM in the finishing section. On the other hand, according to Potsma et al. [14] a higher AM consumption in sows tended to be associated with higher AM consumption from birth until slaughter, and that it was positively associated with the number of pathogens vaccinated against.

The multivariable models presented in Tables 1, 2 and 3 only explained a limited amount of the variation in the data. This shows that many other factors – apart from vaccination – determine the need for AM in a given pig herd. Information about such factors was not available at the time of the study e.g. regarding (1) vaccination protocols applied including age of pigs at time of vaccination (2) initiation and duration of vaccination (3) use of other vaccines that were part of the general vaccination program (4) herd health status including presence of other infections, (5) internal and external biosecurity (6) management practices (7) turnover of animals in each herd (8) export of live animals (where vaccination may be required by the customer). If this information had been available, we would probably have been capable of explaining a larger degree of the variation in the data.

In this study, we focused on MYC, PCV2 and LAW. One reason for only including these three vaccines in the analysis was to avoid that the number of herds representing different combinations of vaccine use would become very low, because this would result in unstable parameter estimates. We did not take into account PRRS vaccination. Although this vaccine only represents 2 % of the vaccines prescribed for pigs in Denmark, it could have been a confounder in the analyses, and it would therefore be of interest to include this in a subsequent analysis. Similarly, it would have been of interest to include also vaccines with an effect on APP. However, this was not done in this analysis due to the limited use (8 % of the prescribed vaccine doses prescribed to Danish swine). It is also possible that vaccination of breeding animals for E. coli to prevent E. coli associated neonatal diarrhea in piglets, could result in higher piglet health at weaning and therefore also affect the medical consumption post weaning. But the contrary is also possible; that herds applying the vaccine do this because they have clinical problems with neonatal diarrhea infections requiring antimicrobial treatment despite the use of vaccination.

This study was a first basic approach to using register data and a cross-sectional design to describe the possible association between vaccinations and AM use in pig herds in Denmark. The vaccine data from VetStat have to the authors' knowledge not been used in analysis of AM use before. It is not possible to elucidate the directions of these associations. A longitudinal study will enable a better understanding of cause and effect and be able to take into account other factors than just vaccination.

More information is needed to assess to which extent vaccinations – and other preventive measures - can in fact reduce the need for the use of AMs. The feasibility of using vaccination as a an alternative to AMs will depend on proper disease diagnostics, the costs of vaccines compared to AM, effectiveness and ease of use [6]. If in the future we get an affirmative answer to this question and farmers can see return on their investment, improvement of pig health and productivity will occur through a wider application of routine vaccination instead of routine AM treatments.

Conclusions

In general, the sow herds applying MYC and PCV2 vaccination had more AMs prescribed for weaners compared to sow herds not using the three studied vaccines – probably as a result of existing health problems in the herds prior to and/or during the use of vaccination. For LAW vaccine there was a trend towards lower or equal amount of prescribed AMs compared to herds not purchasing any of the three vaccines. These results suggest that vaccination alone does not necessarily come along with a low use of AMs, despite being an asset in many regards.

Each herd has its own challenges and several issues need to be taken into account when it concerns alternatives to AM consumption. Further studies need to be carried out to take into consideration other factors regarding prevention of disease, which are of extreme importance, such as biosecurity and management practices within the herds.

Methods
Data
The data used in this study were obtained from two sources. The first was the VetStat database, which contains information about all prescriptions of AM vaccines destined for livestock. VetStat quantifies the AM prescriptions in food animal using the unit animal daily dose (ADD), which is defined as the average maintenance dose per kg live animal for the main indication of an AM in a specified species [27]. This measure takes into account the different potency of the various AM classes. To correct for the large variation in the weight of weaners, the official standard estimate of 15 kg was applied [27, 28].

The second source of data was the Danish CHR register, which contains information about location and size of all livestock herds. All pig herds were selected for the study, if they fulfilled the following inclusion criteria: a) one-site indoor herds b) herds with more than 50 sows and c) herds with more than 200 weaners. In total 1518 herds met these three criteria, and data regarding the prescription of AMs for weaners as well as the number of vaccine doses purchased in 2013 were obtained for each of these herds from VetStat.

Five herds had erroneous (e.g. negative values of recorded AM or vaccine use) or missing data records. All cases were most likely caused by an error in VetStat. As all the herds in the dataset were anonymised, it was not possible to assess the reasons for these data errors. Consequently, these five herds were excluded from the analysis.

For each of the remaining 1513 herds, a variable was created to estimate the average AM consumption per 100 weaners per day. This variable was calculated using the total administered ADD in weaners in year 2013, dividing it by the standard weight of weaners used by VetStat (15 kg). After this first calculation, to have the number of ADD for each weaner, this total was divided by the number weaners (pen places) in each herd. Finally, this total was divided by 3.65, to show the final values in ADD per 100 animals per day – which corresponds to the unit used by VetStat to impose the official AM consumption limits.

Taking into account that weaners may receive more than one type of vaccine, two-way combinations between vaccination groups were constructed to assess the possible association between different vaccinations and AM consumption. Moreover, for the final models,

one variable with eight levels was constructed to take into consideration all combinations of use of the three different vaccines within the herds.

Data analyses

All data analyses were carried out in R (version 3.1.2 of 2014 – The R Foundation for Statistical Computing). Univariable analyses were performed for the total AM consumption (AC-TOTAL), AM consumption with gastrointestinal indication (AC-GI) and AM consumption with respiratory indication (AC-RESP) Figs. 1, 2 and 3). Herd size – measured as number of weaner pen places – was divided into three classes: small (<7500), medium (7500–14,999), and large ($\geq15,000$). AC-TOTAL and AC-GI were square root transformed whereas AC-RESP was log-transformed to normalize the distributions. Regarding vaccination: First we went through a pre-analysis step involving the creation of a vaccination coverage index based on the prescriptions of vaccines in 2013. However, it turned out not very useful, so we decided to assign herds as vaccinated if the respective type(s) of vaccine(s) had been prescribed during 2013 irrespective of the number of doses prescribed.

Initially, a t-test was conducted for each of the three types of vaccination comparing the AM consumption for herds which used the vaccine with herds which did not use the vaccine.

For each of the two-way combinations, a t-test and a one-way ANOVA were conducted. Following the one-way ANOVA, a post hoc comparison – using the TUKEY HSD test – was performed to assess the

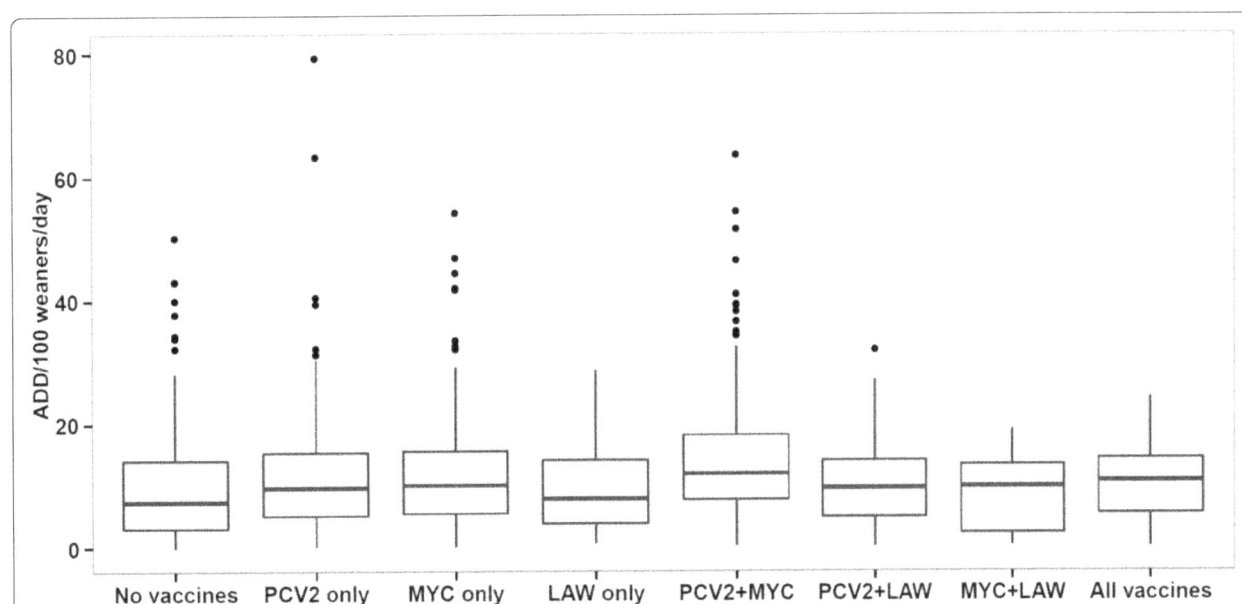

Fig. 1 Total use of antimicrobials – measured as Animal Daily Doses (ADD) per 100 weaners per day – in 1513 Danish sow herds, divided according to the combined use of vaccination against PCV2, *Mycoplasma hyopneumoniae* (MYC), and *Lawsonia intracellularis* (LAW), 2013

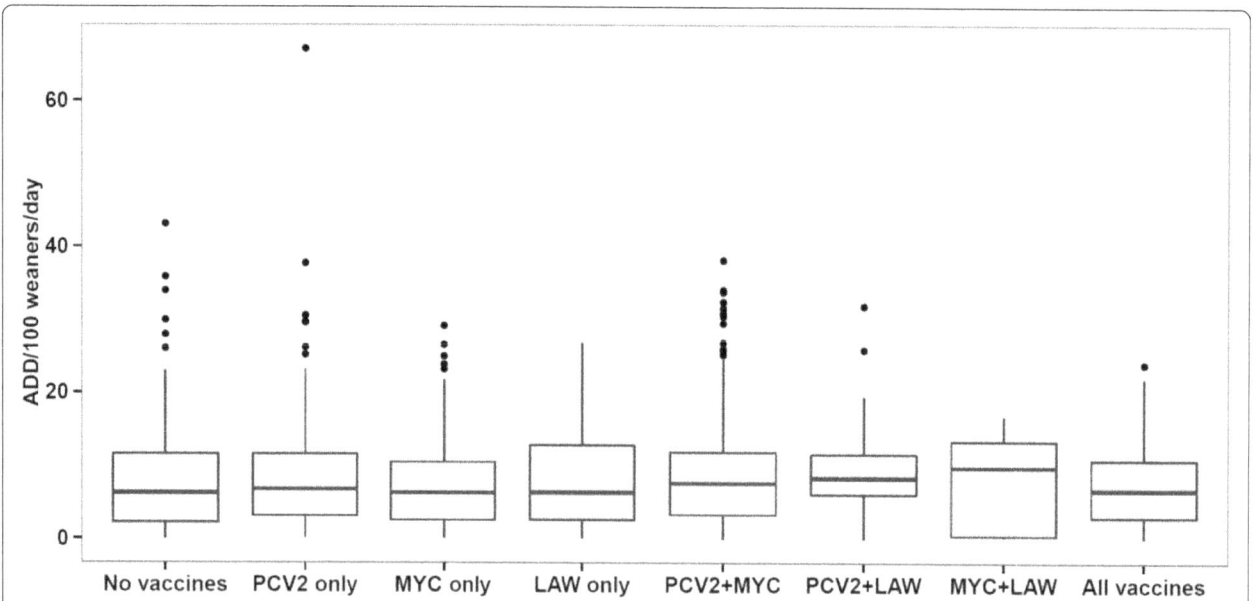

Fig. 2 Use of antimicrobials with gastro-intestinal indication – measured as Animal Daily Doses (ADD) per 100 weaners per day – in 1415 Danish sow herds, divided according to the combined use of vaccination against PCV2, *Mycoplasma hyopneumoniae* (MYC), and *Lawsonia intracellularis* (LAW), 2013

statistical difference between the individual combinations (Data not shown).

Finally, multivariable analyses were conducted for (1) AC-TOTAL, (2) AC-GI and (3) AC-RESP as three separate outputs. The variables herd size and use of vaccine (divided into the eight different combinations of use of the three vaccines) represented the explanatory variables. It was tested whether herd size was significantly associated with the response and whether it acted as a confounder by being associated with the vaccine use. Moreover, a test was made for presence of interaction between

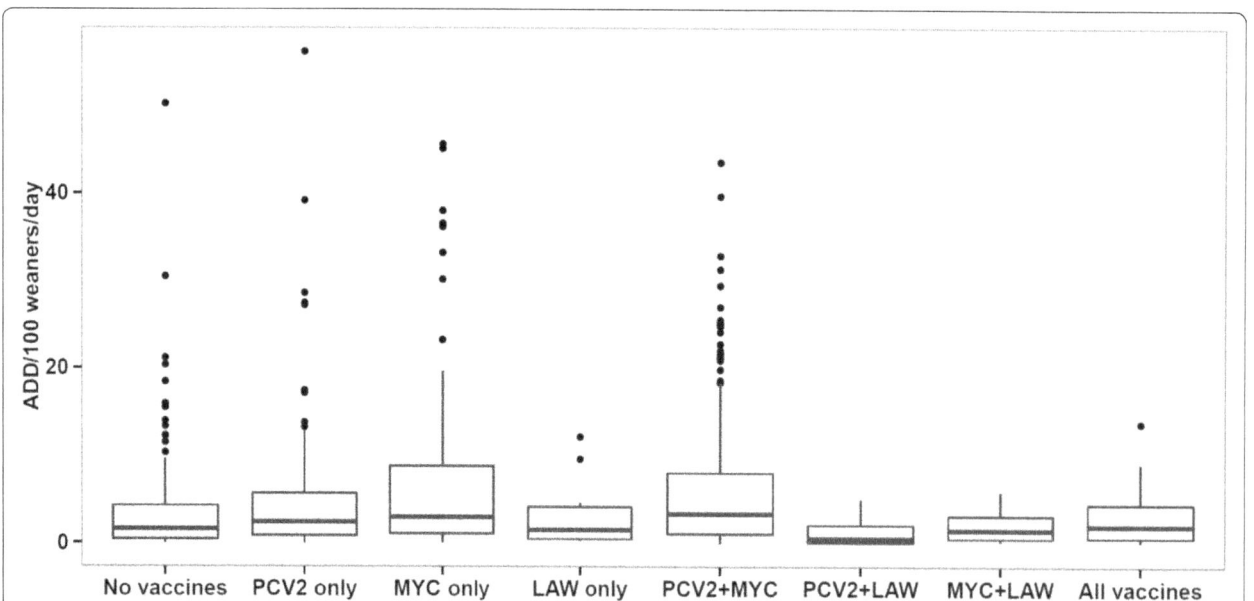

Fig. 3 Use of antimicrobials with respiratory indication – measured as Animal Daily Doses (ADD) per 100 weaners per day – in 836 Danish sow herds, divided according to the combined use of vaccination against PCV2, *Mycoplasma hyopneumoniae* (MYC), and *Lawsonia intracellularis* (LAW), 2013

herd size and vaccine. A *P*-value < 0.05 was used as threshold for statistical significance. As part of model validation, residuals were inspected for normal distribution.

Abbreviations

AC-GI, antimicrobial consumption with gastro-intestinal indication; AC-RESP, antimicrobial consumption with respiratory indication; AC-TOTAL, total antimicrobial consumption; ADD, animal daily doses; AM, antimicrobial; CHR, central husbandry register; LAW, *Lawsonia intracellularis*; MYC, *Mycoplasma hyopneumoniae*; PCV2, porcine circovirus type 2; PCVD, porcine circovirus diseases; PMWS, post-weaning multi-systemic wasting syndrome; PRRS, porcine reproductive and respiratory syndrom

Acknowledgements

Chief Scientist Charlotte Sonne Kristensen, SEGES – The Danish Pig Research Centre, is acknowledged for discussions regarding the planning of the study. Veterinary pig practitioner Frede Keller, LVK, is acknowledged for enabling visits to several pig herds and to provide practical guidance and discussion about use of vaccination and antimicrobials to the first author, which was essential to the development of this work.

Funding

Not applicable.

Authors' contributions

CT contributed to the planning of the study and the analyses. LRN contributed to the planning of the study and the analyses. LA contributed to the planning of the study and the analyses. KSP participated in the planning of the project and performed the data extraction from VetStat. ABK participated in the data analyses and interpretation. All authors contributed to the writing of the manuscript. All authors read and approved the final manuscript.

Authors' information

This work is part of a larger project called UC-CARE. The work was undertaken by Carolina Temtem during her stay in Denmark as part of her veterinary study. Lis Alban and Liza R. Nielsen acted as supervisors for Carolina. Amanda Brinch Kruse was involved in the work as part of her Ph.D.-project.

Competing interests

The authors declare that they have no competing interests.

Author details

[1]Faculty of Veterinary Medicine, University of Lisbon, Avenida da Universidade Técnica, 1300-477 Lisbon, Portugal. [2]Department of Large Animal Sciences, Section for Animal Welfare and Disease Control, University of Copenhagen, Grønnegårdsvej 8, Frederiksberg C DK-1870, Denmark. [3]Danish Agriculture & Food Council, Axeltorv 3, Copenhagen V DK-1609, Denmark.

References

1. Alban L, Dahl J, Andreasen M, Petersen J, Sandberg M. Possible impact of the "yellow card" antimicrobial scheme on meat inspection lesions in Danish finisher pigs. Prev Vet Med. 2013;108:334–41 [Special Issue: SVEPM 2012 - The Cutting-Edge of Animal Disease Control in a Global Environment].

2. Danish Integrated Antimicrobial Resistance Monitoring and Research Programme [DANMAP] 2010. DANMAP 2010: Use of antimicrobial agents and occurence of antimicrobial resistance in bacteria from food animals, food and humans in Denmark. 2011.

3. Grave K, Jensen VF, Odensvik K, Wierup M, Bangen M. Usage of veterinary therapeutic antimicrobials in Denmark, Norway and Sweden following termination of antimicrobial growth promoter use. Prev Vet Med. 2006;75:123–32.

4. Jensen H, Hayes D. Impact of Denmark's ban on antimicrobials for growth promotion. Curr Opin Microbiol. 2014;19:30–6 [Ecology and Industrial Microbiology • Special Section: Novel Technologies in Microbiology].

5. Stege H, Bager F, Jacobsen E, Thougaard A. VETSTAT - the Danish system for surveillance of the veterinary use of drugs for production animals. Prev Vet Med. 2003;57:105–15.

6. Allen H, Levine U, Looft T, Bandrick M, Casey T. Treatment, promotion, commotion: antibiotic alternatives in food-producing animals. Trends Microbiol. 2013;21:114–9.

7. Cheng G, Hao H, Xie S, Wang X, Dai M, Huang L, Yuan Z. Antibiotic alternatives: the substitution of antibiotics in animal husbandry? Front Microbiol. 2014;5:217. doi:10.3389/fmicb.2014.00217. http://journal.frontiersin.org/article/10.3389/fmicb.2014.00217/full.

8. Segalés J, Allan G, Domingo M. Porcine Circoviruses. In: Diseases of Swine. 10th ed. Iowa: Wiley-Blackwell; 2012. p. 1470–522 [Viral Diseases].

9. Thacker E, Minion F. Mycoplasmosis. In: Diseases of Swine. 10th ed. Iowa: Wiley-Blackwell; 2012. p. 2850–923 [Bacterial Diseases].

10. Sibila M, Pieters M, Molitor T, Maes D, Haesebrouck F, Segalés J. Current perspectives on the diagnosis and epidemiology of *Mycoplasma hyopneumoniae* infection. Vet J. 2009;181:221–31.

11. Stege H, Jensen TK, Møller K, Bækbo P, Jorsal SE. Prevalence of intestinal pathogens in Danish finishing pig herds. Prev Vet Med. 2000;46:279–92.

12. Bak H, Rathkjen P. Reduced use of antimicrobials after vaccination of pigs against porcine proliferative enteropathy in a Danish SPF herd. Acta Vet Scand. 2009;51:1.

13. Smith SH, McOrist S. Development of persistent intestinal infection and excretion of *Lawsonia intracellularis* by piglets. Res Vet Sci. 1997;62:6–10.

14. Postma M, Backhans A, Collineau L, Loesken S, Sjölund M, Belloc C, Emanuelson U, Beilage EG, Nielsen EO, Stärk KDC, Dewulf J. Evaluation of the relationship between the biosecurity status, production parameters, herd characteristics and antimicrobial usage in farrow-to-finish pig production in four EU countries. Porc Health Man. 2016;2:9.

15. Raith J, Trauffler M, Firth CL, Lebl K, Schleicher C, Köfer J. Influence of porcine circovirus type 2 vaccination on the level of antimicrobial consumption on 65 Austrian pig farms. Vet Rec. 2016. doi:10.1136/vr.103406

16. Gerber P, Garrocho F, Lana Á, Lobato Z. Serum antibodies and shedding of infectious porcine circovirus 2 into colostrum and milk of vaccinated and unvaccinated naturally infected sows. Vet J. 2011;188:240–2.

17. Tomás A, Fernandes L, Valero O, Segalés J. A meta-analysis on experimental infections with porcine circovirus type 2 (PCV2). Vet Microbiol. 2008;132:260–73.

18. Segalés J, Urniza A, Alegre A, Bru T, Crisci E, Nofrarías M, López-Soria S, Balasch M, Sibila M, Xu Z, Chu H, Fraile L, Plana-Duran J. A genetically engineered chimeric vaccine against porcine circovirus type 2 (PCV2) improves clinical, pathological and virological outcomes in postweaning multisystemic wasting syndrome affected farms. Vaccine. 2009;27:7313–21.

19. Opriessnig T, Meng X, Halbur P. Porcine circovirus type 2–associated disease: update on current terminology, clinical manifestations, pathogenesis, diagnosis, and intervention strategies. J Vet Diagn Invest. 2007;19:591–615.

20. Segalés J, Allan G, Domingo M. Porcine circovirus diseases. Anim Health Res Rev Conf Res Work Anim Dis. 2005;6:119–42.

21. Maes D, Deluyker H, Verdonck M, Castryck F, Miry C, Lein A, Vrijens B, Kruif A. The effect of vaccination against *Mycoplasma hypopneumoniae* in pig herds with a continuous production system. Zentralblatt Für Veterinärmedizin Reihe B J Vet Med Ser B. 1998;45:495–505.

22. Jensen C, Ersbøll A, Nielsen J. A meta-analysis comparing the effect of vaccines against *Mycoplasma hyopneumoniae* on daily weight gain in pigs. Prev Vet Med. 2002;54:265–78.

23. Mateusen B, Maes D, Verdonck M, Kruif A, Goubergen M. Effectiveness of treatment with lincomycin hydrochloride and/or vaccination against *Mycoplasma hyopneumoniae* for controlling chronic respiratory disease in a herd of pigs. Vet Rec. 2002;151:135–40.

24. Thaker MYC, Bilkei G. Comparison of the effects of oral vaccination and different antibiotic prophylactic treatments against *Lawsonia intracellularis*

associated losses in a finishing pig unit with high prevalence of porcine proliferative enteropathy (PPE). Tierärztl Umschau. 2006;61:372–376.

25. Anonymous: Styrket indsats mod ulovlig indførsel af antibiotika til produktionsdyr (Enhanced action against illegal imports of antibiotics for livestock). The Danish Veterinary and Food Administration. 2016. p. 46. http://mfvm.dk/fileadmin/user_upload/MFVM/Publikationer/Rapport_om_styrket_indsats_mod_ulovlig_indfoersel_af_antibiotika_til_produktionsdyr.pdf. Accessed 2 Aug 2016.

26. Danish Integrated Antimicrobial Resistance Monitoring and Research Programme [DANMAP] 2012. DANMAP 2012: Use of antimicrobial agents and occurence of antimicrobial resistance in bacteria from food animals, food and humans in Denmark. 2013.

27. Jensen V, Jacobsen E, Bager F. Veterinary antimicrobial-usage statistics based on standardized measures of dosage. Prev Vet Med. 2004;64:201–15.

28. Dupont N, Stege H. Vetstat - Monitoring usage of antimicrobials in animals. ICAR Tech Ser No 17. 2013:21. [ICAR Technical Series No. 17].

15

Good vaccination practice: it all starts with a good vaccine storage temperature

Frédéric Vangroenweghe ⓘ

Abstract

Background: Recent introduction of strategies to reduce antibiotic use in food animal production implies an increased use of vaccines in order to prevent the economic impact of several important diseases in swine. Good Vaccination Practice (GVP) is an overall approach on the swine farm aiming to obtain maximal efficacy of vaccination through good storage, preparation and finally correct application to the target animals. In order to have a better insight into GVP on swine farms and the vaccine storage conditions, a survey on vaccination practices was performed on a farmers' fair and temperatures in the vaccine storage refrigerators were measured during farm visits over a period of 1 year.

Results: The survey revealed that knowledge on GVP, such as vaccine storage and handling, needle management and injection location could be improved. Less than 10% had a thermometer in their vaccine storage refrigerator on the moment of the visit. Temperature measurement revealed that only 71% of the measured refrigerators were in line with the recommended temperature range of +2 °C to +8 °C. Both below +2 °C and above +8 °C temperatures were registered during all seasons of the year. Compliance was lower during summer with an average temperature of 9.2 °C while only 43% of the measured temperatures were within the recommended range.

Conclusions: The present study clearly showed the need for continuous education on GVP for swine veterinarians, swine farmers and their farm personnel in general and vaccine storage management in particular. In veterinary medicine, the correct storage of vaccines is crucial since both too low and too high temperatures can provoke damage to specific vaccine types. Adjuvanted killed or subunit vaccines can be damaged (e.g. structure of aluminiumhydroxide in adjuvans) by too low temperatures (below 0 °C), whereas lyophilized live vaccines are susceptible (e.g. loss of vaccine potency) to heat damage by temperatures above +8 °C. In conclusion, knowledge and awareness of GVP and vaccine storage conditions are crucial under practical field conditions in swine herds. Focus on a correct on-farm vaccine storage is part of the responsible veterinarians' guidance in order to obtain the required vaccine efficacy.

Keywords: Good vaccination practice, Cold chain, Vaccine storage temperature, On-farm refrigerator

Background

Since 2007, stringent measures to reduce antibiotic consumption by 50% in food producing farm animals, including pigs, were imposed in The Netherlands [1]. In Belgium, the Knowledge Center for Antimicrobial Consumption and Resistance in Animals (AMCRA) has formulated ambitious targets for the reduction of antibiotic use in farm animals by 2020. Due to this antibiotic reduction, a major increase in the use of vaccinations against most currently present swine pathogens, such as *M. hyopneumoniae* (*M.hyo*), Porcine Reproductive and Respiratory Syndrome virus (PRRSv), Porince Circovirus type 2 (PCV-2), *Actinobacillus pleuropneumoniae* (App) and *Haemophilus parasuis* (Hps) has been observed. In the past, vaccinations have contributed to decreasing serious outbreaks by preventing incidence and propagation of contagious diseases in advance [2]. Vaccination programs are cost-effective in preventing outbreaks and spread of vaccine-preventable diseases [3].

To obtain maximal results from the applied vaccination strategies and to ensure optimal potency of vaccines used in veterinary medicine [4], the vaccines have to be handled with care from production through distribution and on-farm storage until application to the target animals under practical field conditions. The

---

Correspondence: vangroenweghe.frederic@telenet.be
Elanco Animal Health, BU Swine & Poultry, Plantijn en Moretuslei 1, 2018 Antwerpen, Belgium

World Health Organisation (WHO) recommends that all vaccines should be stored at between +2 °C and +8 °C at all segments of the cold chain [4]. The need to address this challenge has become increasingly important due to the introduction of new and more expensive combined vaccines that are at risk of damage from heat and/or freeze exposure [5–8].

Maintenance of the cold chain during transport and storage by the end user has been shown to be critically important [4, 9]. In human medicine, several studies were conducted towards general awareness of the importance of cold chain management and the risks of vaccine storage outside the current WHO recommendations of between +2 °C to +8 °C [10]. Depending on the type of vaccine, storage both under too cold (below 0 °C) or too hot (above +8 °C) temperatures can be detrimental for the vaccine potency and its subsequent immunological characteristics following administration to the patient [11]. For adjuvanted vaccines, such as killed (e.g. *M.hyo*, PCV-2, Hps) and subunit (App) vaccines, which are also frequently used in veterinary medicine, storage under 0 °C may cause an irreversible damage to the structure of the adjuvant, resulting in a decreased immunogenicitiy of the vaccine [11–14]. The shake test is the only test with 100% sensitivity, 100% specificity and 100% predictive value to determine whether aluminium-adjuvanted freeze-sensitive vaccines have been affected by freezing [15]. Live vaccines (e.g. PRRSv, *E. coli*), on the other hand, are more prone to damage due to exposure to temperatures above +8 °C, resulting in loss of vaccine potency [11]. Programs focusing on education and improved awareness of the different aspects of vaccine handling and storage by the end users have shown a significant improvement of overall vaccine storage quality [16–18].

Good Vaccination Practice (GVP) is a terminology summarizing the entire procedure from on-farm vaccine receipt until the administration of the vaccine to the target animals, comprising vaccine storage, vaccine preparation for administration and the vaccine administration equipment (including needles, syringes, needleless devices, ...) [19]. Essential elements to check for within the GVP are the refrigerator itself (type, maximal age [20], stable power supply [19]), including accurate knowledge on basic storage principles (first-in first-out (FIFO) principle [19], no vaccine in the door shelves [19], correct range of storage temperature [19], no freezing [11–14]), followed by planning of the vaccination session and vaccine preparation before administration (including the acclimatization of the vaccine to room temperature (+18-20 °C) before administration). For the administration itself several aspects should be taken into account such as needle type (length and diameter adapted to the target animal group) [19] and exact injection location. Subsequent management and conservation of bottles

that have been opened but not entirely used is also an important issue.

The aims of the present study were first to obtain data on the current knowledge of swine farmers of the most important principles of GVP; and second to measure on-farm vaccine storage temperature at the level of the vaccine refrigerator in order to monitor the current vaccine storage situation on swine farms in Belgium and The Netherlands.

Methods

Survey on level of knowledge concerning good vaccination practices

In order to quantify the level of knowledge concerning the key essentials of GVP, a survey of 8 questions on different aspects of GVP was organized on a 3-day farmers' fair in 2015 (LIV Hardenberg, Hardenberg, The Netherlands) (Table 1). The multiple choice questions (Table 2) were presented to 50 sow farmers in The Netherlands with at least 200 sows that were willing to cooperate in the questionnaire. The average respondent had 568 (±80) sows and half of them had additional farm personnel assisting the vaccination process.

On-farm measurement of vaccine storage refrigerator temperature

The actual refrigerator temperature was measured in 126 swine farm vaccine storage refrigerators during a consultative farm visit in Belgium and The Netherlands. The number of farms per season is given in Table 3. Every refrigerator was only measured once, since multiple measurement over time would bias the study data through the increased awareness following the first measurement. The digital thermometer sensor (MOXX Thermometer; TFA® Dostmann GmbH & Co., Wertheim,

Table 1 Survey questionnaire on GVP at a farmers' fair in The Netherlands

N°	Question
1	Are vaccination tasks performed by the swine farmer himself or with the help of other farm personnel?
2	What is the temperature range for storage of vaccines in the refrigerator?
3	What time interval is needed to warm a vaccine from storage temperature to room temperature (18-20 °C)?
4	When freezing of vaccines occurs during storage, what is the consequence?
5	How long can a vaccine bottle after first use still be stored without quality decrease and with full vaccine efficacy?
6	What is the optimal needle management?
7	What is the ideal dimension (length & diameter) for vaccination of piglets during the first week of life?
8	What is the correct injection site for vaccines in the neck region?

Table 2 Questionnaire responses (*n* = 50) on GVP knowledge

N°	Question	Response (%)
1	Are vaccination tasks performed by the swine farmer himself or with the help of other farm personnel?	
	a. Yes	50%
	b. No	50%
2	What is the temperature range for storage of vaccines in the refrigerator?	
	a. 0–5 °C	14%
	b. 2–8 °C	**80%**
	c. Doesn't matter as long as refrigerated	6%
3	What time interval is needed to warm a vaccine from storage temperature to room temperature (18-20 °C)?	
	a. 1 h	76%
	b. 5 h	**18%**
	c. 10 h	2%
	d. The day before vaccination	4%
4	When freezing of vaccines occurs during storage, what is the consequence?	
	a. Antigen in the vaccine damaged	**78%**
	b. No negative effect on immunity	16%
	c. Stronger immune response	6%
5	How long can a vaccine bottle after first use still be stored without quality decrease and with full vaccine efficacy?	
	a. 24 h	**62%**
	b. 1 week	28%
	c. 1 month	4%
	d. Until expiry date	6%
6	What is the optimal needle management?	
	a. Needles until broken	6%
	b. Disposable needle every 10 litters	36%
	c. Disposable needle every litter	**58%**
7	What is the ideal dimension (length & diameter) for vaccination of piglets during the first week of life?	
	a. Length 9 mm, diameter 0.8 mm	**58%**
	b. Length 12 mm, diameter 1.0 mm	22%
	c. Length 16 mm, diameter 0.8 mm	20%
8	What is the correct injection site for vaccines in the neck region?	
	a. In the lower region of the neck	18%
	b. 2 fingers behind the ear	**52%**
	c. Just in front of schoulder	30%

Correct answers are in bold

Germany) was installed in the refrigerator in a standardized way:

1. The sensor was inserted into a cardboard packaging box of a veterinary medicinal product (VMP) present in the refrigerator

2. The VMP package was positioned in the central part of the body of the refrigerator (not the door shelf, not the upper nor lower shelf)
3. Temperature measurement was allowed for at least 45 min
4. The actual refrigerator temperature was noted including date, season and country of measurement.

Additionally, it was registered if a thermometer or other temperature monitoring system was already present in the vaccine storage refrigerators included in the study.

Statistical analysis
Results from the survey were reported as descriptive data with the % of respondents per answer category.

Measured temperatures were categorized based on the season they were measured: S1 (winter; 21/12 – 20/3), S2 (spring; 21/3 – 20/6), S3 (summer; 21/6 – 20/9) and S4 (autumn; 21/9 – 20/12). Since the vaccine storage temperature data were single point measurement of different farms in different seasons, data were reported as descriptive data, including average (± SEM) over season. The distribution of the vaccine storage refrigerator temperatures over the year was plotted in a histogram with intervals of 3 °C.

Results
Survey on level of knowledge concerning good vaccination practices
In total, 50 valid survey responses were collected during the 3-day farmer event. The summary of the responses is shown in Table 2.

The most important observation concerning vaccine storage were that only 80% of the respondents could identify the temperature range of +2 °C to +8 °C as the recommended temperature range for on-farm vaccine storage. There were also 22% of the respondents that did not realize freezing had a significant impact on the subsequent vaccine efficacy. Other questions related to GVP revealed that needle management in general and needle length per animal category and site of injection in particular were not always quite clear to swine farmers. The interval needed to get a vaccine at room temperature (+18 °C) ready for injection was also not very clear.

On-farm measurement of vaccine storage refrigerator temperature
Only 12 (9.5%) vaccine storage refrigerators already had a thermometer present at the moment of the farm visit.

The variation in vaccine storage temperature among the 126 on-farm measurement is shown in Fig. 1. It is apparent that only in 4 cases, the vaccine storage temperature was below the +2 °C, with sub-zero

Table 3 Number of measured farms, average (±SEM) vaccine storage temperature and distribution (%) of on-farm measured refrigerator temperatures in specific temperature category: below +2 °C, between +2 °C and +8 °C, above +8 °C

	# farms per season	Average (± SEM) t° per season	Below +2 °C	Between +2 °C and +8 °C	Above +8 °C
S1, winter	26	6.5 ± 0.64	4	77	19
S2, spring	43	6.4 ± 0.33	0	81	19
S3, summer	23	9.2 ± 1.11	4	43	52
S4, autumn	34	6.5 ± 0.47	6	71	24
Summary	*126*		*3*	*71*	*26*

temperature in 3 cases. In total, 33 cases exceeded the upper range of +8 °C. Most of these events (73%) concerned slight breaches between +8 °C and +11 °C (Fig. 2).

Analysis of seasonal patterns revealed significant differences among season with a statistically higher temperature (9.2 ± 1,1 °C) during the summer (S3) as compared to other seasons. During summer (S3), 52% of the on-farm vaccine storage refrigerators exceeded the upper limit of +8 °C, whereas in other seasons, this percentage varied between 19% (winter; S1 and spring; S2) and 24% (autumn; S4) (Table 3). In total, only 71% of the measured temperatures were within the WHO-recommended range.

Discussion

Even in human medicine, compliance to the WHO recommendations on vaccine storage is a difficult issue [20]. In our survey, 80% of the participants could state the recommended temperature range of between +2 °C and +8 °C. This is much higher than in another study conducted in human medicine, which obtained a score of only 16% [21]. We have to realize that our measurements were performed at a lower level in the cold chain

as compared to most studies performed in a human environment, where vaccine storage refrigerators at the physicians' office were monitored. Nevertheless, we have to emphasize that on-farm vaccine storage is a shared responsibility of both the swine farmer and its veterinarian responsible for on-farm health management and epidemiological surveillance. Two other point of interest in vaccine storage could also be improved this way. First, the fact that frozen vaccines lose their immunological activity and secondly, opened bottles that are not entirely used should not be kept too long under cooled storage after its first use. In this aspect, indication of the date of first use on the bottle would mean a positive evolution.

Another interesting result from our survey is the fact that 76% of the respondents apparently inject the vaccines at a too cold temperature, which might cause injection problems, especially in the case of oil-based vaccines. Current knowledge on the needle specifications for the target animal group to be vaccinated were also quite low (58%) as well as needle management and general hygiene measures to omit transmission of pathogens from one litter to another through injections. It has indeed been shown that e.g. PRRSV can be transmitted among pigs in a swine herd through injection needles [22]. In human

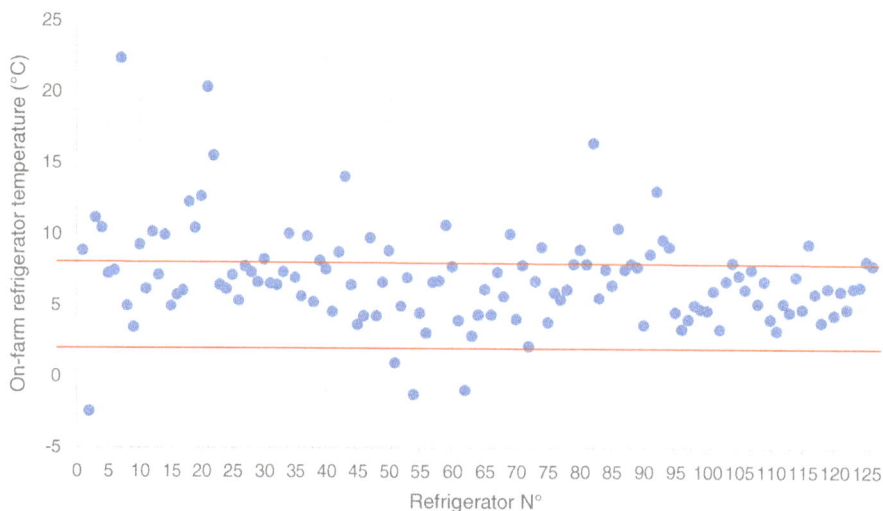

Fig. 1 On-farm refrigerator temperatures (individual data points) measured during 2016-2017 in Belgium and The Netherlands. Red lines indicate lower (+2 °C) and upper (+8 °C) limits of recommended temperature

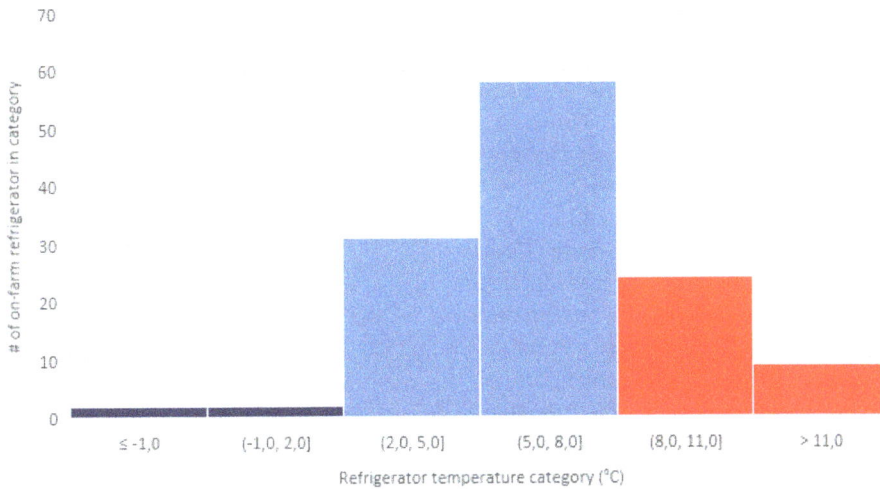

Fig. 2 Distribution of 126 refrigerator temperatures collected on-farm in Belgium and The Netherlands during 2016-2017

medicine, the aspects of needle management and hygiene are quite well defined and carefully followed [19], since stringent protocols are in place to assure maximal prevention of disease between patients [19].

Cold chain monitoring can be performed using different temperature measurement tools, such as cold chain measuring cards [10], digital thermometers [11] including minimum-maximum thermometers and electronic temperature loggers [11]. However, a thermometer only provides a snapshot of the temperature at the point in time when it is checked and can therefore not be considered a long-term appropriate monitoring tool [23], unless outer limits (minimum/maximum) are registered as in the case of a minimum-maximum thermometer. When the temperature is checked and the value is found to be in the range of +2 °C to +8 °C, farmers and vets may erroneously conclude that the vaccine storage on-farm is safe, however, this snapshot measurement is not covering any deviations observed during the rest of the daytime/nighttime period. Therefore, in the present study, we used a minimum-maximum thermometer, in order to provide a tool to the farmer and the veterinarian to emphasize their continuous awareness on the importance of keeping the on-farm vaccine refrigerator within the recommended range (+2 °C till +8 °C) for vaccine storage.

Practices exposing vaccines to both high (> +8 °C) and sub-zero temperatures (< 0 °C) are widespread in both developed and developing countries at all levels of the human health system [8, 21, 24–26]. A recent review on vaccine freezing highlights that accidental freezing is widespread and occurs across all segments of the cold chain [20]. In human medicine, between 14 and 35% of refrigerators or transport shipments were found to have exposed vaccines to temperatures below zero. From our study, it is clear that, although the temperature measurement was a snapshot measurement at the time of the farm visit, only 4% of the refrigerators showed a temperature below the acceptable lower limit of +2 °C at the moment of our visit.

In human medicine, it has been shown that compliance and follow-up of the correct refrigerator temperature was higher when awareness of all stakeholders was kept up-to-date [16, 17, 27]. For example, the knowledge on the fact that heat is harmful to vaccines was rather high (75–100%) [27], whereas the awareness by swine farmers that freezing was also harmful to some vaccines was very low (22.7–44.4%) [27]. From our survey, it is also clear that knowledge and awareness on vaccine storage practices in the broad sense are inadequate. Another point of attention to increase the awareness of continuous monitoring of vaccine storage refrigerator temperature is the daily recording of measured temperature [3, 18].

In our study, 71% of the measured vaccine storage refrigerators were in the recommended temperature range. This is in accordance with other studies in human medicine which showed between 68.1% [27] and 83% [3] of the vaccine refrigerators within the recommended range. The observation that the older the refrigerator, the higher the mean temperature [27], however, bears us some concerns from a veterinary point of view. Personal observations within our area reveal that many refrigerators used for on-farm vaccine storage have been 'recycled' from previous service in home or office kitchens. Therefore, their average age might be well above 12 years, which has been shown to be more likely to result in inappropriate temperatures (52.2% risk) [27]. Unfortunately, we were unable to register the exact age of on-farm vaccine refrigerators in our study, due to lack of reliable data on the farm.

In our study, there were few (< 10%) on-farm vaccine refrigerators which had a thermometer present at the moment of the farm visit. This is somehow in accordance with another study in human medicine where the presence of a thermometer was 11% [27]. However, a more recent study in physicians practices in the same area obtained much higher compliance with an 83% presence of a temperature monitoring device [3].

Another potential solution for improved vaccine efficacy under difficult storage conditions could be the development of more thermostable vaccines by the pharmaceutical industry [28, 29]. However, this possibility is not yet available, and therefore, until then, compliance with the recommended vaccine storage temperatures throughout the entire cold chain remains key to maximize the efficacy of all vaccines used to prevent infectious diseases.

Programs designed to supervise and improve all aspects of vaccine storage management among physicians-professionals have demonstrated significant improvement [16, 17, 27]. Moreover, the appointment of a local responsible person for the vaccine storage resulted in higher odds that refrigerator temperature was kept within the recommended range and the refrigerator was used for vaccine storage only [30].

Taking into consideration the need of compliance with WHO recommendations on vaccine storage, some practical guidelines on vaccine storage on farm level are as following:

- ✓ No vaccine storage in the door compartment to omit the larger temperature variations that occur each time the door is opened [3].
- ✓ No use of refrigerators equipped with an upper freezing compartment.
- ✓ No storage of other materials (food, drinks, …) in vaccine storage refrigerators to reduce the number of times the refrigerator is opened during daytime [3].
- ✓ Use bottles filled with water to reduce the temperature variation within the refrigerator when the volume is not totally filled with vaccines [31].
- ✓ Avoid older refrigerators (> 12 years old) since they have a much higher risk (52.5%) of inappropriate temperatures [27].
- ✓ Position the thermometer in the central part of the refrigerator to continuously monitor the vaccine storage temperature to improve awareness of its importance [16, 17, 27].
- ✓ Perform daily control and monitoring of vaccine storage temperature at the same timepoint [3, 18].

Conclusions

In conclusion, on-farm vaccine storage at swine farms in Belgium and The Netherlands complied in only 71% of the cases with the recommended range between +2 °C

and +8 °C. The general knowledge and awareness on issues concerning vaccine storage and GVP in a broader context show room for improvement through continuous sensibilisation and practical on-farm training of farmers and their farm personnel by the responsible farm veterinarian or other external consultants.

Abbreviations

AMCRA: Knowledge Center for Antimicrobial Consumption and Resistance in Animals; ANOVA: Analysis of variance; App: *Actinobacillus pleuropneumoniae*; FIFO: first-in first-out; GVP: Good Vaccination Practice; Hps: *Haemophilus parasuis*; *M.hyo*: *Mycoplasma hyopneumoniae*; PCV-2: Porcine Circo Virus type 2; PRRSv: Porcine Reproductive and Respiratory Syndrome virus; VMP: Veterinary medicinal product; WHO: World Health Organisation

Acknowledgements

The author greatly acknowledges all the swine farmers and swine veterinarians participating in the study.

Funding

The study was funded by Elanco Animal Health, which facilitated the conduct of the GVP survey and the distribution of the equipment (thermometers) used to measure the vaccine storage refrigerator temperatures during the study.

Authors' contributions

FV coordinated the entire study from study design to data collection and analysis to the manuscript. All authors read and approved the final manuscript.

Authors' information

FV is currently a Sr. Technical Consultant Swine for Benelux within Elanco Animal Health. He holds a DVM and a PhD in Veterinary Sciences, has a specific interest in Good Vaccination Practice in general and vaccine storage management in particular in order for the applied vaccines to be able to work at their maximal efficacy.

Competing interests

The authors declare that they have no competing interests.

References

1. Speksnijder DC, Mevius DJ, Bruschke CJM, Wagenaar JA. Reduction of veterinary antimicrobial use in the Netherlands – the Dutch success model. Zoonoses Public Health. 2015;62(Supp. 1):79–87.
2. Freuling CM, Müller TF, Mettenleiter TC. Vaccines against pseudorabies virus (PrV). Vet Microbiol. 2016. https://doi.org/10.1016/j.vetmic.2016.11.019
3. Gazmararian JA, Oster NV, Green DC, Schuessler L, Howell K, Davis J, Krovisky M, Warburton SW. Vaccine storage practices in primary care physician offices – assessment and intervention. Am J Prev Med. 2002;23:246–53.
4. World Health Organisation. Temperature sensitivity of vaccines: Department of Immunization, Vaccines and Biologicals, WHO; 2006. www.who.int/vaccines-documents/ p. 1–62.

5. Guichard S, Hymbaugh K, Burkholder B, Diorditsa S, Navarro C, Ahmed S, Rahman MM. Vaccine wastage in Bangladesh. Vaccine. 2010;28:858–63.
6. Matthias DM, Robertson J, Garrison MM, Newland S, Nelson C. Freezing temperatures in the vaccine cold chain: a systematic review of literature. Vaccine. 2007;25:3980–6.
7. Nelson C, Froes P, Van Dyck AM, Chavarria J, Boda E, Coca A, Crespo G, Lima H. Monitoring temperatures in the vaccine cold chain in Bolivia. Vaccine. 2007;25:433–7.
8. Wirkas T, Toikilik S, Miller N, Morgan C, Clements CJ. A vaccine cold chain freezing study in PNG highlights technology needs for hot climate countries. Vaccine. 2007;25:691–7.
9. Steinmetz N, Furesz J, Reinhold C, Yarosh W. Storage conditions of live measles, mumps and rubella virus vaccines in Montreal. Can Med Assoc J. 1983;128:162–3.
10. Weltermann BM, Markic M, Thielmann A, Gesenhues S, Hermann M. Vaccination management and vaccination error: a representative online-survey among primary care physicians. PlosOne. 2014;9(8):e105119.
11. Kartoglu U, Milstien J. Tools and approaches to ensure quality of vaccines throughout the cold chain. Expert Rev Vaccines. 2014;13:843–54.
12. Boros CA, Hanlon M, Gold MS, Roberton DM. Storage at −3°C for 24 h alters the immunogenicity of pertussis vaccines. Vaccine. 2001;19:3547–2.
13. Diminsky D, Moav N, Gorecki M, Barenholz Y. Physical, chemical and immunological stability of CHO-derived hepatitis B surface antigens (HBsAg) particles. Vaccine. 1999;18:3–17.
14. Kurzatkowski W, Kartoglu U, Staniszewska M, Górska P, Krause A, Wysocki MJ. Structural damage in adsorbed vaccines affected by freezing. Biologicals. 2013;41:71–6.
15. Kartoglu U, Ozguler NK, Wolfson LJ, Kurzatkowski W. Validation of the shake test for detecting freeze damage to adsorbed vaccines. Bull WHO. 2010b;88:624–31.
16. Lee S, Lim H-S, Kim O, Nam J, Kim Y, Woo H, Noh W, Kim K. Vaccine storage practices and the effects of education in some private medical institutions. J Prev Med Public Health. 2012;45:78–89.
17. Thielmann A, Viehmann A, Weltermann BM. Effectiveness of a web-based education program to improve vaccine storage conditions in primary care (Keep Cool): study protocol for a randomized controlled trial. Trials. 2015;16:301–8.
18. Yakum MN, Ateudjieu J, Water EA, Watcho P. Vaccine storage and cold chain monitoring in the North West region of Cameroon: a cross sectional study. BMC Res Notes. 2015;8:145–52.
19. Vaccine Administration Taskforce. UK guidance on best practice in vaccine administration; 2001. isbn:0-9541497-0-X.
20. Conceição de Oliveira V, Del Pilar Serrano Gallardo M, Arcêncio RA, Laerte Gontijo T, Carvalho Pinto I. Assessment of quality of vaccine storage and conservation in primary health care centers. Ciência Saúde Coletiva. 2014;19:3889–98.
21. Bishai DM, Bhatt S, Miller LT, Hayden GF. Vaccine storage practices in pediatric offices. Pediatrics. 1992;89:193–6.
22. Otake S, Dee SA, Rossow KD, Joo HS, Deen J, Molitor TW, Pijoan C. Transmission of porcine reproductive and respiratory syndrome virus by needles. Vet Rec. 2002;150:114–5.
23. Kartoglu U, Nelaj E, Maire D. Improving temperature monitoring in the vaccine cold chain at the periphery: an intervention study using a 30-day electronic refrigerator temperature logger (Fridge-tag®). Vaccine. 2010a;28:4065–72.
24. Hanjeet K, Lye MS, Sinniah M, Schnur A. Evaluation of cold chain monitoring in Kelantan. Malaysia Bull WHO. 1996;74:391–7.
25. Bell KN, Hogue CJR, Manning C, Kendal AP. Risk factors for improper vaccine storage and handling in private provider offices. Pediatrics. 2001;107:1–5.
26. Jeremijenko A, Kelly H, Sibthorpe B, Attewell R. Improving vaccine storage in general practice refrigerators. BMJ. 1996;312:1651–2.
27. Yuan L, Daniels S, Naus M, Brcic B. Vaccine storage and handling – Knowledge and practice in primary care physician's offices. Can Fam Phys. 1995;41:1169–76.
28. Lloyd J, Cheyne J. The origins of the vaccine cold chain and a glimpse to the future. Vaccine. 2017;35:2115–20.
29. Kristensen DD, Lorenson T, Bartholomew K, Villadiego S. Can thermostable vaccines help address cold-chain challenges? Results from stakeholder interviews in siw low- and middle-income countries. Vaccine. 2016;34:899–904.
30. Bailey HD, Kurinczuk JJ, Kusel MM, Plant AJ. Barriers to immunization in general practice. Austral New Zeal J Public Health. 1999;23:6–10.
31. Lewis JE. Too hot, too cold, or just right? Can Fam Physician. 1995;41:1140–1.

16

Pig castration: will the EU manage to ban pig castration by 2018?

Nancy De Briyne[1]* (iD), Charlotte Berg[2], Thomas Blaha[3] and Déborah Temple[4]

Abstract

Background: In 2010, the 'European Declaration on alternatives to surgical castration of pigs' was agreed. The Declaration stipulates that from January 1, 2012, surgical castration of pigs shall only be performed with prolonged analgesia and/or anaesthesia and from 2018 surgical castration of pigs should be phased out altogether.
The Federation of Veterinarians of Europe together with the European Commission carried out an online survey via SurveyMonkey© to investigate the progress made in different European countries. This study provides descriptive information on the practice of piglet castration across 24 European countries. It gives also an overview on published literature regarding the practicability and effectiveness of the alternatives to surgical castration without anaesthesia/analgesia.

Results: Forty usable survey responses from 24 countries were received. Besides Ireland, Portugal, Spain and United Kingdom, who have of history in producing entire males, 18 countries surgically castrate 80% or more of their male pig population. Overall, in 5% of the male pigs surgically castrated across the 24 European countries surveyed, castration is performed with anaesthesia and analgesia and 41% with analgesia (alone). Meloxicam, ketoprofen and flunixin were the most frequently used drugs for analgesia. Procaine was the most frequent local anaesthetic. The sedative azaperone was frequently mentioned even though it does not have analgesic properties. Half of the countries surveyed believed that the method of anaesthesia/analgesia applied is not practicable and effective. However, countries that have experience in using both anaesthesia and post-operative analgesics, such as Norway, Sweden, Switzerland and The Netherlands, found this method practical and effective. The estimated average percentage of immunocastrated pigs in the countries surveyed was 2.7% (median = 0.2%), where Belgium presented the highest estimated percentage of immunocastrated pigs (18%).

Conclusion: The deadlines of January 1, 2012, and of 2018 are far from being met. The opinions on the animal-welfare-conformity and the practicability of the alternatives to surgical castration without analgesia/anaesthesia and the alternatives to surgical castration are widely dispersed. Although countries using analgesia/anaesthesia routinely found this method practical and effective, only few countries seem to aim at meeting the deadline to phase out surgical castration completely.

Keywords: Piglet castration, Analgesia, Anaesthesia, Animal welfare, Immunocastration, Immunovaccination

Background

Many piglets in Europe are castrated surgically without any anaesthesia or post-operative analgesia. This is allowed by European legislation up to an age of 7 days [1]. Piglets are neurologically mature newborns such as lambs, kids, calves and human infants [2]. Such newborns mature animals usually become conscious within the first few minutes to hours after birth [3]. Castration is a painful and stressful procedure [4]. Some studies report behavioural alterations for several days after the procedure indicating that piglets likely experience post-operative pain [5–7], whereas results based on physiological measures have proven to be more inconsistent as reviewed by [8]. Although the use of anaesthetics [9, 10] would appear to be of benefit during the procedure itself, without the combined use of an analgesic, physiological responses to the procedure post-recovery would seem to indicate that the pain experienced is still great

* Correspondence: nancy@fve.org
[1]Federation of Veterinarians of Europe, Avenue Tervueren 12, 1040 Brussels, Belgium
Full list of author information is available at the end of the article

[4]. Castration of male pigs is hence a substantial animal welfare problem. To tackle this, in 2010, on the initiative of the European Commission and the Belgian Presidency, representatives of European farmers, meat industry, retailers, scientists, veterinarians – represented by the Federation of Veterinarians of Europe (FVE) and animal welfare Non-Governmental Organisations agreed upon the 'European Declaration on alternatives to surgical castration of pigs', from here on referred to as the Declaration [11].

The final goal of this Declaration is to phase out the surgical castration of pigs by 2018 in all European Union (EU) and all European Free Trade Association (EFTA) countries. But the Declaration also requested that from 1 January 2012, surgical castration of pigs shall only be performed with prolonged analgesia and/or anaesthesia.

In September 2015, FVE together with the European Commission decided to analyse the situation with respect to the progress seen in the different countries following up the Declaration. Specific focus was given to getting an overview of the situation regarding surgical castration with prolonged analgesia and/or anaesthesia in the different countries involved.

Methods

This publication is based on an online survey, discussions with regional experts in pig castration and an investigation of (scientific) opinions on the different alternatives existing to surgical pig castration. The online survey on pig castration was designed by FVE and the European Commission, Directorate General for Health and Food Safety via SurveyMonkey©. It was distributed to all national veterinary organisations and to members of the European Association of Porcine Health Management (EAPHM) between 28 September 2015 and 30 October 2015. In total, 44 surveys from 24 countries were received and 40 of them provided usable answers. The final number of respondents per country varied from 1 to 5. Results were expressed at country level. Only consistent answers between respondents of the same country were considered. Each country was asked about the estimated percentage of i) castrated piglets; ii) castrated with analgesia and anaesthesia; iii) castrated with analgesia only; iv) castrated without analgesia or anaesthesia and v) immunocastrated piglets. The surveyed consisted of 3 open questions, 6 dichotomous and 3 multiple-choice questions (Table 1). After the survey, regional experts from 9 countries (pig veterinarians with publications or with known societal involvement in pig castration) were consulted to verify the survey answers and obtain more in-depth information on the situation in the different countries.

Three continuous variables were converted into dichotomous variables to look for possible associations

Table 1 Questions included in the survey on pig castration

Open questions

Percentage of pigs castrated

Percentage of pigs castrated with analgesia and anaesthesia

Percentage of pigs castrated with analgesia only

Percentage of pigs castrated without analgesia or anaesthesia

Percentage of immunocastrated pigs

List the anaesthetics and analgesics used for pigs in "your" country.

What are the main obstacles to reach the goals of the Brussels Declaration in "your" country?

Dichotomous and multiple choice questions

In the last 3–5 years, has the number of male piglets that are being castrated under anaesthesia and/or analgesia gone up in your country? (yes, no)

In the last 3–5 years, has the number of male piglets that are not castrated anymore gone up in your country? (yes, no)

In the last 3–5 years, has the number of male piglets that have been immunocastrated gone up in your country? (yes, no)

F1 - Who is allowed to administer anaesthesia/analgesia in your country? (only a vet, farmer)

F2 - Is the method of anaesthesia/analgesia applied practicable and effective? (yes, no)

F3 - In your country, how do you feel the government and stakeholders are working towards complying with the European declaration on pig castration (0: Little is done to meet the goals of the European declaration of pig castration; 1: Working towards it)

F4 - Has an official deadline to phase out castration been set in your country? (yes, no)

F5 - Economic impact of castration under the use of anaesthesia and/or prolonged analgesia and phasing out pig castration? (0: Neglectable / minor cost in relation to other costs; 1: Serious extra cost)

F6 - Welfare impact of castration under the use of anaesthesia and/or prolonged analgesia and phasing out pig castration? (0: negative; 1: neutral; 2: positive)

between variables. Each country was classified in one of two categories based on expert opinion on the percentages provided by the survey:

i)   surgically castrated piglets (0: 0–20%; 1: 80–100%), twenty three countries classified: Belgium was not considered here for having an intermediate percentage.

ii) castrated with analgesia and anaesthesia (0: 0–6%; 1: 24–99%), twenty four countries classified.

iii) castrated with analgesia only (0: 0–12%; 1: 72–99%). Twenty two countries classified: the Czech Republic and France were not considered here for having intermediate percentages of pigs castrated with analgesia only.

The 'Genmod' procedure for binomial data was applied to detect possible associations between the answers given to those three questions and the variables F1 to F6 present in the survey (Table 1). A *p*-value of 0.05 was considered significant for all analyses.

Results
Percentages of pigs castrated

Table 2 shows the percentage of pigs castrated using different methods, according to the survey. In 18 out of the 24 countries that participated in the survey, 80% or more of male pigs are surgically castrated. In Ireland, Portugal, Spain, the Netherlands and United Kingdom, 20% or less of the male pigs are castrated. Looking at the size of the total pig population, this corresponds to 61% of male pigs being surgically castrated in Europe (Fig. 1). Belgium, France, Germany and Switzerland

reported an increase in the number of entire raised males in the last 3–5 years and the Netherlands a strong increase.

Norway, Switzerland, The Netherlands and Sweden reported 99, 97, 30 and 24% of surgically castrated animals with both anaesthesia and analgesia, respectively. In the other countries and according to the survey, less than 6% of the piglets were castrated using anaesthesia and analgesia.

According to the survey, seven countries castrate surgically more than 70% of the male piglets in their country using analgesia (alone). In France and Czech Republic, 50 and 31% of piglets respectively were castrated surgically using analgesia. The other countries

Table 2 Percentages of entire males, immunocastrated and surgically castrated commercial piglets and methods of castration used in the 24 countries surveyed

Country (number of usable answers)	Entire males	Immuno castrated	Surgical Castration	Break-out surgical castration			Pig population*
				Castrated with analgesia & anaesthesia	Castrated with analgesia only (%)	Castrated without analgesia OR anaesthesia	
	% total	% total	% total	% total surgical	% total surgical	% total surgical	
Austria (2)	5	0	95	1	72	27	2869
Belgium (4)	15	18	67	3	6	91	6351
Czech (2)	5	5	90	6	31	63	1548
Denmark (4)	5	0	95	0	95	5	12402
Estonia (1)	0	0	100	0	10	90	359
Finland (1)	4	0	96	0.5	99	0.5	1258
France (4)	20	0	80	0	50	50	13428
Germany (1)	20	<1%	80	<1%	99	0	28046
Hungary (1)	1	0	99	0	0	100	2935
Iceland (1)	5	0	95	0	95	5	36
Italy (1)	2	5	93	0.5	2.5	97	8561
Ireland (1)	100	0	0	0	0	0	1468
Latvia (1)	0	0	100	0	0	100	368
Luxembourg (1)	1	0	99	0	99	1	90
Netherlands (1)	80	0	20	30	0	70	12013
Norway (1)	1	<1%	99	99	0	1	1644
Portugal (1)	85	2.5	12.5	0	0	100	2014
Romania (1)	0	5	95	2	4	94	5180
Slovakia (1)	0	10	90	0	12	88	637
Slovenia (1)	1	0	99	1	9	90	288
Spain (3)	80	5	15	1	7	92	25495
Sweden (2)	0	6	94	24	76	0	1478
Switzerland (2)	5	2.5	92.5	97	0	3	1573
UK (2)	98	<1%	2	4.5	4.5	91	4383
Europe-24 mean (median)		2.7 (0.2)	78 (95)	11 (0.5)	32 (7.5)	50 (65)	132920
Europe-24 (according to pig population)	36%	3%	61%	5% of the total of surgically castrated pigs	41% of the total of surgically castrated pigs	54% of the total of surgically castrated pigs	

[a] In 1000 heads- data from Eurostat 2013 except Norwegian pig population data from NorwegianNational Bureau of Statistics 2015

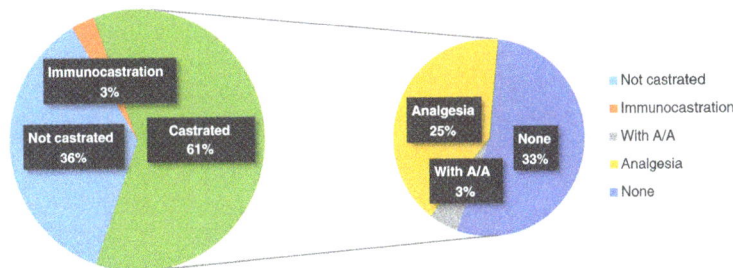

Fig. 1 Percentage of male pigs castrated and methods of castration in the 24 surveyed countries

reported the administration of analgesia in 10% or less of male pigs castrated. In the last 3–5 years, Austria, Denmark, Finland, France, Germany, Iceland and Luxemburg noticed an increase in the number of piglets castrated under anaesthesia and/or analgesia.

The mean percentage of immunocastrated pigs in the countries surveyed was 2.7% (median 0.2%; range = 0–18%) with Belgium having the highest estimated percentage of immunocastrated pigs. Respondents from Belgium, Czech Republic, Norway, Romania, Spain and Sweden reported an increased number of immunocastrated pigs during the last 3–5 years.

Products used for analgesia and anaesthesia in pigs
Using analgesia/anaesthesia: how practical and effective are they?
Respondents were asked whether the method of anaesthesia/analgesia applied is practicable and effective. Overall, in 50% of the countries respondents answered "no" and in 37% they answered "yes". 9% of the countries did not have a consistent answer between the respondents and 4% did not answer.

Nine experts also commented via free text that they felt that the use of analgesia alone (often not prior, but only at the time of the surgery) is insufficient for avoiding stress and pain for the piglets. According to the survey only veterinarians are allowed to administer anaesthesia/analgesia in 67% of the countries. In the Netherlands, Sweden and Switzerland these medicines are used under veterinary prescription but the farmer is allowed to administer them. In some countries (e.g. Sweden), farmers first have to pass a specific training course. In Denmark and France, veterinarians can prescribe analgesia for farmers, who are allowed to administer it, but anaesthetics must be administered by a veterinarian.

Pig castration: how much is it of importance in the different countries?
In respect to how hard the government and stakeholders are working towards complying with the Declaration on pig castration, in 62% of the countries respondents

replied that they felt that the government and stakeholders are working towards complying with the Declaration.

Regarding the question about whether in their country an official deadline on pig castration had been set, no countries, except of Germany and Norway, noted that a national deadline had been set. Respondents from the Czech Republic, the United Kingdom and Switzerland gave different answers. In some countries, experts noted that while the government had set no official date, some farm assurance systems had set deadlines. Several countries also noted that while no date had been set to phase out pig castration, they had a date set demanding analgesia (e.g. Finland has had an industry requirement since 2011, Denmark an industry requirement since 2009 and a legal requirement since 2011) or demanding the use of analgesia and anaesthesia (e.g. Sweden from 1 January 2016).

Regarding the economic impact of castration under the use of anaesthesia and/or analgesia and phasing out pig castration, in 38% of the countries respondents believe that the use of anaesthesia and analgesia causes considerable extra costs.

Regarding the welfare impact of castration under the use of anaesthesia and/or analgesia and phasing out pig castration, respondents from 67% of the countries surveyed were positive or very positive about the animal welfare benefits. One country thought that the welfare impact would be negative. The remaining respondents were either neutral or gave inconsistent answers.

According to the respondents and independently of their country, the main obstacles to reach the goals of the Declaration were the economic implications (mentioned 19 times were that extra costs occur to the farmer which are not be paid back by the consumer), the extra work load caused by using anaesthesia/analgesia (mentioned 11 times), the lack of practical and effective anaesthesia/analgesia protocols (mentioned 10 times), the lack of EU acceptance of entire males both by the market as by slaughterhouses (mentioned 7 times), risk of boar taint in meat (mentioned 3 times) and welfare problems associated with raising entire males (mentioned 2 times).

Associations between variables from the survey

The use of analgesia and anaesthesia in pig castration was significantly associated with whether or not the producer is allowed to administer anaesthesia ($P = 0.02$). From the four countries that uses analgesia and anaesthesia in more than 20% of the pigs castrated, The Netherlands, Sweden and Switzerland allow the producer to administer analgesia and anaesthesia. Norway was the only country where analgesia and anaesthesia was frequently used to castrate piglets (99% castrated with analgesia and anaesthesia) but where the producer could not administer such products. The four countries that have experience in using analgesia and anaesthesia found this method practical and effective ($P = 0.005$).

The use of analgesia was associated with whether or not the country is working towards complying with the EU legislation ($p = 0.03$). The countries where respondents agreed that "little is done to meet the goals of the Declaration" did not use analgesic to castrate the majority of the piglets.

Discussion of the survey results

For most countries, reliable statistical data on the amount of pigs castrated and on the methods used to castrate them is not available. The present survey by the FVE relied upon the answers of experts in pig production from different countries. Therefore, while the results presented in this document indicate the situation of each country in terms of pig castration, it should be recognised that this might not reflect the situation in the whole of Europe, nor give a complete picture.

Ireland, United Kingdom, Spain and Portugal have a history in producing entire males. In the Netherlands, now also the great majority of pigs produced are entire males (80%). The remaining 19 countries that participated to the survey castrated more than 80% of their male pig population. The ultimate goal of the Declaration [11], namely to phase out surgical pig castration, is therefore far from being reached by 2018.

Several countries agreed on deadlines with respect to banning surgical castration without analgesia and/or anaesthesia (Table 3). No country, however, has set a deadline to completely phase out surgical castration.

On average 5% of the male pig population surgically castrated across the 24 European countries surveyed was castrated with anaesthesia and analgesia; 41% with analgesia (alone) and 54% was castrated completely without any anaesthesia or analgesia. In 2010, it was estimated that 79% of the piglets were castrated without anaesthesia or analgesia [12].

Based on these results, there is still a major bottleneck in the use of the combination of anaesthesia and analgesia, the anaesthesia being the biggest constraint. Results from the PIGCAS project published in 2009 [13]

Table 3 Overview of deadlines in a selected number of countries

Country	Year	Deadline content
Denmark	2009, 2011	Ban on surgical pig castration without analgesia, industry requirement since 2009, legal requirement since 2011
Germany	2019	Ban on surgical pig castration without anaesthesia
Netherlands	2009	Ban on surgical pig castration without anaesthesia
Norway	2002	Ban on surgical pig castration without analgesia and anaesthesia
Sweden	2016	Ban on surgical pig castration without analgesia and anaesthesia
Switzerland	2010	Ban on surgical pig castration without anaesthesia

indicated as well that in most countries, anaesthesia was not used and that analgesia was used even more seldom than anaesthesia. The use of analgesics (alone) for male pig castration has hence increased in the last few years.

Expert opinion on surgical castration with analgesia and anaesthesia

The number of authorised and licensed analgesics and anaesthetics for pig castration is limited and differs largely between countries as can be seen in Table 4. For surgical castration of male piglets to be used at farm level, the method must be easy to run without requiring expensive equipment while resulting in a significant reduction of pain for the piglets [14].

Procaine was the most cited local anaesthetic among the countries surveyed. Even though lidocaine is by far the most common local anaesthetic tested in experimental studies [8], this local anaesthetic was only mentioned in Italy, Norway and Sweden. Local administration of lidocaine has been shown to reduce the cortisol level measured 20 min after castration and has shown to reduce the movements and intensity of vocalisation during castration [15]. The anaesthetic effectiveness of lidocaine under experimental conditions has been reviewed [8] and found not to be immediate and limited in duration. In case of the use of intratesticular injection of lidocaine with adrenaline, it takes the lidocaine 3 min to reach the testicular cordons [16]. Lidocaine does not readily diffuse through the tunica vaginalis and in the cremaster muscle which can explain the nociceptive response to surgical castration under local anaesthesia [17]. In our survey, meloxicam, ketoprofen and flunixin were the most frequently cited analgesics across countries. Those three drugs are non-steroidal anti-inflammatory drugs (NSAIDs). Their effectiveness in alleviating pain during male pig castration is questionable. Some studies show that pre-emptive administration of meloxicam, 30 min

Table 4 Overview of the products used for analgesia and/or anaesthesia in pigs in the different countries according to the answers collected in the survey

Country	Trade name	Active substance	Marketing authorization holder
Austria	Finadyne	flunixin meglumine	MSD Animal Health
	Melovem	meloxicam	Dopharma
	Metacam	meloxicam	Boehringer Ingelheim
	Narketan	ketamine	Vétoquinol AG
	Stresnil	azaperone	Provet AG
Belgium	Metacam	meloxicam	Boehringer Ingelheim
	Ketamidor	ketamine	Richter farma
	Stresnil	azaperone	Eli Lilli
	Novocain	procaine hydrochloride, Procaine + adrenaline	Kela laboratoria/VMD
Czech Republic	Narketan	ketamine	Vetoquinol, Bioveta
	Stresnil	azaperone	Eli Lilli
	Procamidor	procaine	Richter Pharma AG
Denmark	Finadyne	flunexin	MSD Animal Health
	Melovem	meloxicam	Sacnvet
	Ketador	ketamine	Salfarm
	Procamidor	procaine hydrochloride	Salfarm
	Coxofen	ketoprofen	Dechra
	Romefen	ketoprofen	Merial
	Rifen	Ketoprofen	Salfarm
	Metacam	meloxicam	Boehringer Ingelheim
	Meloxidolor	meloxicam	Huvepharma
Estonia	Porcamidor	procaine	Richter pharma
France	Stresnil	azaperone	Eli Lilly
	Metacam, Melovem	meloxicam	Boehringer Ingelheim
	Imalgene	ketamine	Merial
	Finadyne	Flunixine	MSD Animal Health
	Procamidor	procaine hydrochloride	Richter farma
Germany	Ursotamin	ketamine	Medistar Arzneimittelvertrieb
	Stresnil	azaperone	Elanco animal Health
	Metacam	meloxicam	Boehringer Ingelheim, Vetmedica
Hungary	Finadyne	flunixin	Intervet
	Melovem	meloxicam	Dopharma International
	Minocain	procaine	Kon-Pharma
	Ketofen, Ketolodor, Ketanest, Ketamidor, Ketink	ketoprofenum	Merial, Le Vet Beheer B.V., Bela-pharm GmbH and Co.KG, Richter Pharma, Industrial Veterinaria S.a.
	Stresnil	azaperone	Eli Lilly Benelux N.V.
Iceland	Metacam	meloxicam	Boehringer Ingelheim
	Procamidor	procaine hydrochloride	Boehringer Ingelheim
Ireland	Metacam	meloxicam	
	Tolfine	tolfenamic	Vetoquinol
	Anaestamine Ketamidor	ketamine	Le Vet Beheer B.V Richter Pharma
	Stresnil	azaperone	Elanco

Table 4 Overview of the products used for analgesia and/or anaesthesia in pigs in the different countries according to the answers collected in the survey *(Continued)*

	Flunazine	flunixine	Cross Vetpharm Group Limited
Italy	Metacam	meloxicam	Boehringer Ingelheim
	Tolfedine	tolfenamic acid	Vetoquinol
	Stresnil	azaperone	Elanco animal Health
		lidocaine	
	Alivios	flunixin meglumine	Fatro
Latvia	Ketofen Ketodolor Dinalgen Ketink Rifen	Ketoprofenum	Merial Le Vet Laboratorios Dr. Esteve Industrial Veterinaria. - Richter Pharma
	Aniketam Ketamidor	ketamine	Le Vet Beheer B.V Richter Pharma AG
	Alfacilline Procamidor	procaine hydrochloride	Alfasan International Richter Pharma
	Sodium Salicyl	sodium salicylate	Dopharma Research
	Novasul	metamizole	Richter Pharma
	Pracetam	paracetamol	Ceva Sante Animale
Luxembourg	same as Belgium		
Netherlands	Novem	meloxicam	Boehringer Ingelheim
	Castralgin	metamizole	Interchemie de Adelaar
	Gas	CO2 O2	
	Anaestamine Ketamidor Narketan	ketamine	Le Vet Beheer B.V Richter Pharma Vetoquinol
	Procamidor Pronestesic	procaine hydrochloride	Richter Pharma Fatro S.P.A.
Norway	Lidokain 20 mg/ml- adrenalin 5	lidocaine	NAF Apotek
	Lidokel-Adrenalin vet		Kela
	Procamidor	procaine hydrochloride	Richter pharma
	Metacam	meloxicam	Boehringer Ingelheim
	Loxicom	meloxicam	Norbrook
Romania	Stresnil	azaperone	Janssen Pharmaceutica
Slovakia	Stresnil	azaperone	Janssen Pharmaceutica
Slovenia	Bioketan	ketamine	Vetconsult
	Novasul	metamizole	Vetconsult
Spain	Ketolar	ketamine	Parke-Davis
	Zoletil	tiletamine + zolazepam	Virbac
	Stresnil	azaperone	Esteve
	Valium	diazepam	Roche
	Metacam	meloxicam	Mylan Pharmaceuticals
	Meloxidyl	meloxicam	Ceva
	Procamidor	procaine hydrochloride	Richter pharma
	Ketoprofeno	ketoprofen	
Sweden	Melovem	meloxicam	Salfarm Scandinavia
	Metacam	meloxicam	Boehringen Ingelheim
	Xylocain	Lidocaine	AstraZeneca

Table 4 Overview of the products used for analgesia and/or anaesthesia in pigs in the different countries according to the answers collected in the survey *(Continued)*

Switzerland	Metacam	meloxicam	Boehringer Ingelheim
	Stresnil	azaperone	Ketavet, Janssens
	Janssen	ketamine	Graeub
	Dolorex	butorphanol	Intervet
	Narketan	ketamine	Vétoquinol
	Isoflurane	isoflurane	
UK	Ketamidor	ketamine	Richter Le Vet Beheer B.V.
	Stresnil	azaperone	Eli Lilly
	Solacyl	sodium salicylate	Dechra, Eurovet
	Finadyne, Allevinix, Pyroflam, Flunixin	flunixine	Intervet, Merial, Norbrook
	Kefotem	ketamine	
	Meloxidyl Metacam, Novem Inflacam, Rheumacam Recocam Melovem Emdocam Meloxidolor Loxicom Contacera	meloxicam	Ceva Boehringer Ingelheim Chanelle Cross VetPharm Dopharma Emdoka Le Vet Norbrook Zoetis

Some products may be missing and some products are used off-label

before the procedure, gives some post-operative analgesia after surgical castration [18]. However, others [10] reported very limited effects of meloxicam in reducing pain related to pig castration. SUIVET [19], an organisation of pig veterinarians in Italy, proposed a protocol for pig castration using a combination of meloxicam and procaine. To give the product time to become efficient, they suggest giving the injection first to 5 litters, after which to come back to castrate the piglets. In order to limit the number of injections, they suggest to combine it with the iron injection usually provided anyway [19]. Ketoprofen did not show any effect on pain responses during castration, but postoperative pain was reduced in these piglets in terms of scratching, tail wagging and isolating themselves on the day after castration [20].

General anaesthesia can be induced by use of inhalation agents or injection. The use of inhalation agents was mentioned by the Netherlands (Carbone dioxide) and Switzerland (Isoflurane). The availability of injection anaesthetics for general anaesthesia was mentioned in several countries. General anaesthesia has advantages but is difficult to practice at the farm level and present some major drawbacks [15, 21]. The use of CO_2 is very controversial. Piglets castrated under CO2 anaesthesia display more interactive behaviours during the 8 day observation period, however the piglets that were castrated under anaesthesia also displayed behaviours indicative of pain and discomfort up 6 days after castration [22].

Although CO_2 is very commonly used for pre-slaughter stunning, due to a lack of alternatives, CO_2 produces strong aversion (irritation and asphyxia) in pigs before they lose consciousness [23, 24]. Isoflurane inhalation was found in one large scale study to only have given sufficiently anaesthesia in 77% of the piglets [25].

The sedative azaperone was frequently mentioned. Sedation makes the piglets easier to handle, however it is not effective at all in relieving pain. It may be used as premedication to local and general anaesthesia such as in combined use with ketamine [26].

Half of the countries surveyed believe that the method of anaesthesia/analgesia applied is not practicable and effective. Extra cost, extra work load and the lack of practical and effective protocols were 3 main constraints identified by the respondents. One study [20] estimated that local anaesthesia prior to castration increase the labour demand by 39 to 52%. Still, countries that have some experience in using analgesia and anaesthesia (Norway, Switzerland, The Netherland and Sweden) found their method practical and effective. Furthermore, based on the survey, that a producer is allowed to administer anaesthesia and analgesia seems to facilitate the use of such products in a routine basis to castrate piglets. In the Netherlands, Sweden and Switzerland the farmer is allowed to administer anaesthesia and analgesia. In Norway, farmers cannot use analgesia and anaesthesia. In some other countries as Denmark and

France, veterinarians can prescribe analgesia to be administered by farmers, but anaesthetics must be administered by a veterinarian. In Sweden, a farmer may inject local anaesthesia and analgesia to perform pig castration, when he has attended both a course in handling pharmaceuticals and a course in correct administration of scrotal local anaesthesia. According to FVE's Veterinary Act [27] and most national Veterinary Acts, administering anaesthesia and doing surgery entering a body cavity is a task that can only be performed by veterinarians. Potential complications associated with surgical castration include haemorrhage, excessive swelling or oedema, infection, poor wound healing, and failure to remove both testicles and risks involved with anaesthesia when used [28]. Therefore, FVE, the Federation of veterinarian of Europe, is of the position that pig castration should always be performed by a veterinarian under general or local anaesthesia with additional prolonged analgesia [29]. It should also be noted that some anaesthetics such as ketamine in many countries is upon strict regulation due to illicit use.

As a priority to make further progress, a series of mutually agreed, practical and effective analgesia and/or anaesthesia protocols should be agreed at a national or EU level. These protocols should be cost effective, produce minimum stress and pain both during and after castration and be safe for both the handler and the piglet. The method should also ensure a quick recovery to minimize the risk of the piglet being crushed by the sow.

In 2016, a European consortium on the basis of a call of the European Commission (SANCO/2014/G3/026) started a study on methods of pig castration – called 'CASTRUM'. More specifically the study will try to identify available methods for the use of anaesthesia and/or prolonged analgesia and specifically look into alternatives to surgical castration for 'heavy' pigs used in traditional products. The outcome of this study should become available in 2017.

Expert opinion on immunocastration
The estimated average percentage of immunocastrated pigs in the countries surveyed was 2.7% (median = 0.2%), where Belgium presented the highest estimated percentage of immunocastrated pigs (18%). Respondents from Czech Republic, Norway, Romania, Spain and Sweden reported a slight increase in immunocastrated pigs in the last 3–5 years. Immunocastration has been permitted in the EU since 2009, but while it is used to a great extend in some countries abroad such as Australia [30], it seems still difficult to break through in Europe. Immunocastration is used in a higher proportion of pigs in Belgium mainly due to the impact of a major Belgian retailer (Colruyt) who since end 2010 only accepts pork from pigs castrated by vaccination. At this moment

Zoetis is the only company which has a Gonadotrofine Releasing Factor vaccine on the market (Improvac R). In terms of feasibility, the vaccine requires two doses, at least 4 weeks apart, with the second dose being given ideally 3–4 weeks before slaughter. Pigs slaughtered at a higher slaughter weight may need more than two doses. A single effective shot of the "vaccine" is being investigated at the moment [31]. Immunocastration eliminates the acute pain experienced by surgically castrated piglets; however welfare concerns still arise due to the fact that immuno-castrated pigs behave as entire males until the second vaccination. The main limitation to immunocastration is linked to market issues and human error (vaccinating outside the recommended time period, missing a dose [32]. Most retailers do not accept pork from immunocastrated pigs being afraid for poor public acceptance. However, in the case of Belgium, the acceptance of immunocastration led to a better welfare-friendly image of the retailer and large scale surveys conducted in European countries, showed that over 60% of surveyed consumers informed about the issue preferred immunocastration to surgical castration with anaesthesia [33].

From an animal-ethical point of view, not all alternatives to pig castration are equal [34, 35]. Immunocastration may give the greatest benefit to the animals, while raising entire males can still lead to pigs suffering from aggressive behaviour amongst each other and giving pain relief are seen as less animal-friendly alternative [34].

Expert opinion on entire males
Entire males' production is another main alternative to surgical castration. From an animal welfare perspective, raising entire males has benefits but also disadvantages [30]. In Ireland, Portugal, Spain and the United Kingdom less than 20% of the pigs were surgically castrated. Most countries do not rear entire male pig due to the incidence of boar taint. There is so far no international accepted and validated on-line method available for the measurements of boar taint in carcasses that throughout fulfils the requirement for a highly streamlined industry at the slaughterhouses [36]. Ireland and the United Kingdom address the incidence of boar taint by slaughtering at low weight and before sexual maturity. According to de Roest [37], the raising of entire males can be an interesting option for many countries, except for countries and production systems with a high age at slaughtering. The costs and benefits of this alternative will depend on the percentage of males with boar taint at slaughtering. Raising entire males should not generate more than 2.5% of boar taint among slaughter pigs, in order to maintain the considerable economic benefits of better feed efficiency of entire males with respect to castrate [37].

Conclusions

The deadline of 1 January 2012, which marks the day after which all castrated piglets reared in the EU and EFTA countries have to be treated with prolonged analgesia and/or anaesthesia, is far from being met in the majority of the 24 countries we surveyed. Analgesia alone is now used in several countries, probably partly due to the Declaration, but the effectiveness of this method to alleviate the pain during male piglet castration is questionable. There is still a major bottleneck in the use of the combination of anaesthesia and analgesia among the majority of the countries surveyed, the anaesthesia appearing to be the biggest constraint at the farm level.

The percentage of male pig population immunocastrated is still very low. Still, it appears as a promising alternative to surgical castration in countries such as Belgium. In Ireland, United Kingdom, Spain and Portugal, the production of entire males has been for long used as the main type of pig meat and a further increase is foreseen in other countries. In our survey Belgium, France, Germany, the Netherlands and Switzerland reported an increase in the number of pigs raised as entire males. Depending of the country, immunocastration and entire male production are foreseen as valuable alternatives to surgical castration.

As a priority to make further progress, a series of practical and effective analgesia and/or anaesthesia protocols should be mutually agreed at a national or EU level.

It is the apprehension of the authors that given the current economic climate, it is unlikely that pig producers will be able to follow the Declaration on pig castration unless it becomes mandatory in one way or another.

Abbreviations

Declaration: European Declaration on alternatives to surgical castration of pigs; EAPHM: European Association of Porcine Health Management; EU: European Union; FVE: Federation of Veterinarians of Europe.

Acknowledgements

Our thanks goes to the European Commission, Directorate General for Health and Food Safety, for the assistance with the survey design and all members of the Federation of Veterinarians of Europe (FVE) and the European Association of Porcine Health Management (EAPHM) for spreading the survey. Our special thanks to all porcine health experts who completed the survey and provided expert opinion.

Funding

No funding was provided.

Authors' contributions

NDB study design, data collection, and draft of manuscript. DT data analysis, statistical analysis, and support drafting manuscript. CB draft of manuscript, data collection. TB draft of manuscript, data collection. All authors reviewed, edited and approved the final manuscript.

Competing interests

The authors declare that they have no competing interests.

Author details

[1]Federation of Veterinarians of Europe, Avenue Tervueren 12, 1040 Brussels, Belgium. [2]Department of Animal Environment and Health, Swedish University of Agricultural Sciences, POB 234, Skara SE-532 23, Sweden. [3]German Veterinary Association for Animal Welfare, Wiesenweg 11, 49456 Bakum, Germany. [4]Universitat Autònoma de Barcelona, Veterinary School, Farm Animal Welfare Education Center, 08193 Bellaterra, Barcelona, Spain.

References

1. European Union. Council Directive 2008/120/EC of 18 December 2008 laying down minimum standards for the protection of pigs. OJ L 47, 18.2. 2009.
2. Mellor DJ, Stafford KJ. Animal welfare implications of neonatal mortality and morbidity in farm animals. Vet J. 2004;168:118–33.
3. Mellor DJ, Gregory NG. Responsiveness, behavioural arousal and awareness in fetal and newborn lambs: experimental, practical and therapeutic implications. N Z Vet J. 2003;51:2–13.
4. Marchant-Forde JN, Lay Jr DC, McMunn KA, Cheng HW, Pajor EA, Marchand-Forde JN. Postnatal piglet husbandry practices and well-being: The effects of alternative techniques delivered separately. J Anim Sci. 2009;87:1479–92.
5. Wemelsfelder F, van Putten G. Behaviour as a possible indicator for pain in piglets, Report B-260. Zeist, The Netherlands: Instituut voor Veeteeltkundig Onderzoek 'Schoonoord'; 1985.
6. Hay M, Vulin A, Genin S, Sales P, Prunier A. Assessment of pain induced by castration in piglets: behavioral and physiological responses over the subsequent 5 days. Appl Anim Behav Sci. 2003;82:201–18.
7. Hansson M, Lundeheim N, Nyman G, Joansson G. Effect of local anaesthesia and/or analgesia on pain responses induced by piglet castration. Acta Vet Scand. 2011;53:34. doi:10.1186/1751-0147-53-34.
8. Rault JL, Lay Jr DC, Marchant-Forde JN. Castration induced pain in pigs and other livestock. Appl Anim Behav Sci. 2011;135:214–25.
9. Horn TT, Marx G, et al. Behavior of piglets during castration with and without local anaesthesia. Deutsche tierärztliche Wochenschrift. 1999;106: 271–4.
10. Kluivers-Poodt M, Hopster H, Spoolder H. Castration under anaesthesia and/or analgesia in commercial pig production. Report 85. Animal science Group 2007. Wageningen-UR, The Netherlands.
11. European Commission. European Declaration on alternatives to surgical castration of pigs. https://ec.europa.eu/food/sites/food/files/animals/docs/aw_prac_farm_pigs_castalt_declaration_en.pdf. Accessed 26 July 2016.
12. Backus G, et al. First progress report from the European declaration on alternatives to surgical castration of pigs. 2014. http://ec.europa.eu/dgs/health_food-safety/information_sources/docs/ahw/20150226_ahw_pig-castration_pres_9_en.pdf. Accessed 26 Oct 2016.
13. Fredriksen B, Furnols MFI, Lundstrom K, Migdal W, Prunier A, Tuyttens FAM, Bonneau M. Practice on castration of piglets in Europe. Anim. 2009;3:1480–7.
14. Prunier A, Bonneau M, von Borell EH, Cinotti S, Gunn M, Fredriksen B, Giersing M, Morton DB, Tuyttens FAM, Velarde A. A review of the welfare consequences of surgical castration in piglets and the evaluation of non-surgical methods. Anim Welf. 2006;15:277–89.
15. Kluivers-Poodt M, Houx B, Robben S, Koop G, Lambooij E, Hellebrekers L. Effects of a local anaesthetic and NSAID in castration of piglets, on the acute pain responses, growth and mortality. Animal. 2012;6:1469–75.
16. Haga HA, Ranheim B. Castration of piglets: the analgesia effects of intratesticular and intrafunicular lidocaine injection. Vet Anaesth Analg. 2005;32:1–9.
17. Ranheim B, Haga HA. Local anaesthesia for pigs subject to castration. Acta Vet Scand. 2006;48:S13.
18. Keita A, Pagot E, Prunier A, Guidarini C. Pre-emptive meloxicam for postoperative analgesia in piglets undergoing surgical castration. Vet Anaesth Analg. 2010;37:367–74.
19. SUIVET. Castration protocols. www.suivet.it. Accessed on 26 Oct 2016.

20. Courboulay V, Hemonic A, Gadonna A, Prunnier A. Castration avec anesthésie locale ou traitement anti-inflammatoire : quel impact sur la douleur des porcelets et quelles conséquences sur le travail en élevage? JRP. 2010;27.

21. McGlone JJ, Hellman JM. Local and general anesthesic effects on behavior and performance of two- and seven-week-old castrated and uncastrated piglets. J Anim Sci. 1988;66:3049–58.

22. Van Beirendonck S, Driessen B, Verbeke G, Geers R. Behavior of piglets after castration with or without carbon dioxide anesthesia. J Anim Sci. 2011;89:3310–7.

23. Raj ABM, Gregory NG. Welfare implications of gas stunning of pigs. Stress of induction of anaesthesia. Anim Welf. 1996;5:71–8.

24. Llonch P, Rodriguez P, Jospin M, Dalmau A, Manteca X, Velarde A. Assessment of unconsciousness during exposure to nitrogen and carbon dioxide mixtures for stunning in pigs. Animal. 2013;7:492–8.

25. Schwennen C, Kolbaum N, Waldmann KH, Höltig D. Evaluation of the anaesthetic depth during piglet castration under an automated isoflurane-anaesthesia at farm level. Berl Munch Tierarztl Wochenschr. 2016;129:40–7.

26. Nussbaumer I. Azaperone, Butorphanol and Ketamine: Anaesthetic concept for castration of young pigs. 2012. Veterinary Science Development; volume 2:e9 file:///C:/Users/nansd/Downloads/3983-27173-2-PB.pdf. Accessed on 26 July 2016.

27. Federation of Veterinarians of Europe FVE. European Veterinary Act. 2013. www.fve.org, Accessed on 26 Oct 2016.

28. American Veterinary Medical Association, AVMA. Literature Review on the Welfare Implications of Swine Castration. 2014. https://www.avma.org/KB/Resources/LiteratureReviews/Documents/swine_castration_bgnd.pdf. Accessed on 26 Oct 2016.

29. Federation of Veterinarians of Europe FVE. FVE position paper on pig castration. 2009. www.fve.org. Accessed on 26 Oct 2016.

30. European Food Safety Agency EFSA. Welfare aspects of the castration of piglets. Scientific Report of the Scientific Panel for Animal Health and Welfare on a request from the Commission related to welfare aspects of the castration of piglets European Food Safety Authority 2004 AHAW/04-087. (http://www.efsa.europa.eu/en/efsajournal/pub/91). Accessed 26 Oct 2016.

31. De Briyne N. Personal communication. 2016.

32. Fredriksen B, Hexeberg C, Dahl E, Nafstad O. Vaccination against boar taint – control regimes at the slaughter house [abstract]. Proceedings of the European Federation of Animal Science– 62nd Annual Meeting. Stavanger, Norway; 2011, p. 256.

33. Vanhonacker F, Verbeke W. Consumer response to the possible use of a vaccine method to control boar taint v. physical piglet castration with anaesthesia: a quantitative study in four European countries. Anim. 2011;5:1107–18.

34. Blaha T. Der Ausstieg aus der betäubungslosen Kastration des Schweines – Eine Bewertung der Alternativen aus der Sicht der Tierethik. (Phasing out the surgical castration of pigs without analgesia/anesthesia – evaluating the alternatives from an animal-ethical standpoint). 2016; Deutsche TBl. 6, 836.

35. Whitford A. Derecho Animal. 2014. http://www.derechoanimal.info/images/pdf/Whitfort-Ethics-Paper-Castration-of-Piglets.pdf. Accessed on 26 Oct 2016.

36. Danish Centre for Food and Agriculture. Alternatives to surgical castration in Danish pig production - a position review, DCA report no. 042. 2014. http://web.agrsci.dk/djfpublikation/djfpdf/dcarapport42.pdf. Accessed on 26 Oct. 2016.

37. de Roest K, Montanari C, Fowler T, Baltussen W. Resource efficiency and economic implications of alternatives to surgical castration without anaesthesia. Animal. 2009;11:1522–31.

17

Relationships between colostrum supply of suckling piglets and *Salmonella* prevalence in piglet rearing

Anton Schulte zu Sundern[1*], Carolin Holling[2], Karl Rohn[3], Josef Schulte-Wülwer[4], Ansgar Deermann[4] and Christian Visscher[1]

Abstract

Background: Despite years of effort, the proportion of serologically *Salmonella*-conspicuous pig farms has not been significantly reduced. Incoming piglets are considered to be a significant source of *Salmonella* for feeder-to-finish-farms. Therefore it is important for farrow-to-feeder-farms to deliver *Salmonella*-inconspicuous piglets. The aim of the present study was to establish a possible link between an inadequate colostrum supply as a side effect of steadily increasing number of piglets born alive and weaned per sow and increasing *Salmonella* seroprevalence in piglet rearing on *Salmonella*-conspicuous farms.

Methods: Twenty four farms in total were selected for this study. Half of the farms ($n = 12$) had been detected as *Salmonella*-conspicuous in previous serological tests on piglets (25 kg) and remaining farms (n = 12) had appeared *Salmonella*-inconspicuous. Every farm was visited once 24–28 h after the main day of farrowing. For sampling, four sows were randomly selected on each farm. The parity, the litter weight and the litter size were recorded. The sow and six of her piglets were selected for blood sampling (two light-weight, two medium-weight and two heavy-weight piglets respectively). In addition, the colostrum supply of newborn piglets was estimated by using the immunocrit.

Results: The lightest piglets on *Salmonella*-inconspicuous and *Salmonella*-conspicuous farms showed a significant difference ($p < 0.0339$) in the colostrum supply (estimated by immunocrit). While light-weighted piglets in *Salmonella*-inconspicuous farms had an average immunocrit of 0.100 ($\pm$0.04) light-weighted piglets in *Salmonella*-conspicuous farms had an average immunocrit of 0.087 ($\pm$0.04). There was no significant difference ($p > 0.05$) in the factors body weight, litter weight, parity and litter size.

Conclusion: The study provides preliminary evidence that when comparing *Salmonella*-inconspicuous farms with *Salmonella*-conspicuous ones, the colostrum supply may be a critical factor that needs to be considered. The fact that there is no difference in body weight between the two groups of farms suggests that there may be differences in farrowing management and especially colostrum management. Further studies are now required to investigate what causes the various colostrum supply on the respective farms and what long-term effects the individual colostrum supply might have on *Salmonella* prevalence at abattoir.

Keywords: *Salmonella*, Health status, Fertility, Piglet rearing, Monitoring, Colostrum

* Correspondence: anton.schulte.zu.sundern@tiho-hannover.de
[1]Institute for Animal Nutrition, University of Veterinary Medicine Hannover, Foundation, Bischofsholer Damm 15, D-30173 Hannover, Germany
Full list of author information is available at the end of the article

Background

In 2016, human salmonellosis was the second most common foodborne zoonosis in the European Union as a whole as well as in Germany [1, 2]. Although the absolute number of human salmonellosis cases reported by the Robert Koch Institute (RKI) in Germany decreased from more than 70,000 patients in 2001 to 12,962 in 2016 [3], pork received attention as being the cause of human salmonellosis [1]. *Salmonella* Typhimurium (*S.* Typhimurium) pork-associated human salmonellosis accounted for the second largest percentage of all RKI-reported cases (36%) [3]. The *Salmonella* monitoring programme, which was started in 2003 and adapted in 2007 to the Pig-Salmonella Regulation, obliges all pig farmers to participate in the Quality and Safety GmbH (QS) system. Sampling in this programme is usually carried out in abattoirs and classifies fattening farms into risk classes [4]. This can lead to marketing disadvantages and price reductions. Despite intensive efforts, the percentage of *Salmonella*-conspicuous farms in Germany could not be significantly reduced [5]. The QS - statistics have shown an almost unchanged picture in the last ten years. The percentage of farms classified into category III (> 40% positive samples) decreased only slightly from 5.4% in 2006 to 3.4% in 2017. The percentage of category II farms (21–40% positive samples) even increased in the same period from 14.7% to 20.0% [6, 7]. Experience from various field studies in which also hygienic well-managed farms were included, suggests that improving hygiene as the sole means of reducing *Salmonella* is not the only priority [8]. Of greatest significance for the entry and distribution of *Salmonella* in pig herds are carrier pigs [9]. The association between *Salmonella* seroprevalence in sows and the direct detection of *S.* Typhimurium in rearing piglets is well known, as is the association between the direct detection of *S.* Typhimurium in rearing pigs and increased *Salmonella* seroprevalence in fattening pigs [10, 11]. These findings suggest that a reduction in *Salmonella* prevalence can only be successful if the piglet producers are involved. In recent years, they have been able to achieve an enormous increase in reproductive performance. For example, an analysis performed among northern German piglet producers showed an increase from 11.10 live born piglets per litter in the marketing year 2006/07 to 13.91 in the marketing year 2015/16 [12]. This also presents piglet producers with new challenges. Increasingly large litters with low average birth weights require intensive care and good management. Schulte zu Sundern et al. [13] were able to demonstrate in comparative analysis of results of a health screening and results of computer-supported sow planning that farms with an above-average fertility performance (live born or weaned piglets) often do not belong to the farms with the lowest

Salmonella seroprevalence of ready-to-sell piglets. It was also shown that the average number of weaned piglets had a greater influence on the *Salmonella* seroprevalence than the average number of piglets born alive. This suggests that management from birth to weaning could be critical for *Salmonella* prevalence on the farm. The focus of many studies is the colostrum supply in the first days of life. Quesnel et al. [14] were able to prove that the litter size is not directly related to the amount of colostrum which is produced. For very large litters, there may be a gap between the amount of colostrum produced and the amount that would be necessary for a sufficient supply of all piglets. This condition is intensified by the fact that the amount of colostrum produced varies between 2.8 kg / d and 8.5 kg / d [15]. The aim of the present study was to establish a possible link between an inadequate colostrum supply as a side effect of steadily increasing reproductive performance and increasing *Salmonella* seroprevalence in piglet rearing on *Salmonella*-conspicuous farms.

Methods

The study was carried out in cooperation with EVH-Select GmbH, an association of six northern German piglet producer communities in which more than 250 piglet producers are organised. The data from a health status monitoring programme organised by EVH-Select GmbH was used retrospectively for this field study. Under the organisation of EVH-Select GmbH, this monitoring has taken place every six months since 2014 on the farms and provides information about the health status of the piglets to the feeder-to-finish-farms. Participation is voluntary. For sampling, ten piglets weighing 25 kg are used for each screening. The animals used for the sampling are randomly selected within an age group. Obviously sick and nursed animals are not selected. *Salmonella* LPS antibodies were detected by Herdcheck® *Salmonella* ELISA (IDEXX Laboratories, Hoofddorp, the Netherlands). The samples were considered "positive" if the optical density (OD) was ≥10%. The direct test for *Salmonella* is not part of this health-status-monitoring. On the basis of the available health-status-monitoring results, farms (*n* = 12) were selected (Table 1) that had been experiencing an increased *Salmonella* seroprevalence of ready-to-sell piglets for a longer period of time and that had consulted veterinarians for advice. For every single *Salmonella*-conspicuous farm one farm was selected (n = 12) comparable in hygiene, management, performance, farm size and veterinary care but inconspicuous in *Salmonella* seroprevalence. The farms C and F were assessed as *Salmonella*-inconspicuous despite striking health-status-monitoring results. The relatively high average values could be explained by very high individual values in older health-status-monitoring results.

Table 1 Results of the voluntary health-status-monitoring from 2014 to 2017 on *Salmonella*-inconspicuous and *Salmonella*-conspicuous farms

Salmonella-inconspicuous farms					Salmonella-conspicuous farms				
Farm	Average Salmonella - OD	Number of tests	Proportion of postive piglets	Proportion of postive piglets [%]	Farm	Average Salmonella - OD	Number of tests	Proportion of postive piglets	Proportion of postive piglets [%]
A	1.4	4	0/40	0	M	16.26	5	19/50	38
B	2.83	4	2/40	5	N	19.71	4	14/40	35
C	6.14	4	7/40	18	O	18.41	5	22/50	44
D	0.32	1	0/10	0	P	9.62	1	2/10	20
E	0.94	4	1/40	3	Q	18.08	5	21/50	42
F	22.35	7	16/70	23	R	14.73	7	24/70	34
G	1.64	5	2/50	4	S	8.01	5	13/50	26
H	1.84	5	1/50	2	T	9.09	5	17/55	31
I	1.00	3	0/30	0	U	11.57	7	26/70	37
J	2.38	5	4/50	8	V	15.01	6	22/60	36
K	3.00	4	4/40	10	W	22.28	5	29/50	58
L	0.39	6	0/60	0	X	16.05	5	18/50	36

Animals

All participating piglet producers (*n* = 24) were located in the federal state of Lower Saxony in the districts of Emsland, Grafschaft Bentheim and Osnabrück. Only a small proportion of farms (*n* = 2) were farrow-to-finish farms. The remaining farms were exclusively piglet producers. The average number of sows kept was 309 sows (*Salmonella*-inconspicuous farms: 280, *Salmonella*-conspicuous: 339, respectively). The average number of piglets born alive and weaned per litter (Ø 12 month before sampling) was 13.87 and 11.98. (*Salmonella*-inconspicuous farms: 13.99 and 11.99, *Salmonella*-conspicuous: 13.76 and 11.97, respectively). The majority of the farms used sows from breeding lines of DanAvl® (*n* = 10). The remaining farms used sows from the breeding lines of the Bundes Hybrid Zucht Programm, Ellringen, Germany (BHZP®, *n* = 7), Topig's Norsvin®, Senden, Germany (*n* = 3) or Pig Improvement Company Deutschland GmbH, Hannover, Germany (PIC®, *n* = 4).The large proportion of farms produced at three-weekly intervals (*n* = 9), followed by those producing at fortnightly intervals (*n* = 6), at weekly intervals (n = 4) and others (*n* = 5). The average suckling time was 25.25 days (*Salmonella*-inconspicuous 24.91 days, *Salmonella*-conspicuous 25.58 days). The sows selected for the study had on average 5.03 parities (*Salmonella*-inconspicuous 4.78 ± 2.48, *Salmonella*-conspicuous 5.27 ± 2.14, respectively). The following boar lines were used, listed in decreasing order of importance PIC® 408 (*n* = 8), db.77® (n = 6), German Pietran® (*n* = 3), Topigs® (*n* = 3). Four farms used different boar lines.

Sample collection

All farms (*n* = 24) were visited once depending on their production rhythm 24–48 h after the main farrowing day. On each farm, four sows were randomly selected from all sows already farrowed. A uniform selection of sows was not possible. Due to different herd sizes the total number of sows (24-48 h after farrowing) was totally different. But if possible one of the selected sows was first parity. Foster-mother sows and sows with unfamiliar piglets were not included in the selection. Recorded were the parity, the litter size and the total weight of the litter. For blood sampling, six piglets per litter were selected. The selection of the piglets was made in such a way that two light-weight, two medium-weight and two heavy-weight piglets were always used for sampling in relation to the litter. The individual weight of the selected piglets was recorded, too. On 19 farms blood sampling also included the respective maternal sows (*n* = 71); (12 *Salmonella*-inconspicuous farms, seven *Salmonella*-conspicuous farms). In order to ensure the comparability of the serological results despite different sample numbers, seven additional pairs were formed between the categories (seven *Salmonella*-inconspicuous farms, seven *Salmonella*-conspicuous farms). For the sample collection Serum Monovette with coagulation activator were used (Monovette 9 mL, Sarstedt AG & Co., Nümbrecht, Germany). The collected blood samples were refrigerated, transported to the laboratory and centrifuged at 2000 x g for 10 min, and the serum samples stored at – 20 °C until further analysis.

Analysis

The samples were serologically examined using standardised methods in an accredited laboratory (Vaxxinova diagnostics GmbH, Leipzig, Germany). The detection of *Salmonella* LPS antibodies was carried out as in the health-status-monitoring using Herdcheck® *Salmonella* ELISA (IDEXX Laboratories, Hoofddorp, the Netherlands).

The cut-off for the examined sows was carried out in accordance with the requirements of the Pig *Salmonella* Regulations for slaughter pigs. The samples of the examined sows were regarded as "serologically positive" if the optical density (OD) was ≥40%. The suckling piglets were not classified into "serologically positive" or "serologically negative" groups. The quantification of the colostrum supply of the piglets was carried out by means of the immunocrit method [16]. For this, 50 µL of serum were mixed with 50 µL of 40% (wt / vol) ammonium sulphate. The Ig present in the serum was precipitated. This was followed by centrifugation at 12000×g in a hematocrit capillary (disposable microhaematocrit capillary tubes 75 mm / 75 µL, Hirschmann Laborgeräte GmbH & Co. KG, Eberstadt, Germany) for 10 min. The resulting precipitate in relation to the total volume allows the colostrum supply to be estimated.

Statistical analysis

The statistical analysis of the data was carried out with the statistical analysis program SAS®9.4 for Windows, using the SAS® Enterprise Guide®, Client Version 7.1 (SAS Institute Inc. Cary, USA). By means of the Shapiro-Wilks test, the quantitative parameters were checked for normal distribution. For the normally distributed parameters immunocrit and body weight, possible differences between inconspicuous and conspicuous farms for the three weight categories were tested by the t-test for independent samples. The comparison between inconspicuous and conspicuous farms for non-normally distributed *Salmonella* antibody results was performed using the Wilcoxon 2-Sample test. A significance level α of 5% ($p <$ 0.05) was determined. For the correlation analysis of normally distributed data the correlation coefficient of Pearson was used. For non-normally distributed data sets, the Spearman rank correlation coefficient was calculated. Interpreting the correlation coefficient Rho was determined as follows: $0.0 \leq r \leq 0.2$ = no to low correlation; $0.2 < r \leq 0.5$ = weak to moderate relationship; $0.5 < r \leq 0.8$ = clear relationship; $0.8 < r \leq 1.0$ = high to perfect correlation.

Results

Serology

In the serological examination and the detection of *Salmonella* antibodies the average OD in the examined sows showed a significant difference ($p < 0.0451$) between those of *Salmonella*-inconspicuous and *Salmonella*-conspicuous farms. The average OD of sows selected for sampling was 45.43% (± 26.89) for the 12 *Salmonella*-inconspicuous farms. In the seven farms that were previously classified as *Salmonella*-conspicuous by sampling the ready-to-sell piglets, the average OD of the tested sows was 32.88% (± 21.96). When considering only the results of the sows of the 14 farms (seven

Salmonella-inconspicuous farms, seven *Salmonella*-conspicuous farms), the difference was even greater ($p < 0.0153$). The mean OD of the sows on the seven *Salmonella*-inconspicuous farms was 50.85% (± 29.34) and on the seven *Salmonella*-conspicuous farms 32.88% (± 21.96). On evaluating the study results of the 14 farms, no serologically positive sow was detected on five farms (Table 2). Although there was a significant difference in the *Salmonella* seroprevalence of the sows, the serological results of the piglets were similar on *Salmonella*-inconspicuous and *Salmonella*-conspicuous farms (Table 3).

Colostrum supply

On both the *Salmonella*-inconspicuous and *Salmonella*-conspicuous farms, the two selected light-weight piglets per litter had a significantly lower colostrum supply (estimated by the immunocrit) than their medium-weight and heavy-weight littermates. It was also shown in this study that on *Salmonella*-conspicuous farms the colostrum supply of the light-weight piglets in the litter was significantly worse ($p < 0.0339$) than in the group of the light-weight piglets on *Salmonella*-inconspicuous farms. While light-weighted piglets in *Salmonella*-inconspicuous farms had an average immunocrit of 0.100 (±0.04) light-weight piglets in *Salmonella*-conspicuous farms had an average immunocrit of 0.087 (±0.04). There was no significant difference between *Salmonella*-inconspicuous and *Salmonella*-conspicuous farms, in the colostrum supply of medium-weight and heavy-weight piglets. The average weights of the light-weight, medium-weight and heavy-weight piglets did not differ in the two categories (Table 3). It was also shown that the colostrum supply on *Salmonella*-conspicuous farms was weak to moderate dependent ($r = 0.220$) from piglet weight. No correlation could be found on *Salmonella*-inconspicuous farms between bodyweight and colostrum intake ($r = 0.097$). Furthermore there were no significant differences between Salmonella-inconspicuous and Salmonella-

Table 2 On 14 farms (seven Salmonella-inconspicuous and seven Salmonella-conspicuous farms) four sows were tested by Salmonella antibodies

Farm	"Positiv"– tested sows on *Salmonella*-inconspicuous farms	Farm	"Positiv"-tested sows on *Salmonella*-conspicuous farms
A	2	M	1
B	4	N	1
D	4	P	1
G	0	S	1
H	0	T	2
I	0	U	0
J	1	W	0

The samples were regarded as "serologically positive" if the optical density (OD) was ≥40%

Table 3 Body weight (BW), Immunocrit value and Salmonella-OD of the tested piglets 24–48 h post natum (p.n.) divided into light-, medium- and heavy-weight piglets, Salmonella-inconspicuous and Salmonella-conspicuous farms

		Body weight [kg]		immunocrit		Salmonella - OD	
		Salmonella-inconspicuous farms	Salmonella-conspicuous farms	Salmonella-inconspicuous farms	Salmonella-conspicuous farms	Salmonella-inconspicuous farms	Salmonella-conspicuous farms
BW category	n-animals/ BW category	88	96	88	96	88	96
Light-weight		1.05 (±0.25)	1.05 (±0.29)	0.100[a] (±0.04)	0.087[b] (±0.04)	35.85 (± 38.66)	36.18 (± 39.31)
Medium-weight		1.38 (±0.25)	1.36 (±0.27)	0.107 (±0.03)	0.098 (±0.03)	38.71 (± 40.12)	37.59 (± 37.51)
Heavy-weight		1.69(±0.27)	1.78(±0.31)	0.114 (±0.03)	0.111(±0.03)	43.65 (± 41.88)	41.77 (± 38.55)

[a,b]averages differ significantly within a row ($p < 0.05$)

conspicuous farms in recorded litter weight, parity and litter size (Table 4).

Discussion
Classifying the farms
Classifying the farms into Salmonella-inconspicuous and Salmonella-conspicuous was based on a retrospective evaluation of health-status-monitoring. This monitoring was not performed on sows but on piglets (25 kg) and included only the indirect detection of Salmonella antibodies and not direct cultural Salmonella detection. The already established health-status-monitoring is based on the desire of the feeder-to-finish-farms to obtain information on the Salmonella status of the farrow-to-feeder farms. Comparing the inconspicuous ($n = 12$) and the conspicuous ($n = 12$) farms, it was found that the percentage of serologically positive sows was higher on those farms classified as inconspicuous (40.9%) than on those classified as conspicuous (29.6%). Furthermore, the average OD of the examined sows was higher on those farms classified as inconspicuous (OD 40.43%) than on those farms classified as conspicuous (OD 32.88%). These results raise the question whether the previous monitoring results, which focused on the sampling of piglets, provide a realistic picture of Salmonella prevalence for the entire herd (and the classification) into inconspicuous and conspicuous farms. In a pan-European study on Salmonella prevalence, Bole-Hribovšek et al. [17] found Salmonella on 31.8% of all studied farrow-to-feeder farms by direct detection. Meyer et al. [18] achieved similar results. In their study, carried out among northern German piglet producers of

various forms of husbandry, they found at least one positive seroreactors among the sows examined in 71.8% of all conventional piglet producers studied. Overall, 12.3% of all sows tested were seropositive. The detection of Salmonella positive seroreactors on those farms classified as Salmonella inconspicuous farms is therefore not surprising. The spread of Salmonella in pig herds can be considered ubiquitous.

Selection of animals
The animals selected for sampling were, two light-weight, two medium-weight and two heavy-weight piglets. The selection referred to the respective litter. A small percentage of individual animals were selected with a body weight of less than 1 kg. Some of these underweight animals, which had received only an insufficient amount of colostrum, were not successfully weaned and thereby played no role in the Salmonella distribution in the flat deck. Ferrari et al. [19] investigated the influence of birth weight and colostrum uptake (in g) on suckling pig mortality. While piglets with a birth weight of 1.40–1.45 kg and a colostrum intake of 250–300 g had a suckling pig mortality of 6.0% and 4.7% respectively, the mortality rate in 1.10–1.15 kg piglets and a colostrum intake of ≤150 g had a suckling pig mortality of 12.2% and 23.1%, respectively. High-performance farms are also able to raise the proportionately larger numbers of pigs, which are less developed at birth, through intensive management [20]. Despite losses among light or underserved piglets, many of these piglets are successfully weaned and could play a role in the infection in the flat deck. This is also supported by the findings of Schulte zu Sundern et al. [13] in a

Table 4 Average litter size, litter weight, parity and Salmonella-OD of the tested sows

	Salmonella-inconspicuous farms	Salmonella-conspicuous farms
Litter size	13.65 (± 2.10)	13.57 (± 2.91)
Litter weight [kg]	18.94 (± 3.99)	18.93 (± 3.51)
Parity	4.78 (± 2.48)	5.27 (± 2.14)
Salmonella - OD – Sow	45.43 (± 26.89)	32.88 (± 21.96)

retrospective analysis of health status monitoring results and a comparison with data from computer-supported sow planning. They were able to prove that the most productive piglet producers were not among those with the lowest *Salmonella*-seroprevalence.

Possible causes of a different colostrum supply

Both on the *Salmonella*-inconspicuous and *Salmonella*-conspicuous farms, the medium-weight and heavy-weight piglets in a litter were better supplied with colostrum than their light-weight littermates. The impact of birth weight on colostrum intake and the critical role played by light-weight piglets compared to their heavier littermates have been demonstrated in numerous studies ([16, 19, 21]). There was a significant difference ($p = 0.033$) in the colostrum supply of the lightest piglets between the *Salmonella*-inconspicuous and *Salmonella*-conspicuous farms. While the light-weight piglets on *Salmonella*-inconspicuous farms had an average immunocrit of 0.100 ($\pm$ 0.04), the lightest piglets on *Salmonella*-conspicuous farms had only an average immunocrit of 0.087 ($\pm$ 0.04). In the medium-weight and heavy-weight piglets, the difference between the inconspicuous and conspicuous farms was not significant ($p = 0.199$ and $p = 0.591$, respectively). In the data on litter weight and litter size, which also influence the colostrum supply as does birth weight ([15, 16]), no significant differences were found between the *Salmonella*-inconspicuous and *Salmonella*-conspicuous farms (Table 4). As the aforementioned biological factors do not cause the differing amounts in the colostrum supply it would appear that the farrowing-management or unrecorded factors play a decisive role therein. This is supported by the fact that, in our comparative analysis, the influence of weight on the colostrum supply on *Salmonella*-inconspicuous farms did not seem to be decisive ($r = 0.097$) whereas this factor was at least mild to moderate on *Salmonella*-conspicuous farms ($r = 0.220$). Factors that may explain the differences in colostrum supply of the light-weight piglets on *Salmonella*-inconspicuous and *Salmonella*-conspicuous farms are numerous. Declerck et al. [22] were able to show that the use of Oxytocin at birth and a long interval between births correlated negatively with the colostrum supply. Farmer and Quesnel [23] found numerous other factors in their review. In particular, the impact of on-demand sow feeding in the near-term and stress had a negative impact on colostrum formation. Finding the weak point in management for individual farms would be subject for further studies.

Maternal-transmitting antibodies as effective protection against *Salmonella*

In our experiment, we found that every farm, both *Salmonella*- inconspicuous and *Salmonella*-conspicuous

farms, a large percentage of the sows had *Salmonella* antibodies. This indicates a common spread of *Salmonella* on the farms. Effective protection of the piglets from *Salmonella* infection by vaccination of the sows was the aim of numerous experiments. The effectiveness thereof could be proved, for example [24]. In this previous study piglets from five sows were orally infected with a field strain on the fourth day of life and euthanised three days later. Two of the accompanying sows were vaccinated with an inactivated strain. Two more sows were classified as *Salmonella* negative by ELISA. The fifth selected sow had a high *Salmonella* antibody titer despite no vaccination. After piglet euthanasia, cultural studies on *Salmonella* were carried out. The piglets of the sows, which had either been vaccinated or, had high *Salmonella* antibody titers, showed a significantly lower number of *Salmonella* in the tested tissue. These findings are supported by the investigations by Roesler et al. [25]. Here, the use of an inactivated *Salmonella* vaccine in 25 sows also showed an effective reduction in *Salmonella* prevalence in piglet rearing. A similar result was found by Hur and Lee [26]. When considering the *Salmonella* antibodies detected by ELISA, it can be stated that despite differing amount of colostrum supply (measured by immunocrit), no significant differences in the average OD between the *Salmonella*-inconspicuous and *Salmonella*-conspicuous farms could be recognized. The complexity of the protection given by the colostrum intake does not appear to be fully ensured by sole consideration of the ELISA results. In addition to the immunoglobulins transmitted by the colostrum, other substances also appear to provide protection against *Salmonella* infection. Blais et al. [27] demonstrated a positive effect of colostrum-containing whey in their in vitro experiments. Their experiments utilised a porcine-intestinal-epithelial-cell (IPEC-J2) model, bovine colostrum and heat-killed (HK) *Salmonella* Typhimurium. The colostrum in the model was able to reduce the inflammatory processes caused by *Salmonella*, making it difficult to attach to the intestinal cells.

Conclusion

The results of this field study suggest that in comparative investigations of *Salmonella*-inconspicuous and *Salmonella*-conspicuous piglet producers, inadequate colostrum supply of light-weight piglets could be a factor in increased *Salmonella* seroprevalence of piglets (25 kg) on *Salmonella*-conspicuous farms. Furthermore, no differences in birth weight, litter size, litter weight and parity between the *Salmonella*-inconspicuous and *Salmonella*-conspicuous farms could be determined. This suggests that there must be differences in management, especially between birth, weaning and sale. Based on this presumption, it must be examined in subsequent follow-up studies whether piglets with insufficient colostrum supply, at the end of rearing or slaughtering, appear conspicuous in their *Salmonella*-prevalence or whether piglets with sufficient colostrum supply appear inconspicuous at the same time in their *Salmonella* prevalence.

Abbreviations
BW: Bodyweight.; HK: Heat-killed.; Ig: Immunoglobulin.; IPEC-J2 : Porcine-intestinal-epithelial-cell.; LPS: Lipopolysaccharide.; OD: Optical density.; RKI: Robert Koch Institute

Acknowledgements
We would like to thank the farmers who provided the animals for taking samples and Frances Sherwood-Brock for editing the manuscript to ensure correct English.

Funding
This study was supported by EIP-Agri (Agriculture & Innovation), European Agricultural Fund for Rural Development (Project 276 03 454 035 0521).

Authors' contributions
CV, AD and JSW and were the initiators of the idea. CV, ASZS designed the study. ASZS and CH visited the farms. ASZS and CH took the samples. ASZS made the analyses. ASZS and KR did the statistics. ASZS wrote the paper. All authors read and approved the final manuscript.

Competing interests
The authors declare that they have no competing interests.

Author details
[1]Institute for Animal Nutrition, University of Veterinary Medicine Hannover, Foundation, Bischofsholer Damm 15, D-30173 Hannover, Germany. [2]Swine Health Service, Chamber of Agriculture Lower Saxony, Sedanstr. 4 D-26121, Oldenburg, Germany. [3]Institute for Biometry, University of Veterinary Medicine Hannover, Foundation, Bünteweg 2, D-30559 Hannover, Germany. [4]EVH Select GmbH, An der Feuerwache 14, D-49716 Meppen, Germany.

References
1. Anonym. EFSA scientific committee-scientific opinion on a quantitative microbiological risk assessment of salmonella in slaughter and breeder pigs. EFSA J. 2010:1547.
2. Pfennigwerth N: Bericht des Nationalen Referenzzentrums (NRZ) für gramnegative Krankenhauserreger. 2017.
3. Anonym. Berichte zur Lebensmittelsicherheit 2016: Zoonosen-Monitoring. In: Bundesamt für Verbraucherschutz und Lebensmittelsicherheit; 2016.
4. Anonym: Verordnung zur Vermeidung der Salmonellenverbreitung durch Schlachtschweine (Schweine-Salmonellen-Verordnung vom 13. März 2007 (BGBl. I S. 322)), die zuletzt durch Artikel 137 des Gesetzes vom 29. März 2017 (BGBl. I S. 626) geändert worden ist. 2007.
5. Rostalski A. Salmonella in pig farms. Limitations of counselling and alternatives to the exclusive control of slaughter pigs *Tierärztl Prax*. 2015;43:305–11.
6. Römer R. Salmonellenmonitoringprogramm für die Fleischerzeugung-Aktuelle Trends und Herausforderungen für die Zukunft. In bpt Kongress Hannover 2016 Hannover bpt Akademie GmbH. 2016:92–6.
7. May T: Salmonellenmonitoring. QS Qualität und Sicherheit GmbH; 2017.
8. Roesner P, Eisenberg T, Hornstein O, Gebele U, Schulte-Wuelwer J, Schulze-Horsel T: Salmonellen beim Schwein-Beratungsempfehlungen der Schweinegesundheitsdienste. 2014.
9. Ahrens A: Epdemiologische Untersuchungen zum Vorkommen von Salmonellen bei sächsischen Mastschweinen mittels Fleischsaft-ELISA - Technik und bakteriologischer Untersuchungsmethodik nach der Amtlichen Sammlung von Untersuchungsverfahren nach § 35 LMBG. Universität Leipzig, Institut für Lebensmittelhygiene der Veterinärmedizinischen Fakultät; 2003.
10. Kranker S. Bacteriological and serological examination and risk factor analysis of salmonella occurence in sow herds, including risk factors for high salmonella seroprevalence in receiver finishing herds. Berl Munch Tierarztl Wochenschr. 2001;114:350–2.
11. Hill AA, Simons RR, Kelly L, Snary EL. A farm transmission model for salmonella in pigs, applicable to EU member states. Risk Anal. 2016;36:461–81.
12. Anonym: Emslandauswertung 2016 - Ergebnisse und Auswertungen der Sauenplanerauswertung und Betriebszweigauswertung - Beratungsringe aus den Regionen Emsland, Grafschaft Bentheim und Ostfriesland; 2016.
13. Schulte zu Sundern A, Rohn K, Holling C, Deermann A, Schulte-Wuelwer J, Visscher C. Influence of increased fertility on the salmonella prevalence in piglets in pig-holding farms. Praktischer Tierarzt. 2017;98:1060–8.
14. Quesnel H, Farmer C, Devillers N. Colostrum intake: influence on piglet performance and factors of variation. Livest Sci. 2012;146:105–14.
15. Vadmand C, Krogh U, Hansen C, Theil P. Impact of sow and litter characteristics on colostrum yield, time for onset of lactation, and milk yield of sows. J Anim Sci. 2015;93:2488–500.
16. Vallet J, Miles J, Rempel L. A simple novel measure of passive transfer of maternal immunoglobulin is predictive of preweaning mortality in piglets. Vet J. 2013;195:91–7.
17. Bole-Hribovšek V, Chriél M, Davies R, Fanning J, van de Giessen AW, Palancar LP, Ricci A, Rose N, Snow L: Analysis of the baseline survey on the prevalence of salmonella in holdings with breeding pigs in the EU, 2008: part a: salmonella prevalence estimates. European Food Safety Authority; 2008.
18. Meyer C, große Beilage E, Krieter J. Untersuchungen zur Salmonella-Seroprävalenz in unterschiedlichen Produktionssystemen beim Schwein. Tierarztl Prax Ausg G. 2005;33:104–12.
19. Ferrari C, Sbardella P, Bernardi M, Coutinho M, Vaz I, Wentz I, Bortolozzo F. Effect of birth weight and colostrum intake on mortality and performance of piglets after cross-fostering in sows of different parities. Preventive veterinary medicine. 2014;114:259–66.
20. Boulot S, Quesnel H, Quiniou N. Management of high prolificacy in French herds: can we alleviate side effects on piglet survival? In: Proceedings of the 2008 Banff pork seminar; University of Alberta; 2008. p. 213–20.
21. Quesnel H. Colostrum production by sows: variability of colostrum yield and immunoglobulin G concentrations. Animal. 2011;5:1546–53.
22. Declerck I, Sarrazin S, Dewulf J, Maes D. Sow and piglet factors determining variation of colostrum intake between and within litters. Animal. 2017;11:1336–43.
23. Farmer C, Quesnel H. Nutritional, hormonal, and environmental effects on colostrum in sows. J Anim Sci. 2009;87:56–65.
24. Matiasovic J, Kudlackova H, Babickova K, Stepanova H, Volf J, Rychlik I, Babak V, Faldyna M. Impact of maternally-derived antibodies against salmonella enterica serovar typhimurium on the bacterial load in suckling piglets. Vet J. 2013;196:114–5.
25. Roesler U, Heller P, Waldmann KH, Truyen U, Hensel A. Immunization of sows in an integrated pig-breeding herd using a homologous inactivated salmonella vaccine decreases the prevalence of salmonella typhimurium infection in the offspring. J Veterinary Med Ser B. 2006;53:224–8.
26. Hur J, Lee J. Immunization of pregnant sows with a novel virulence gene deleted live salmonella vaccine and protection of their suckling piglets against salmonellosis. Vet Microbiol. 2010;143:270–6.
27. Blais M, Fortier M, Pouliot Y, Gauthier S, Boutin Y, Asselin C, Lessard M. Colostrum whey down-regulates the expression of early and late inflammatory response genes induced by Escherichia coli and salmonella enterica typhimurium components in intestinal epithelial cells. Br J Nutr. 2015;113:200–11.

18

Vaccination of 1-day-old pigs with a porcine reproductive and respiratory syndrome virus (PRRSV) modified live attenuated virus vaccine is able to overcome maternal immunity

Monica Balasch[1][*] ⓘ, Maria Fort[1], Lucas P. Taylor[2] and Jay G. Calvert[2]

Abstract

Background: The objective of the study was to evaluate the influence of maternally derived antibodies (MDA) on the efficacy of a PRRSV-1 based attenuated vaccine, when administered in 1 day-old piglets by the intramuscular route. The protective immunity of the modified live virus vaccine was evaluated in pigs born from seropositive sows, vaccinated at 1 day of age, upon inoculation with a PRRSV-1 isolate. The animals were challenged when the levels of MDAs detected by seroneutralization test (SNT) in the non-vaccinated control group became undetectable (10 weeks after vaccination).

Results: A protective effect of vaccination was observed since a significant reduction of viral load in serum compared to the control group was detected in all sampling days after challenge; efficacy was supported by the significant reduction of nasal and oral shedding as well as in rectal temperatures. Clinical signs were not expected after the inoculation of a PRRSV-1 subtype 1 challenge strain. However, the challenge virus was able to develop fever in 61% of the control pigs. Vaccination had a positive impact on rectal temperatures since the percentage of pigs that had fever at least once after challenge was reduced to 31% in vaccinated animals, and control pigs had significantly higher rectal temperatures than vaccinated pigs 3 days post-challenge. The lack of a vaccination effect in body weight gain was probably due to the short evaluation period after challenge (10 days). In the vaccinated group, 9/16 pigs (56%) experienced an increase in ELISA S/P ratio from the day of vaccination to 67 days post-vaccination. All vaccinated pigs were seropositive before challenge, indicating the development of an antibody response following vaccination even in the face of MDAs. In contrast to ELISA results, only 2/16 vaccinated pigs developed neutralizing antibodies detectable by a SNT that used a subtype 1 MA-104 adapted strain. Even in the absence of SN antibodies, vaccinated pigs were protected from challenge with a heterologous strain. The role of cell-mediated immunity should be considered, if protection was not mediated by SN antibodies only.

Conclusions: The efficacy of the attenuated PRRSV-1 vaccine in 1-day-old pigs seropositive to PRRSV prior to a PRRSV-1 challenge was demonstrated by improvement of clinical, virological and immunological variables. With the current experimental design, maternal immunity did not interfere with the development of a protective immune response against a PRRSV-1 challenge, after vaccination of 1 day-old pigs. Confirmation of these results under field conditions will be needed.

Keywords: Porcine reproductive and respiratory syndrome, Modified live vaccine, Maternal-derived immunity

* Correspondence: monica.balasch@zoetis.com
[1]Zoetis Manufacturing & Research Spain S.L., Ctra. Camprodon s/n, Finca La Riba, 17813, Girona, Vall de Bianya, Spain
Full list of author information is available at the end of the article

Background

Porcine Reproductive and Respiratory Syndrome Virus (PRRSV) is the causative agent of a disease that affects pigs worldwide and produces large economic losses to the swine industry [1]. It belongs to the genus Arteriviridae and two different species are now recognized: PRRSV-1 (formerly genotype 1), grouping European isolates, and PRRSV-2 (formerly genotype 2), grouping North American and Asian isolates [2]. The disease is characterized by reproductive disorders in sows and respiratory disorders in pigs. Weaner and grower pigs show mainly varying degrees of respiratory distress, and up to 20% of pigs may die. The incidence of other infectious diseases is increased and these may include meningitis caused by *Streptococcus suis*, bacterial bronchopneumonia and Glässer's disease [3, 4].

PRRSV usually becomes endemic in infected herds and clinical disease is then observed in highly susceptible groups like weaned pigs in which passive immunity has waned, or naïve pigs introduced into the herd such as gilts and young boars [5]. Having immunity in place when piglets are weaned can protect them from early infections; early infections are apparently increasing in recent years in some specific countries [6]. Due to the effect of maternally derived immunity in newborns, vaccination is usually delayed until 3–4 weeks of age. The duration of maternal derived antibodies (MDA) has been described to be in the range of 6 and 11 weeks [7, 8]. Consequently, many pigs are vaccinated while still having maternal immunity in place. Most of the vaccines commercialized in Europe have a specific warning regarding interference by maternal-derived antibodies; thus, the protection induced by these vaccines according to the current vaccination practice in piglets may be compromised.

Once pigs are vaccinated, the onset of immunity against PRRSV can take 3 to 4 weeks to develop [9, 10]. Moreover, in animals with high maternal antibody titers, the post-vaccination immune response may be hampered for at least 4 weeks [8]. Due to this, piglets can have a period of risk for PRRSV infection, in which maternal immunity is no longer acting, and vaccine immunity has not yet been developed.

In Europe, the interference of maternal immunity with vaccine efficacy has been demonstrated at both the immunological and virological levels [8, 11, 12]. In a study conducted in France, it was demonstrated that pigs vaccinated when maternal antibody titers were high presented a delayed development of vaccine-related immunity, measured by both total antibody titers and neutralizing antibody titers [8]. However, whether this impairment of vaccine-related immunity development resulted in a lack of protection against exposure to a wild type virus was not investigated. In a second study conducted in France, it was demonstrated that pigs vaccinated when maternal

antibody titers were high had a lower percentage of seroconversion, and, after challenge, viremia was not reduced, compared to non-vaccinated and challenged animals [12]. However, the level of neutralizing antibodies in non-vaccinated animals at challenge was not known, and if they had not declined there is the possibility that the challenge did not take and the absence of differences was due to this fact. In a study conducted in Italy, it was demonstrated that pigs vaccinated when maternal antibody titers were high presented PRRSV viremia values that were similar to non-vaccinated pigs, when a wild type virus circulated in the farm [11]. Since this study evaluated the effect of PCV2 and PRRSV vaccination on the clinical outcome of field exposure to multiple infectious agents at farm level, it was not possible to determine if clinical differences attributable to PRRSV infection were observed between vaccinated and control pigs. In Korea, lack of interference of maternal immunity with early vaccination has been demonstrated, using a MLV vaccine based in a PRRSV-2 strain, at the clinical and immunological level, but not at the virological level [6]. Thus, additional studies are needed to characterize the potential interference of maternal immunity with attenuated PRRS vaccines.

Early vaccination of piglets, when lack of interference by maternal immunity can be demonstrated, can be used in those situations in which early circulation of PRRSV occurs after weaning. The usefulness and lack of interference of 1-day-old piglet vaccination has already been demonstrated with a PRRSV-2 based modified life virus (MLV) vaccine [6]. The objective of the present study was to investigate the potential interference of vaccination of pigs from 1 day of age with a commercial PRRSV-1 based attenuated vaccine (Suvaxyn PRRS MLV) in presence of maternal immunity. Immunological, virological and clinical parameters were used to evaluate the outcome of vaccination in an experimental challenge model.

Methods

Experimental design

To produce PRRSV MDA positive piglets, six pregnant seronegative sows (coming from a PRRSV naïve farm) were vaccinated with a PRRSV-1 based attenuated vaccine (Suvaxyn PRRS MLV) at maximum release dose ($10^{5.2}$ $TCID_{50}$/dose) during the first half of gestation (45 days of pregnancy). The day before the expected farrowing date, parturition was induced with an intramuscular injection of cloprostenol (Cyclix® Porcino, Virbac). All sows farrowed the next day.

Thirty-four one day-old piglets born from PRRSV-seropositive sows were used. Before farrowing, sows were randomly assigned to two rooms. Treatments were randomly assigned to sows within rooms using a completely randomized design. Immediately after birth and prior to vaccination, piglets were cross-fostered such that piglets were randomized and spread as even as possible over all sows. At weaning sows were removed and piglets were moved into three rooms. Cross-fostered litters were randomly assigned to rooms and crates such that all animals from the same treatment were housed in the same room. Prior to challenge, animals were comingled within four pens such that original litters were kept together and all treatments were represented within each pen.

At 1 day of age, 16 pigs were administered a single 2 mL dose of vaccine via the intramuscular route (T02). Eighteen pigs from the control group (T01) received 2 mL intramuscular and 2 mL intranasal of saline solution. At the age when the MDA levels detected by serum neutralization test (SNT) in the T01 group were negative (SNT titer $\leq1:2$) all pigs were challenged with PRRSV Olot/91 and at 10 days later they were euthanized and necropsied (Table 1). PRRSV viral load in serum, lung lesions, rectal temperatures, nasal and oral shedding, clinical signs and body weight were evaluated.

Vaccination

Piglets of 24 ± 12 h were used. A PRRSV-1 based attenuated vaccine (Suvaxyn PRRS MLV) was used for T02, below the minimum immunizing dose ($10^{2.1}$ TCID$_{50}$/dose). At day 0, piglets of T02 were injected intramuscularly in the right side of the neck. Piglets of T01 received 2 mL intramuscular and 2 mL intranasal of saline solution.

Challenge

At 67 days post-vaccination all pigs were challenged intranasally with the PRRSV-1 subtype 1 isolate Olot/91 [13], at a dose of $10^{4.3}$ CCID$_{50}$/pig. The challenge virus was a passage 8 in PAM and shared only 90.6% genomic nucleotide identity with the vaccine strain.

Sampling

Sows were bled at farrowing and sera were tested by ELISA and by SNT to a subtype 1 field strain, to confirm the seropositive status of sows to PRRSV.

Before vaccination, at day 0, piglets were bled to be tested by SNT to the vaccine strain, with the aim to detect MDA interference with vaccination.

After vaccination, control pigs were bled at day 52, to be tested by SNT to the vaccine strain, with the aim to determine the MDA decay and establish the day of challenge.

All pigs were bled just before challenge and sera tested by SNT to a MA-104 adapted subtype 1 strain, with the aim to determine the presence of NA that could be directed to the challenge strain. The challenge strain itself could not be used in this assay due to the fact that, in the testing laboratory, is not adapted to MA-104.

Before challenge (day 67) and after challenge, all pigs were bled and nasal and oral swabs were taken at days 3, 6, 8 and 10 (study days 70, 73, 75 and 77).

Blood was collected in the adequate containers to obtain serum. Nasal and oral swabs were placed in 1 mL of PBS. Samples were tested by PRRSV RT-qPCR to quantify PRRSV load.

Clinical observations and body weight

At the same days of sampling, clinical observations including general condition, depression, sneezing, coughing, respiratory distress and others (if present) were made. Rectal temperatures were also taken those days. Body weight was measured at birth, the day of challenge and the day of necropsy.

Macroscopic lung lesion scoring

After euthanasia, lungs were extracted from the thoracic cavity. Lung macroscopic lesions were immediately scored using the following method: the percentage of consolidation for each lobe (left cranial, left middle, left caudal, right cranial, right middle, right caudal and accessory) was scored and recorded as percent of lobe observed with lesions. Percentage of total lung with lesions was calculated using the following formula: Percentage of total lung with lesions = (0.10 x left cranial) + (0.10 x left middle) + (0.25 x left caudal) + (0.10 x right cranial) + (0.10 x right middle) + (0.25 x right caudal) + (0.10 x accessory).

PRRSV ELISA test

Sow sera at farrowing, and piglet sera collected before vaccination (D0), before challenge (D67) and at necropsy (D77) was tested for antibodies to PRRSV using a PRRSV ELISA test (IDEXX PRRS X3), following the manufacturer's instructions.

Table 1 Experimental design

Group	Treatment	Dose	N° pigs	Day of vaccination	Day of challenge (DC)	Sampling days	Necropsy
T01	Saline solution	2 mL IM + 2 mL IN	18	D0 (1 day-old)	D67 (10-week-old)	D70, D73, D75, D77 (DC + 3, DC + 6, DC + 8, DC + 10)	D77 (DC + 10)
T02	Suvaxyn PRRS MLV	2.1 log$_{10}$ CCID$_{50}$/2 mL	16				

PRRSV serum neutralization assays

Both SNT described below have been adapted from a previously described method [14].

SNT to vaccine strain: Heat inactivated serum samples were two-fold diluted (1:2 to 1:4096) in 96-well plates. One-hundred $CCID_{50}$ of the vaccine strain 96 V198 were added to each well and plates were incubated for 1 h at 36–38 °C. A BHK21-CD163 expressing cell suspension containing $2.5\text{-}3 \times 10^5$ cells/mL was prepared and 100 μL were added to each well in a new plate. Fifty microliters of the sample + virus mix was transferred to the plate containing cells. The mixture was incubated at 37 °C ± 1 °C and 5% CO_2 for five days. A direct immunofluorescence assay technique using SDOW-17 FITC conjugated as primary antibody was performed. The neutralizing antibody (NA) titer was determined as the inverse of the last dilution of serum that inhibited the immunofluorescence signal.

SNT to MA-104 adapted subtype 1: Heat inactivated serum samples were two-fold diluted (1:2 to 1:4096) in 96-well plates. One hundred $CCID_{50}$ of the subtype 1 strain were added to each well and plates were incubated overnight (18–24 h) at 2–8 °C. An MA-104 cell suspension containing $2.5\text{-}3 \times 10^5$ cells/mL was prepared and 100 μL were added to each well. The mixture was incubated at 37 °C ± 1 °C and 5% CO_2 for one week. The NA titer was determined as the inverse of the last dilution of serum that inhibited the cytopathic effect.

PRRSV RT-qPCR

RNA was purified from serum and nasal swab samples using a commercial kit and a semi-automatic system (Biosprint 96 DNA Blood kit). Viremia was measured by means of a Reverse Transcription (RT) qPCR. In brief, viral RNA was purified from 200 μl of sample. Elution was performed in 100 μl. Five μl of RNA were used as template, reverse transcribed at 50 °C for 30 min, and denatured at 95 °C for 5 min. The PCR program consisted of 40 cycles of denaturation at 95 °C for 20 s and annealing/extension at 53 °C for 40 s. The RT-qPCR was conducted in a thermocycler (7500 Real-Time PCR System).

The sequences of primers and probe were the following:

Forward primer (Lelystad F): 5′-GCACCACCTCACCC AGAC-3′ (Final concentration 0.5 μM).
Reverse primer (Lelystad R): 5′-CAGTTCCTGCGCCT TGAT-3′ (Final concentration 0.5 μM).
Probe (Lelystad S): 5′-6-FAM- CCTCTGCTTGCAAT CGATCCAGAC –TAMRA-3′ (Final concentration 0.6 μM).

To quantify the viral load, the number of RNA copies obtained per 5 μl of reaction were × 100 and the result was expressed as number of RNA copies/mL of sample.

Data analysis

Data summaries and analyses of data were performed with a centralized data management system (SAS/STAT User's Guide Version 9.3 or higher, SAS Institute, Cary, NC). Only post challenge data (once animals were comingled) were analyzed. Pre-challenge data was summarized with descriptive statistics. Prior to statistical analysis results were transformed, where necessary, using an appropriate logarithm transformation. For viral load analysis, negative samples were given a value of 1.7 $\log_{10}$ RNA copies/mL, which is half the limit of quantification of the technique.

Viral load, serology, body weight, and rectal temperature were analyzed with a generalized linear repeated measures mixed model with fixed effects: treatment, time point, and treatment by time point interaction, and random effects: pen, block within pen, and animal within block, pen, and treatment, which is the animal term. Linear combinations of the parameter estimates were used in a priori contrasts after testing for a significant ($P \le 0.05$) treatment effect or treatment by time point interaction. Comparisons were made between treatments at each time point. The 5% level of significance ($P \le 0.05$) was used to assess statistical differences. Least squares means (back transformed for viral load and serology), standard errors, 95% confidence intervals of the means and ranges were calculated for each treatment and time point.

The percent of positive piglets was analyzed with a general linear mixed model with fixed effect treatment and random effect pen and block within pen. Pair-wise treatment comparisons were made if the treatment main effect was significant ($P \le 0.05$). Fisher's Exact test was used for analysis if the mixed model did not converge.

The arcsine square root transformation was applied to the percentage of total lung with lesions prior to analysis. Transformed percentage of total lung with lesions was analyzed with a general linear mixed model with fixed effects, treatment, and random effects pen and block within pen. Linear combinations of the parameter estimates were used in a priori contrasts after testing for a significant ($P \le 0.05$) treatment effect. Comparisons were made between treatments. The 5% level of significance ($P \le 0.05$) was used to assess statistical differences. Least squares means (back-transformed), standard errors, 95% confidence intervals of the means and ranges were calculated for each treatment.

All hypothesis tests were conducted at the 0.05 level of significance using two-sided tests.

Results
Sow serology
All sows were seropositive to PRRSV at farrowing, with ELISA S/P ratios ranging between 0.887 and 2.204 and NA titers ranging from < 1:2 to 1:8 (Table 2).

Table 2 Sow serology at farrowing (ELISA and NA titers)

Sow ID	ELISA S/P ratio	Inverse NA titer
302	1.140	< 2
517	1.222	NT
336	2.023	3
343	0.887	3
513	2.204	8
511	0.955	4

ELISA positive: S/P ratio ≥ 0.4; SNT positive ≥2; *NT*: not tested

Piglet serology (SNT)

Sera collected from control pigs at day 52 was used to determine if MDA had decayed enough to proceed to challenge. All sera tested negative (< 1:2) to a MA-104 adapted subtype 1 strain. Based on these results, it was considered that the levels of MDA in the control T01 group were low enough to ensure a successful challenge take.

Sera collected from all pigs at day 0 and 67 were evaluated for the presence of PRRSV-specific neutralizing antibodies by means of an SNT to the vaccine strain (day 0) and to a MA-104 adapted subtype 1 strain (day 67) (Fig. 1).

Just before vaccination, once all piglets had suckled colostrum, NA titers were ranging from < 1:2 to 1:11 in control pigs (15 out of 18 pigs with NA titers ≥1:2) and < 1:2 to 1:8 in vaccinated pigs (10 out of 16 pigs with NA titers ≥1:2).

Just before challenge, NA titers were negative (< 1:2) in all control pigs and were ranging from < 1:2 to 1:45 in vaccinated pigs (2 out of 16 pigs with NA titers of 1:2 and 1:45).

Piglet serology (ELISA)

All pigs had presence of PRRSV-specific MDA prior to vaccination as detected by ELISA (S/P ratio ≥ 0.4). The mean S/P ratio was 1.662 in the control group and 1.836 in the vaccinated group (Table 3, Fig. 2).

At challenge (D67), all (100%) vaccinated pigs (T02) were seropositive to PRRSV by ELISA. In the control group (T01), 7/18 pigs (39%) had also detectable PRRSV antibodies before challenge. The mean S/P ratio was 0.279 in the control group and 1.803 in the vaccinated group.

Ten days after challenge (D77), all pigs were seropositive to PRRSV.

The levels of PRRS antibodies detected before challenge (67 days post-vaccination) in the vaccinated group were significantly higher ($p < 0.0001$) compared to the levels detected in the control group.

Clinical observations and body weight

No clinical observations (general condition, depression, respiratory distress, cough, sneeze or other) were recorded for any pig during the whole observation period.

Before challenge, the least squares mean rectal temperatures was significantly lower in T02 group compared to T01. However, none of the pigs from any group had fever (rectal temperature ≥ 40.5 °C) at that time. After challenge, the percentage of pigs that had fever at least once was 61%, and 31%, in control and vaccinated groups, respectively. Comparison between groups showed that pigs from the control T01 group had significantly higher ($p = 0.0005$) rectal temperature than pigs from T02 group at day 70 (3 days post-challenge).

Regarding body weight, the mean for T01 at birth was 1.4 kg and for T02 was 1.3 kg. Comparison of least squares means between groups at D67 (challenge) and D77 (necropsy) showed no significant differences between groups, although the least squares mean starting weight at challenge was 28.7 kg for T01 and 28.1 kg for T02, and the least squares mean weight at necropsy was 31.0 for T01 and 32.0 for T02.

Viremia

All pigs were found RT-qPCR PRRSV negative in serum before vaccination (D0) and all pigs from the T01 group remained so until challenge. In contrast, 8/16 (50%) piglets from the T02 group were RT-qPCR PRRSV positive at challenge (67 days post-vaccination).

After challenge, 100% of pigs from the T01 group became viremic at D70 (3 days post-challenge) and remained positive until the end of the study at 10 days post-challenge. In the vaccinated group T02 all pigs were detected PRRSV positive at least once; however, by the end of the study (DC + 10), only 11/16 T02 pigs (68.8%) were still viremic (Table 4).

Pigs from the T02 group had significantly lower viral load in serum than pigs from the T01 control group at all sampling days post-challenge (Table 4, Fig. 3).

Nasal and oral shedding

All pigs were found RT-qPCR PRRSV negative in nasal swabs before challenge, and all but one (belonging to T02 group) were found RT-qPCR PRRSV negative in oral swabs.

After challenge, the percentage of pigs that ever shed PRRSV by nasal route in the T01 group was significantly higher compared to T02 (100% vs.75%) (Table 4). All pigs (T01 and T02) became oral shedders, except one pig from T02 group that was negative at all sampling points post-challenge.

The amount of virus shed by the nasal and oral routes was significantly lower in the T02 group compared to T01 group at day 70, corresponding to 3 days post-challenge (Figs. 4 and 5). At day 73 (6 days post-challenge) the amount of virus shed by the nasal route was significantly lower in the T02 group compared to T01 (Table 4).

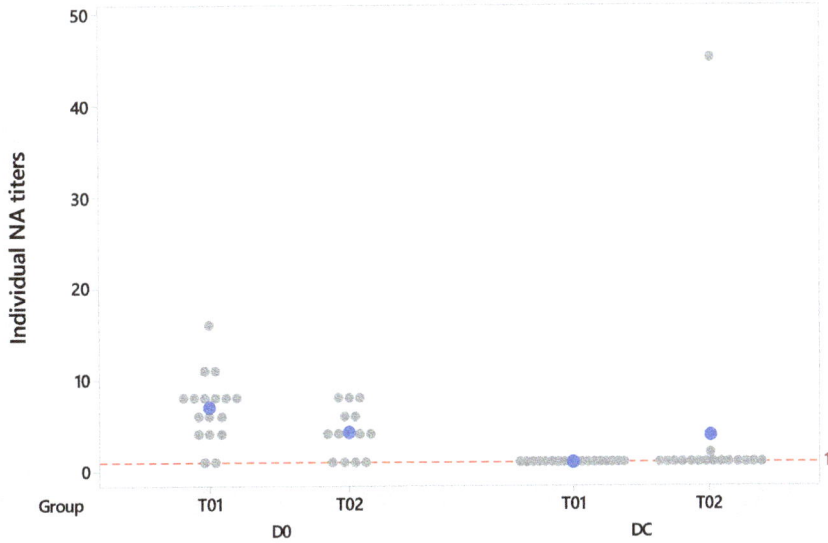

Fig. 1 Neutralizing antibody titers to vaccine strain (D0, day of vaccination) and to field-type heterologous strain (DC, day of challenge); positive > 1,0

Macroscopic lung lesions

At necropsy, 13/18 pigs (72%) from the control group T01 had a positive lung visual score, indicating that PRRSV challenge was successful in inducing lung lesions. In the T02 group, 7/16 (44%) pigs scored positive as well (Fig. 6).

Comparison between treatment groups showed no significant differences (p = 0.092) in the % of lung with lesions (4.3% in control pigs vs 1.3% in vaccinated pigs).

Discussion

Early vaccination of piglets against PRRSV, when non-interference with passively acquired immunity can be demonstrated, is a useful tool to control PRRSV-related disease in young animals. The objective of the present study was to evaluate the effect of maternally derived immunity on the efficacy of a PRRSV-1 based MLV, when administered in 1 day-old piglets by the intramuscular route. Efficacy was evaluated in seropositive pigs vaccinated at 1 day of age upon inoculation with a

pathogenic PRRSV-1 isolate, heterologous to the vaccine strain, as a respiratory challenge. The animals were challenged when the levels of MDAs detected by SNT in the control group became undetectable, to guarantee challenge take in control animals and the ability to detect differences between the treatment groups.

Historically PRRSV-1 subtype 1 isolates, the most predominant in Western Europe, have showed a very limited ability to induce respiratory clinical signs compared to PRRSV-2 and subtypes 2 and 3 of PRRSV-1. However, some recent isolates (e.g. from Italy, Belgium, and Austria) may indicate a trend towards increasing virulence of subtype 1 [15–17]. The challenge strain used in this study, Olot/91, has been shown to be very aggressive when used in a reproductive model [13] but induces a mild disease in young pigs [18]. Consequently, other variables must be selected as primary variables to evaluate the outcome of infection. Viremia is the most frequently used parameter to verify PRRSV infection outcome in pigs [7, 19]. In the present study, a protective effect of vaccination

Table 3 Summary of ELISA results (S/P ratio) in piglets

Treatment Number	Day of Study	Geometric Mean/LSM[a]	SE	Range	% of seropositive
T01	Day 0	1.662	0.437	0.609 to 2.641	100.0
T02	Day 0	1.836	0.358	0.967 to 2.632	100.0
T01	Day 67	0.279	0.015	0.021 to 0.747	38.9
T02	Day 67	1.803	0.101	1.151 to 2.310	100.0
T01	Day 77	1.517	0.111	0.543 to 2.070	100.0
T02	Day 77	1.794	0.096	1.187 to 2.343	100.0

[a]Day 0 results are expressed with the Geometric Mean and Days 67 and 73 with the Back transformed – Least Square Mean (LSM); SE: standard error; ELISA positive: S/P ratio ≥ 0.4

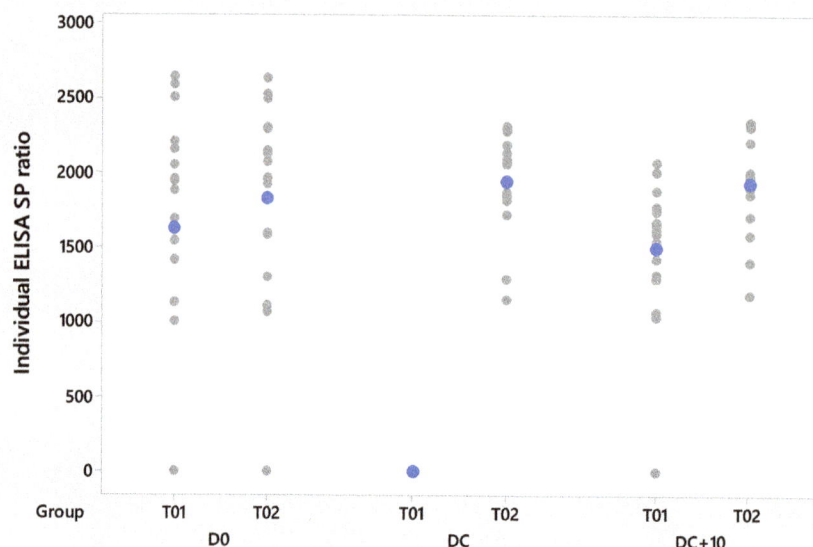

Fig. 2 Mean ELISA S/P ratio at vaccination (D0), at challenge (DC) and at necropsy (DC + 10); ELISA positive: S/P ratio ≥ 0,4

was observed when comparing viral load in serum between the vaccinated and control groups. The vaccinated group had significantly lower viral titers compared to the control group at all sampling days post-challenge. The vaccine strain was still detected at low levels in some vaccinated animals before challenge; consequently, the amount of virus detected in this group in the following days was probably a mixture of vaccine strain and challenge strain. Since the values obtained were analyzed as being all due to challenge, the results could not favor the interpretation of vaccine efficacy.

The protection conferred following vaccination was supported by the significant reduction in the percentage of nasal shedders as well as in the amount of virus detected

in nasal and oral secretions in the vaccinated group in relation to the control group. These results are in contrast of those recently reported [12]; in that case, a clear interference of maternally derived neutralizing antibodies with PRRSV vaccination was described (no significant differences in viremia reduction and lower transmission rate estimated for pigs vaccinated with low antibody titers than for pigs vaccinated with high antibody titers).

It has been described that the ability of PRRSV attenuated vaccines to control the disease (measured by reduction of viremia) appears to be much lower in the field than under experimental conditions [11, 20]. In these studies, the same PRRSV attenuated vaccine performed differently when used under laboratory conditions

Table 4 Least squares mean (±standard error) viral load in serum and nasal/oral swabs, and percentage of RT-qPCR positive pigs (in brackets). Results from RT-qPCR are expressed as $\log_{10}$ RNA copies/mL of serum. A positive result is considered when > 1.7 $\log_{10}$ RNA copies/mL (limit of quantification)

	Treatment	Day of study					
		D0	D67 (Ch)	D70 (Ch + 3)	D73 (Ch + 6)	D75 (Ch + 8)	D77 (Ch + 10)
Viremia	T01	≤ 1.7 (0%)	1.65 ± 0.20 (0%)	6.60 ± 0.20 (100%)	6.39 ± 0.20 (100%)	5.32 ± 0.20 (100%)	5.29 ± 0.20 (100%)
	T02	≤ 1.7 (0%)	2.25 ± 0.36 (50%)	2.87 ± 0.36 (50%)	5.18 ± 0.36 (94%)	4.18 ± 0.36 (100%)	2.96 ± 0.36 (69%)
	T01 vs T02 (p value)	NT	0.1495	< 0.0001	0.0043	0.0071	< 0.0001
Nasal shedding	T01	NT	≤ 1.7 ± 0.19 (0%)	3.91 ± 0.19 (100%)	3.98 ± 0.19 (100%)	2.27 ± 0.19 (61%)	1.90 ± 0.19 (22%)
	T02	NT	≤ 1.7 ± 0.20 (0%)	1.81 ± 0.20 (12%)	2.72 ± 0.20 (50%)	2.35 ± 0.20 (44%)	1.70 ± 0.20 (0%)
	T01 vs T02 (p value)	NT	0.9986	< 0.0001	< 0.0001	0.7576	0.4654
Oral shedding	T01	NT	1.70 ± 0.03 (0%)	3.34 ± 0.21 (83%)	3.68 ± 0.23 (94%)	2.57 ± 0.19 (67%)	2.28 ± 0.20 (39%)
	T02	NT	1.75 ± 0.03 (6%)	2.32 ± 0.22 (56%)	3.62 ± 0.25 (81%)	2.30 ± 0.20 (50%)	1.80 ± 0.22 (12%)
	T01 vs T02 (p value)	NT	0.1978	0.0009	0.8800	0.3243	0.1096

NT: not tested

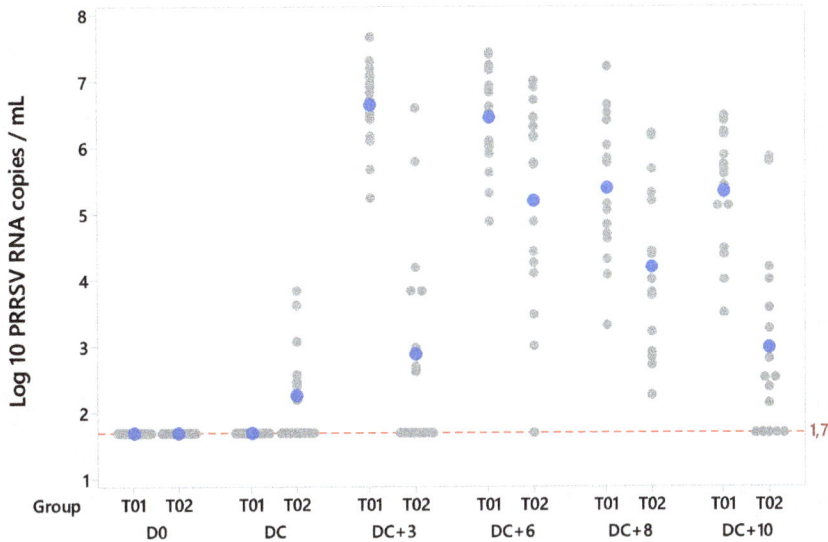

Fig. 3 PRRSV viral load in serum during the post-challenge phase; PRRSV RT-qPCR positive > 1.7 PRRSV RNA copies/mL

(significant reduction of the magnitude and duration of viremia) and under field conditions (no significant reduction of viremia). Although it has been suggested that this could be linked to the influence of maternal derived antibodies, this could not be used as a universal explanation, since in some cases this effect has been observed in piglets that were seronegative at vaccination [21]. Moreover, when 1-day-old piglets were vaccinated in the presence of maternal antibodies [6], a very limited effect in reduction of wild type virus viremia was observed.

However, the efficacy of vaccination was demonstrated by improved growth performance and reduced mortality. Thus, any demonstration of PRRSV vaccination interference by maternal antibodies should be verified under both laboratory and field conditions.

Clinical signs, mainly respiratory signs, were not expected after the inoculation of the challenge strain Olot/91, as described in previous reports [18]. However, the challenge virus was able to induce fever in 61% of the control pigs. Vaccination had a positive impact on

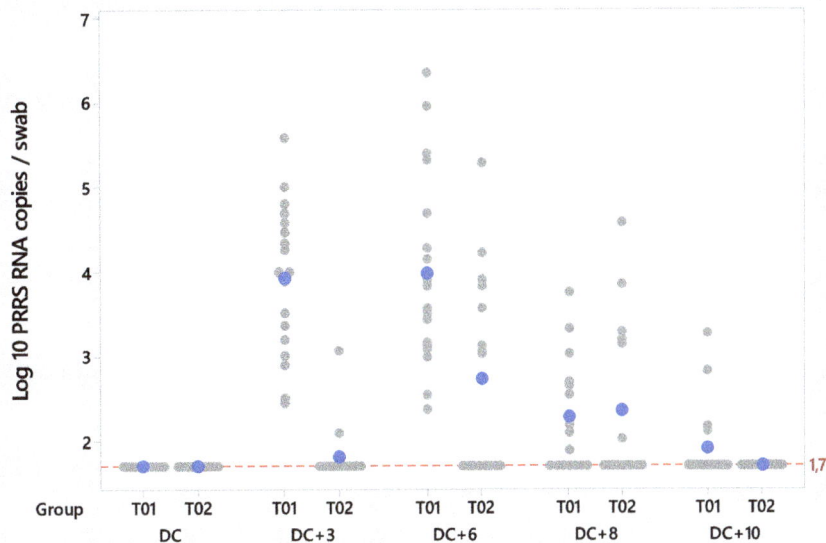

Fig. 4 PRRSV viral load in nasal swabs during the post-challenge phase; PRRSV RT-qPCR positive > 1.7 PRRSV RNA copies/mL

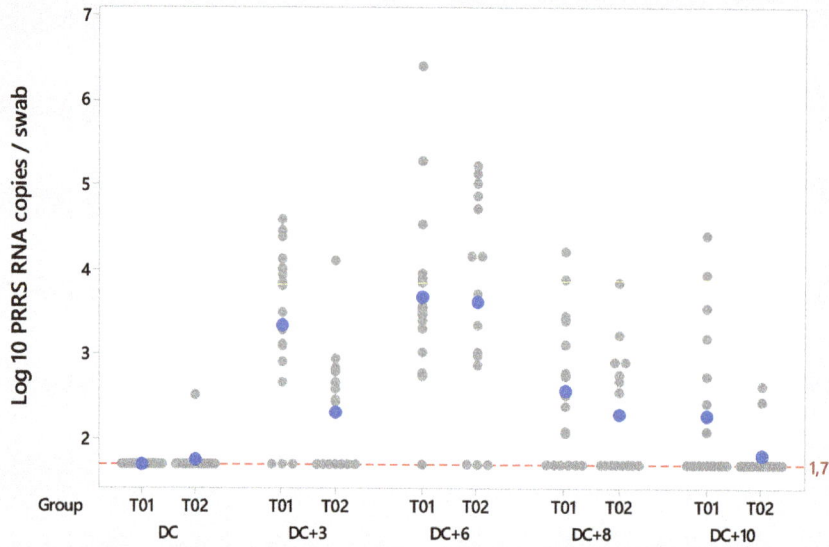

Fig. 5 PRRSV viral load in oral swabs during the post-challenge phase; PRRSV RT-qPCR positive > 1.7 PRRSV RNA copies/mL

rectal temperatures since the percentage of pigs that had fever at least once after challenge was reduced to 31% in vaccinated animals, and control pigs had significantly higher rectal temperatures than vaccinated pigs 3 days post-challenge. The lack of a positive vaccination effect in body weight gain was probably due to the short evaluation period after challenge (10 days). Those reports demonstrating improved daily weight gain after vaccination have considered much wider periods of analysis [6, 11, 21]. The difference in body weight

between birth and challenge was not statistically analyzed because during the post-vaccination phase the treatment groups were not commingled. The difference of 0.6 kg between vaccinated and control groups (in favor of the control group) was overcome by the vaccinated group after challenge.

At necropsy, 13/18 pigs (72%) from the control group had developed macroscopic lung lesions compatible with PRRSV infection. In contrast, only 7/16 (44%) vaccinated pigs developed lesions. Comparison between treatment

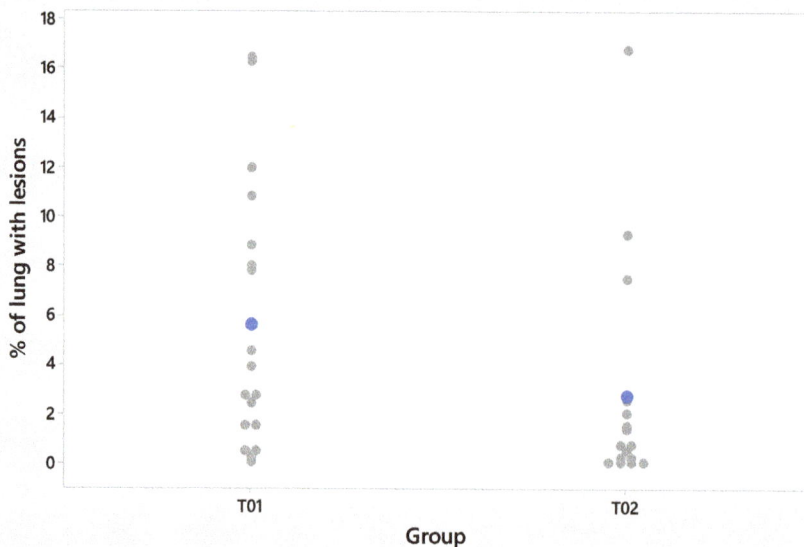

Fig. 6 Distribution of the individual lung macroscopic lesion scores

groups showed no significant differences in the % of lung with lesions. However, the differences observed were close to significance ($p = 0.092$), indicating that these differences might have a biological relevance. Taken together the clinical, virological and pathological data clearly indicate that vaccinated animals were able to better respond to PRRSV infection than non-vaccinated animals.

All pigs had PRRSV-specific antibodies before vaccination as measured by ELISA (S/P ratio ≥ 0.4), thus complying with the inclusion criteria. Before challenge (67 days post-vaccination), 39% of the pigs in the control group were still seropositive, indicating the presence of remaining MDAs at that time (mean S/P ratio: 0.279). However, the fact that all pigs from the control group developed viremia after challenge and that 13/18 had also a positive lung score at necropsy indicates that the remaining MDA detected by ELISA did not interfere with the challenge take. In fact, when the levels of PRRSV-specific NA were determined in those pigs by means of an SNT, all T01 pigs were below the level of detection before challenge (Day 52).

In the vaccinated group, 9/16 pigs (56%) experienced an increase in the ELISA S/P ratio from the day of vaccination to 67 days post-vaccination and all of them were seropositive before challenge (mean S/P ratio: 1.803), indicating the development of an antibody response following vaccination even in the face of MDAs. These results are in agreement with those recently reported [12], in which 44% of piglets vaccinated in presence of maternal immunity seroconverted 4 weeks later. In contrast to ELISA results, only 2/16 vaccinated pigs developed serum NA detectable by a SNT that used a subtype 1 field strain. Since the strain used in the SNT was not the challenge strain (although both were subtype 1 strains), the low number of pigs having NA could be due to the previously described effect of the use of a heterologous strain in the assay [14, 22]; if that was the case, NA could have been under-detected. Even in the absence of NA antibodies, vaccinated pigs were partially protected from challenge with a heterologous strain (as demonstrated by virological and clinical variables). The role of cell-mediated immunity should be considered, if protection was not mediated by NA only. It has been suggested that protection against PRRSV infection is not based on humoral immunity only, and that a combination of NA and virus-specific IFN-γ secreting cells is needed to achieve clearance of PRRSV infection [23].

The NA titers detected before vaccination were considered moderate to low, below the demonstrated level of interference in seroconversion [8] and below the proposed limit of protection [19], which has been set at 1:8. However, they were generated using the most stringent conditions possible: vaccination of sows with the maximum antigen titer according to label (to achieve maximum level of MDAs in the newborn piglets). To achieve higher titers before vaccination, repeated vaccination of sows should be considered for future studies. The combination of sow vaccination with maximum antigen titer and piglet vaccination with the same strain as sows, homologous to the one that elicited the MDAs, represents the worse-case scenario for demonstrating the potential for maternal immunity interference with vaccination in terms of affinity of NA with the vaccine strain. However, in field conditions the scenario may be even more challenging for overcoming immunity, when sows are repeatedly vaccinated and exposed to different field strains.

Although both vaccine and challenge strains are PRRSV-1 subtype 1, they are far from being homologous, since they share 90.6% of nucleotide identity only. Studies with more divergent strains would be needed to confirm the results of the present study.

The reasons the outcomes of the current study are different from a similar study carried out in France [12] are not known. There are obvious differences in study design that might affect the outcomes of the two studies. The age of the pigs at vaccination, the vaccine used, and the timing of challenge administration are important factors that may have influenced the results. On the other hand, the results obtained in the current study are in agreement with those reported for a similar vaccine based on a PRRSV-2 strain, which demonstrated that vaccination may overcome maternal immunity yielding an improvement of growth performance in 1 day-old vaccinated pigs [6].

Conclusions

The efficacy of an attenuated PRRSV-1 vaccine (Suvaxyn PRRS MLV) in 1-day-old seropositive pigs was demonstrated by an improvement in clinical, virological and immunological variables. Thus, with the current experimental design, maternal immunity did not interfere with the development of a partially protective immune response against a PRRSV-1 challenge, after vaccination of 1 day-old pigs. Confirmation of these results under field conditions will be needed.

Abbreviations

CCID$_{50}$: Cell Culture Infectious Dose 50%; ELISA: Enzyme linked immunosorbent assay; FITC: Fluorescein isothiocyanate; IFN-γ: Interferon gamma; MDA: Maternally Derived Antibodies; MLV: Modified Live Vaccine; NT: Not tested; PBS: Phosphate Buffered Saline; PCV2: Porcine Circovirus Type 2; PRRSV: Porcine Reproductive and Respiratory Syndrome Virus; RNA: Ribonucleic acid; RT-qPCR: Quantitative Reverse-Transcription Polymerase Chain Reaction; S/P: Sample to Positive; SNT: Serum Neutralization Test; TMB: 3,3',5,5'-Tetramethylbenzidine

Funding

Zoetis Inc. funded the study.

Authors' contributions

MB and MF were the investigators of the study, analysed the results and wrote the manuscript; MF was the clinician of the study; LT performed the biometrics analysis; JC reviewed the manuscript. All authors read and approved the final manuscript.

Competing interests

The authors declare that they have no competing interests.

Author details

[1]Zoetis Manufacturing & Research Spain S.L., Ctra. Camprodon s/n, Finca La Riba, 17813, Girona, Vall de Bianya, Spain. [2]Zoetis Inc., 333 Portage St, Kalamazoo, MI 49007, USA.

References

1. Nathues H, Alarcon P, Rushton J, Jolie R, Fiebig K, Jimenez M, Geurts V, Nathues C. Cost of porcine reproductive and respiratory syndrome virus at individual farm level - an economic disease model. Prev Vet Med. 2017;142: 16–29.

2. Adams MJ, Lefkowitz EJ, King AM, Harrach B, Harrison RL, Knowles NJ, Kropinski AM, Krupovic M, Kuhn JH, Mushegian AR, Nibert M, Sabanadzovic S, Sanfaçon H, Siddell SG, Simmonds P, Varsani A, Zerbini FM, Gorbalenya AE, Davison AJ. Ratification vote on taxonomic proposals to the international committee on taxonomy of viruses (2016). Arch Virol. 2016; 161(10):2921–49.

3. Kefabber KK. Reproductive failure of unknown etiology. Am Assoc Swine Pract Newsl. 1989;1:1–10.

4. Keffaber KK, Stevenson G, Van Alstine W, Kanitz C, Harris L, Gorcyca D, Schlesinger K, Schultz R, Chladek D, Morrison R. SIRS virus infection in nursery/grower pigs. Am Assoc Swine Pract Newsletter. 1992;4:38–9.

5. Stevenson GW, Van Alstine WG, Kanitz CL, Keffaber KK. Endemic porcine reproductive and respiratory syndrome virus infection of nursery pigs in two swine herds without current reproductive failure. J Vet Diagn Investig. 1993;5:432–4.

6. Jeong J, Kim S, Park KH, Kang I, Park SJ, Yang S, Oh T, Chae C. Vaccination with a porcine reproductive and respiratory syndrome virus vaccine at 1-day-old improved growth performance of piglets under field conditions. Vet Microbiol. 2018;214:113–24.

7. Chung WB, Lin MW, Chang WF, Hsu M, Yang PC. Persistence of porcine reproductive and respiratory syndrome virus in intensive farrow-to-finish pig herds. Can J Vet Res. 1997;61(4):292–8.

8. Fablet C, Renson P, Eono F, Mahé S, Eveno E, Le Dimna M, Normand V, Lebret A, Rose N, Bourry O. Maternally-derived antibodies (MDAs) impair piglets' humoral and cellular immune responses to vaccination against porcine reproductive and respiratory syndrome (PRRS). Vet Microbiol. 2016; 192:175–80.

9. Mateu E, Díaz I. The challenge of PRRS immunology. Vet J. 2008;177(3): 345–51.

10. López OJ, Osorio FA. Role of neutralizing antibodies in PRRSV protective immunity. Vet Immunol Immunopathol. 2004;102(3):155–63.

11. Martelli P, Ardigò P, Ferrari L, Morganti M, De Angelis E, Bonilauri P, Luppi A, Guazzetti S, Caleffi A, Borghetti P. Concurrent vaccinations against PCV2 and PRRSV: study on the specific immunity and clinical protection in naturally infected pigs. Vet Microbiol. 2013;162(2–4):558–71.

12. Renson P, Fablet C, Andraud M, Mahe S, Dorenlor V, Le Dimna M, Eveno E, Eono F, Paboeuf F, Rose N, Bourry O. Maternally derived

13. Plana J, Vayreda M, Vilarrasa J, Bastons M, Rosell R, Martínez M, San Gabriel A, Pujols J, Badiola JL, Ramos JA, Domingo M. Porcine epidemic abortion and respiratory syndrome (mystery swine disease). Isolation in Spain of the causative agent and reproduction of the disease. Vet Microbiol. 1992;33(1–4):203–11.

14. Yoon IJ, Joo HS, Goyal SM, Molitor TW. A modified serum neutralization test for the detection of antibody to porcine reproductive and respiratory syndrome virus in swine sera. J Vet Diagn Investig. 1994;6:289–92.

15. Sinn LJ, Klingler E, Lamp B, Brunthaler R, Weissenböck H, Rümenapf T, Ladinig A. Emergence of a virulent porcine reproductive and respiratory syndrome virus (PRRSV) 1 strain in Lower Austria. Porcine Health Manag. 2016;2:28.

16. Frydas IS, Trus I, Kvisgaard LK, Bonckaert C, Reddy VR, Li Y, Larsen LE, Nauwynck HJ. Different clinical, virological, serological and tissue tropism outcomes of two new and one old Belgian type 1 subtype 1 porcine reproductive and respiratory virus (PRRSV) isolates. Vet Res. 2015;46:37.

17. Canelli E, Catella A, Borghetti P, Ferrari L, Ogno G, De Angelis E, Corradi A, Passeri B, Bertani V, Sandri G, Bonilauri P, Leung FC, Guazzetti S, Martelli P. Phenotypic characterization of a highly pathogenic Italian porcine reproductive and respiratory syndrome virus (PRRSV) type 1 subtype 1 isolate in experimentally infected pigs. Vet Microbiol. 2017;210:124–33.

18. Rovira A, Balasch M, Segalés J, García L, Plana-Durán J, Rosell C, Ellerbrok H, Mankertz A, Domingo M. Experimental inoculation of conventional pigs with porcine reproductive and respiratory syndrome virus and porcine circovirus 2. J Virol. 2002;76(7):3232–9.

19. Lopez OJ, Oliveira MF, Garcia EA, Kwon BJ, Doster A, Osorio FA. Protection against porcine reproductive and respiratory syndrome virus (PRRSV) infection through passive transfer of PRRSV-neutralizing antibodies is dose dependent. Clin Vaccine Immunol. 2007;14(3):269–75.

20. Martelli P, Cordioli P, Alborali LG, Gozio S, De Angelis E, Ferrari L, Lombardi G, Borghetti P. Protection and immune response in pigs intradermally vaccinated against porcine reproductive and respiratory syndrome (PRRS) and subsequently exposed to a heterologous European (Italian cluster) field strain. Vaccine. 2007;25(17):3400–8.

21. Martelli P, Gozio S, Ferrari L, Rosina S, De Angelis E, Quintavalla C, Bottarelli E, Borghetti P. Efficacy of a modified live porcine reproductive and respiratory syndrome virus (PRRSV) vaccine in pigs naturally exposed to a heterologous European (Italian cluster) field strain: clinical protection and cell-mediated immunity. Vaccine. 2009;27(28):3788–99.

22. Martínez-Lobo FJ, Díez-Fuertes F, Simarro I, Castro JM, Prieto C. Porcine reproductive and respiratory syndrome virus isolates differ in their susceptibility to neutralization. Vaccine. 2011;29(40):6928–40.

23. Murtaugh MP, Xiao Z, Zuckermann F. Immunological responses of swine to porcine reproductive and respiratory syndrome virus infection. Viral Immunol. 2002;15(4):533–47.

19

Efficacy of a one-shot marbofloxacin treatment on acute pleuropneumonia after experimental aerosol inoculation of nursery pigs

Doris Hoeltig[1]* ⓘ, Judith Rohde[2], Birgit Brunner[3], Klaus Hellmann[3], Erik Grandemange[4] and Karl-Heinz Waldmann[1]

Abstract

Background: Porcine pleuropneumonia, caused by *Actinobacillus pleuropneumoniae*, is a bacterial respiratory disease of swine. Acute outbreaks of the disease are often accompanied by high mortality and economic losses. As severe cases of the disease frequently require parenteral antibiotic treatment of the animals, the efficacy of a single, high dose of marbofloxacin was compared to a three-time application of a dose of enrofloxacin under experimental conditions.

Methods: A blinded, controlled, randomized and blocked dose confirmation study was conducted to test the efficacy and safety of a single dose of 8 mg/kg marbofloxacin (160 mg/ml, Forcyl® Swine, Vetoquinol SA, France) to treat acute porcine pleuropneumonia after experimental aerosol inoculation of pigs with *A. pleuropneumoniae* serotype 2. The results were compared to a three consecutive day treatment of 2.5 mg/kg enrofloxacin and a mock (saline) treatment. Criteria for the assessment of efficacy were severity of lung lesions, bacteriological cure and the course of clinical disease after treatment.

Results:: Thirty six nursery pigs were divided into three treatment groups: marbofloxacin (T1), enrofloxacin (T2) and mock (T3). Statistically significant superiority ($p < 0.05$) of marbofloxacin and enrofloxacin compared to the mock-treated group was demonstrated for all efficacy criteria. The need of rescue euthanasia due to severity of symptoms was significantly reduced in both treatment groups (T1: 1 pig; T2: 0 pigs; vs. T3: 8 pigs). On day 6 after treatment initiation, clinical cure was observed in 10 (T1), 10 (T2) but only 1 of the piglets in T3. Extent of lung lesions (mean of lung lesion score T1: 3.9, T2: 6.0, T3: 21.1) and bacteriological isolation from lung tissue (on day 6 after treatment initiation: T1 = 0 pigs; T2 = 1 pig; T3 = all pigs) were also significantly reduced within both treatment groups. There were no adverse events linked to the drug administration and no injection site reactions were observed.

Conclusions: Both applied antimicrobial treatments were proven safe and efficacious for the treatment of acute porcine pleuropneumonia. No statistically significant differences were detected between the antibiotic treatments.

Keywords: Enrofloxacin, Marbofloxacin, Respiratory disease, Swine, Bacteriological cure, Fluoroquinolone, Concentration-dependent activity, Pig, *Actinobacillus pleuropneumoniae*

* Correspondence: doris.hoeltig@tiho-hannover.de
[1]Clinic for Swine, Small Ruminants, forensic Medicine and Ambulatory Service, University of Veterinary Medicine Hannover, Foundation, Bischofsholer Damm 15, D-30173 Hannover, Germany
Full list of author information is available at the end of the article

Background

Porcine pleuropneumonia is a respiratory disease caused by the gram-negative bacterium *Actinobacillus* (*A.*) *pleuropneumoniae*. This germ is distributed worldwide and is considered obligate pathogenic and can therefore cause severe respiratory disease without additional co-infections [1–3]. The severity of disease depends on several factors such as involved serotype, infection dose, co-infections, immune status and genetic background of the animal and other environmental factors [4–6]. The disease occurs predominantly in pigs under six months of age but pigs of all ages can be affected [7, 8]. In the last few years, an increase in clinical cases, especially in nursery pigs and replacement sows has been observed throughout Germany and in other European countries [9]. Acute outbreaks of the disease have a major impact on animal welfare as well as on profitability of the pig farms. Carcass trimming and condemnation as well as costs due to animal losses in cases of high mortality, treatment, reduced daily weight gain and a prolonged fattening period lead to high direct as well as indirect economic losses [10–12].

Currently control and prevention of the disease are mainly achieved with the administration of antimicrobials and by vaccination. However, vaccination efficacy is often hampered by limited cross-serovar protection. Furthermore, it does not prevent the colonization of the lungs. This means that pigs may still carry the pathogen and remain an important source of contagion for the spreading of the infection [13–17]. The antimicrobial treatment of pigs also has some disadvantages. One disadvantage is that despite an antibiotic treatment *A. pleuropneumoniae* might not be completely cleared from the lungs of colonized animals as was demonstrated for tulathromycin treatment [18]. Another disadvantage of antimicrobial treatments is the risk of resistance development towards antibiotic substances. Highest rates of resistance of *A. pleuropneumoniae* were detected against tetracyclines followed by sulfonamides, ampicillin and trimethoprim, whereas the lowest levels of resistance were seen against fluoroquinolones, cephalosporins and florfenicol [19–24]. Fluoroquinolones and 3rd generation cephalosporins are classified as critically important antimicrobials in human medicine [25]. Therefore their use should be limited to an inevitable minimum, administered only to diseased animals that are expected to respond poorly to other classes of antibiotics based on susceptibility testing results [26–29]. One approach for the reduction of antibiotic use is the treatment of the individual diseased animal in contrast to the treatment of the whole group. This approach is controversial, as all animals of the group might be at risk of developing the disease. Nevertheless, the individual, parenteral treatment is often necessary, especially during acute outbreaks of porcine pleuropneumonia where suffering animals may be too weak for sufficient water or feed intake leading to inadequate intake of antibiotics that are administered in the feed or drinking water. Many antibiotic products including fluoroquinolones, which are registered for the parenteral treatment of porcine pleuropneumonia, require an administration of at least three or more consecutive days [8, 30]. Fluoroquinolones have a concentration-dependent mode of action and it has been shown that a high dose given as a single injection has good efficacy against *A. pleuropneumoniae* infection [31–33]. The aim of this study was to investigate the efficacy of a one-shot 8 mg/kg marbofloxacin treatment on the development of clinical signs, lung lesions and colonisation of the lungs of piglets inoculated with *A. pleuropneumoniae*, in comparison to a mock and to a standard 3-day enrofloxacin treatment protocol to obtain marketing authorization approval for a product containing marbofloxacin.

Methods

Study design

The study was a blinded, controlled, randomized and blocked dose confirmation study to test the efficacy of a single dose of 8 mg/kg marbofloxacin (160 mg/ml, Forcyl® Swine, Vetoquinol SA, France) as treatment for acute porcine pleuropneumonia after experimental aerosol inoculation of piglets. The experimental and treatment unit was the individual animal.

Animals and animal housing

A total of 36 nursery pigs, aged eight weeks were included in this study. All pigs were German hybrid pigs, male castrates, vaccinated against *M. hyopneumoniae* and PCV-2. All piglets originated from the same *A. pleuropneumoniae* free piglet producer farm and had been transferred to the experimental farm at the age of four weeks. The pigs were kept and cared for according to the principles for Protection of Vertebrate Animals used for Experimental and other Scientific Purposes European Treaty Series, nos. 123 and 170 (http://conventions.coe.int/treaty/EN/treaties/html/123.htm; http://conventions.coe.int/treaty/EN/treaties/html/170.htm).

The study design and housing conditions were approved by the local governmental ethics committee (Commission for ethical estimation of animal research studies of the Lower Saxonian State Office for Consumer Protection and Food Safety; approval number: 33.9–42,502-05-14A447). The pigs were kept under standardized level 2 conditions with $8m^2$ floor space per 12 pigs and fed a standardized commercial diet.

The piglets arrived at the research unit 28 days prior to inoculation, to ensure that they were thoroughly acclimatized to the new environment, diet and clinical examination procedure. After arrival blood samples for serological testing were drawn and a physical examination was performed. From the day of arrival until day of inoculation, general health status observations of the pigs were conducted twice a day. On the day prior to inoculation, all pigs were weighed and examined. All animals entering the study were tested serologically negative for *A. pleuropneumoniae* and considered to be clinically healthy. Serological screening of the pigs was conducted using ApxIV-ELISA (IDEXX APP-ApxIV Ab Test®, Co. IDEXX Laboratories, Maine, USA).

Experimental inoculation

The experimental inoculation was performed via aerosol following the procedure described by Jacobsen et al. [6]. Briefly, the pigs were driven calmly into an aerosol chamber in groups of six animals. The animals were nebulized with 13 ml of a suspension of *A. pleuropneumoniae* serotype 2 strain C3656 containing $5,2 \times 10^7$ colony forming units (cfu). The total time of exposure was 30 min. The Minimal Inhibitory Concentrations (MIC) of marbofloxacin and enrofloxacin were determined prior to infection. For both antibiotics the MIC was 0.125 μg/ml. Thus the challenge strain was considered susceptible to fluoroquinolone antibiotics according to the CLSI clinical breakpoint of ≤0.25 μg/ml for susceptibility in *A. pleuropneumoniae* from respiratory samples from pigs [34].

Assignment to treatment groups and inclusion criteria

Only animals that fulfilled all inclusion criteria were enrolled for treatment. Inclusion criteria were pyrexia with rectal temperature > 40.3 °C and a respiratory score ≥ 2 and a depression score ≥ 1 after the experimental inoculation. Table 1 presents the description of scoring schemes. Each individual pig that fulfilled the inclusion criteria was immediately randomized and treated directly. The randomization allocation is shown in Table 2. Randomized

blocking, arranging the experimental units in groups (blocks) that were equal, was used to reduce the experimental error. Blocking size was 3 at the ratio of 1:1:1, blocking factor was sex of the pigs.

Treatments (antibiotics and/or mock) were administered on Day 0, Day 1 and Day 2 (Table 2). Enrofloxacin was chosen as a reference product for the positive control with a dose of 2.5 mg/kg/day, administered on three consecutive days. Animals in the mock treatment group (T3) received administrations of saline per kg bodyweight at the same volume as the animals treated with marbofloxacin (T1) at the same time interval. For blinding purposes, all clinical examinations and the drug administrations were carried out by different members of staff. This ensured that the person responsible for the evaluation of the clinical symptoms, and therefore efficacy of the treatment, was not aware of the treatment group the pigs were assigned to.

Clinical examination

Starting four hours after inoculation and thereafter every two hours over the following 24 h period, the pigs were clinically examined for signs of respiratory disease until they fulfilled the inclusion criteria and received the first dose of treatment. After this first treatment administration, the pigs were examined 4, 8, 12 and 24 h ± one hour. Thereafter the clinical signs were recorded twice a day until day 7 post inoculation. The clinical examination of pigs consisted of the assessment of general appearance (including posture, behavior, feed intake, rectal temperature, presence of vomiting) and clinical signs of respiratory disease (breathing type, respiratory frequency, coughing). Results of the examination were transformed into a respiratory and a depression score (Table 1) on a scale from 0 to 3. Clinical cure was defined as a rectal temperature < 40.0 °C and absence of clinical signs of respiratory disease and no depression on

Table 1 Scoring schemes for the assessment of clinical signs

Scoring Points	Respiratory Score	Depression score
0	No clinical signs of respiratory disease	Active, alert, normal feed intake
1	Breathing frequency of 35–45/min and / or occasional coughing	Calm, alert, reduced feed intake
2	Breathing frequency of 46–70/min and/ or multiple coughing periods within 10 min and dyspnea	Dull, increased recumbence, increased reaction time, still moving to the feeding trough but without or only minimal feed intake or dull, sitting like a dog, increased reaction time, still moving to the feeding trough but no or only minimal feed intake
3	Breathing frequency > 70/min and cyanosis or gasping or open-mouth breathing or breathing frequency > 70/min and cyanosis and gasping or open-mouth breathing	Apathetic, no reaction to stimulation and/or shaky movements without lying down and / or standing with head down without lying down and/or vomiting and / or foam around nostrils and mouth

Table 2 Assignment to treatment groups and treatment procedures

Treatment Group	Active Ingredients	Application Route	Dosage [unit/kg]	Duration of treatment[a]	Number of animals[b]
T1	Marbofloxacin	IM	8 mg/kg	Day 0[c]	11
T2	Enrofloxacin	IM	2.5 mg/kg	Days 0, 1, 2	12
T3	Saline 0.9%	IM	1 ml/20 kg	Days 0, 1, 2	11

[a]after fulfilling the inclusion criteria for treatment
[b]Intention to treat populations
[c]animals of this group received 0.9% NaCl solution (1 ml/20 kg) on days 1 and 2 after first treatment

study day 6 (D6). Using the body weight taken prior to inoculation and on the day of removal, the average daily weight gain of the pigs was calculated.

Additional criteria for euthanasia were determined to reduce the level of stress and suffering of the pigs. Criteria for euthanasia were multifold (Table 3). Animals that were removed prior to D6 due to severity of disease were counted as not cured.

On day 7 post inoculation, or earlier in cases of withdrawal on humane grounds, the pigs were euthanized by lethal intravenous injection of 80 mg/kg pentobarbital (Euthadorm® 500 mg/ml; Co. CP Pharma GmbH, Burgdorf, Germany). Necropsy was performed directly after the death of each animal.

Bacteriological lung examination

For the bacteriological examination, 7 lung tissue samples (approximately 1cm²) collected from defined areas, located in the outer third of each of the seven lung lobes (one from each lobe), were collected and examined for the presence of *A. pleuropneumoniae*. Samples were plated on Columbia sheep blood agar, chocolate agar supplemented with 0.001% NAD and *A. pleuropneumoniae*-selective blood agar [35] using the quadrant streaking method. Abundance of growth was assessed semi-quantitatively. Bacterial isolates were identified as *A. pleuropneumoniae* by amplification of the apxIV gene [36].

Necropsy

During necropsy the macroscopic extent of the developed lung lesions was assessed. For an objective assessment the lung lesion score (LLS) specified by the European Pharmacopoeia (3rd edn. EDQM, Council of Europe, Strasbourg, France) for the testing of *A. pleuropneumoniae* vaccines [37] was used. The score is based on the recording of lung lesions after palpation and macroscopic evaluation of the lung on a schematic map of the lungs. On this map the lung is split into equal sized triangles. According to the size of the lesions a number of triangles is marked. The maximum score of each lung lobe is five, leading to a total maximum score of 35.

Statistical analysis

All collected data were entered into a database, based upon MS Access® 2010 (Microsoft Corporation, Dublin, Ireland). Verification was assured by double data entry. All statistical operations were carried out using SAS® statistical analysis software version 9.3 (SAS Institute Inc., Cary, NC, USA). Primary criterion for efficacy testing was the assessment of the developed lung lesion. Secondary criteria for the analysis were bacteriological cure, clinical cure on day D6, evolution of clinical scores, rectal temperature, withdrawals related to respiratory disease after inoculation and daily weight gain. The safety of the treatments was analyzed based upon percentage of adverse events and percentage of injection

Table 3 Criteria for euthanasia of animals prior to end of study

Code	Description of criteria
E1	Respiratory score of 3
E2	Depression score of 3
E3	Rectal body temperature > 42.0 °C
E4	Rectal body temperature < 37.5 °C and respiratory score > 1
E5	Rectal body temperature < 37.5 °C and depression score > 1
E6	Rectal body temperature > 40.3 °C and respiratory score > 1 on more than 2 consecutive days after day 3 post inoculation
E7	Rectal body temperature > 40.3 °C and depression score > 1 on more than 2 consecutive days after day 3 post inoculation
E8	Any unpredictable event, reaction to treatment or disease leading to a moderate to severe reduction of general condition for more than 48 h
E9	Any unpredictable event, reaction to treatment or disease inducing pain for more than 48 h

site reactions. For all continuous variables sample size, mean (m), standard deviation (SD), median, quartiles, minimum and maximum were calculated. Categorical or binary variables were displayed as absolute and relative frequencies. For the analyses ANOVA, Fisher's exact test and Mantel-Haenszel chi- square statistics were used. The data of the LLS were log-transformed as the non-transformed data were expected to be not normally distributed. The applied level of significance was 5% ($p < 0.05$).

Results

An overview of the main clinical data characteristics and results is given in Table 4.

Clinical data and inclusion for treatment

Prior to inoculation all pigs had a respiratory score and a depression score of 0 and a body temperature ≤ 40.0 °C. The last clinical examination prior to inoculation was performed one hour before the start of the experimental inoculation. Of the 36 nursery pigs included in this study, 35 animals developed typical clinical signs of porcine pleuropneumonia after challenge. One pig stayed clinically

healthy without any signs of disease and another one met the criteria for euthanasia prior to treatment. These two pigs were therefore not treated, leaving 34 pigs for the intention to treat population (ITT); 11 pigs in group T1, 12 pigs in group T2 and 11 pigs in group T3. Two pigs were treated despite not fulfilling all inclusion criteria (respiratory scores of 1 instead of 2). Therefore they were excluded from the final primary efficacy criterion analyses. These pigs belonged to treatment groups T1 and T3.

The mean body weight of the ITT population prior to inoculation was 12.1 kg with an SD of 2.5 (T1: 12.0 ± 2.4; T2: 12.6 ± 2.9; T3: 12.1 ± 2.4). The median time between challenge and treatment was 5.9 h for T1, 6.6 for T2 and 5.9 for T3 with no statistical significant differences between the three treatment groups. All pigs of the ITT population had a rectal temperature ≥ 40.3 °C prior to treatment (no statistical significant differences between treatment groups). The depression score was 1 for 79.4% (27 pigs) of all included animals and 2 for 20.6% of the pigs (T1:1 pig, T2: 2 pigs and T3: 4 pigs; no statistical significant differences between the treatment groups). Seven pigs in group T3 and one in group T1 met the criteria for euthanasia and were euthanized

Table 4 Overview of results of comparative treatment analysis including main data characteristics

	Treatment Group T1	Treatment Group T2	Treatment Group T3	p-Values for Differences
Active component	Marbofloxacin	Enrofloxacin	0.9% saline	
Number of animals	12	12	12	
Average body weight of the animals	12.0 ± 2.4	12.6 ± 2.9	12.1 ± 2.4	
Intention to treat population (number of animals)	11	12	11	
Number of animals included for primary efficacy criterion analysis	10	12	10	
Number of animals included for secondary efficacy criteria analyses	11	12	11	
Number of removals due to euthanasia criteria (mortality %)	1 (8.3%)	0 (0.0%)	8 (66.7%)	T1:T2 = > 0.05
				T2:T3 = < 0.001
				T1:T3 = 0.008
Lung Lesion Score[a]				T1:T2 = 0.34
mean	3.9 ± 4.1	6.0 ± 5.1	21.1 ± 7.7	T2:T3 = < 0.0001
Min-Max	0.0–14.9	0.5–20.1	10.2–35.0	T1:T3 = < 0.0001
Number of animals bacteriologically cured[b] (%)	11 (100%)	1 (91.7%)	0 (0%)	T1:T2 = > 0.05
				T2:T3 = < 0.001
				T1:T3 = < 0.001
Numbers of animals clinically cured[b] (%)	10 (90.9%)	10 (83.3%)	1 (9.1%)	T1:T2 = > 0.05
				T2:T3 = < 0.001
				T1:T3 = < 0.001
Daily weight gain[b]: infection to removal (kg)	1.81 ± 0.774	1.83 ± 0.606	0.69 ± 1.335	T1:T2 = < 0.05
				T2:T3 = < 0.05
				T1:T3 = < 0.05

[a]Primary efficacy criterion
[b]Secondary efficacy criterion

prior to day D6. One pig in group T3 died due to the severity of the infection. An overview of the most important clinical data is shown in Table 4.

Four hours after the first treatment, no animal in group T2, one pig in group T1 and seven in T3 had met the criteria for euthanasia. On day 2, one more pig in group T3 fulfilled the criteria for euthanasia and was removed, whereas no pig in group T1 or T2 showed any signs of clinical disease from 24 h after the first treatment onwards. On day 6 the respiratory score of one of

the remaining pigs in group T3 was still 1 (Fig. 1). Overall, 8.3% (1 pig) belonging to group T1, 0.0% belonging to group T2 and 66.7% (8 pigs) belonging to group T3 were euthanized (Table 4).

A depression score of 2 was observed in none of the animals in T1, in two animals (16.7%) in group T2 and in all four remaining animals (100.0%) in group T3, four hours after treatment initiation. Eight hours after the first treatment, none of the animals in group T1 and T2 and one pig in group T3 showed a depression

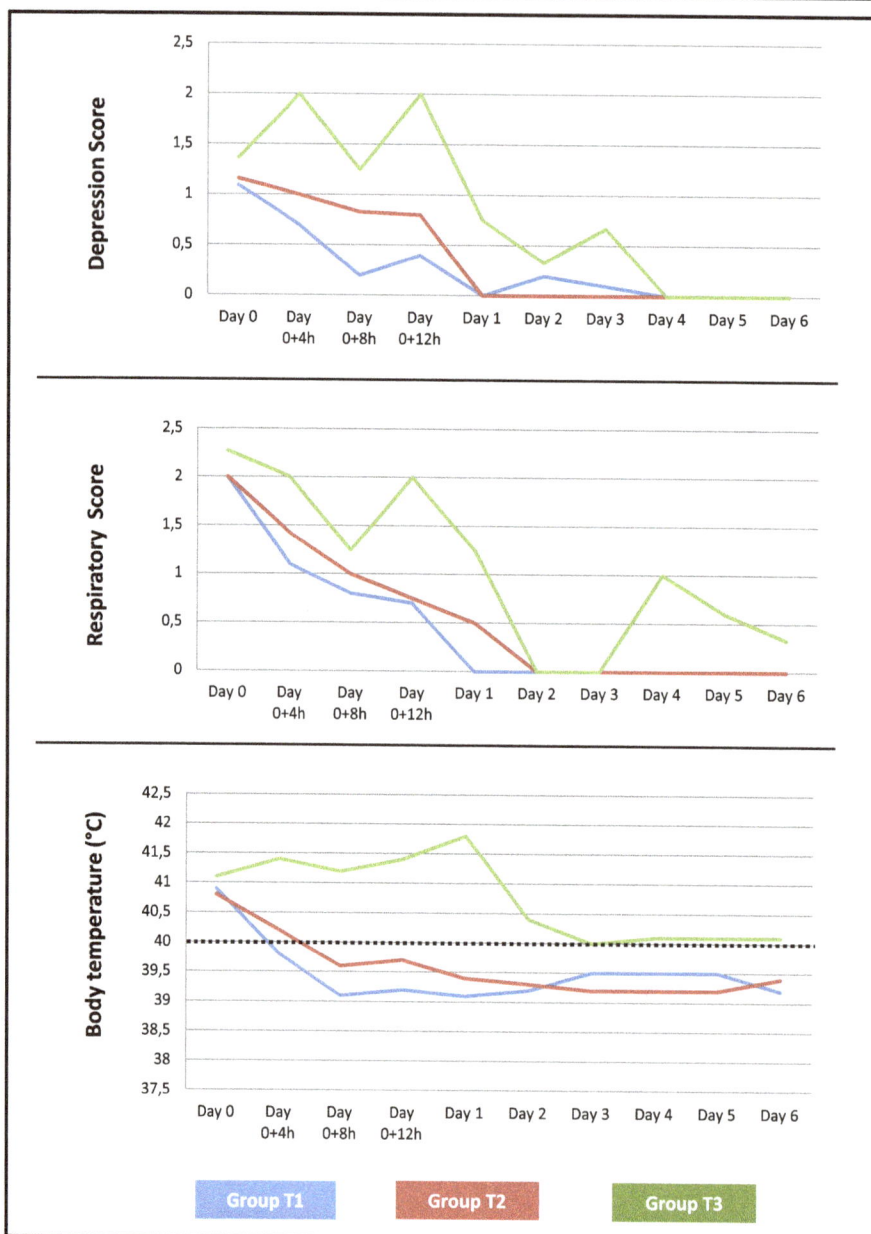

Fig. 1 Clinical course of disease after treatment. Group T1: 8 mg/kg marbofloxacin, one-shot treatment, 11 pigs at Day 0, 10 pigs from Day 0 + 4 h onwards; Group T2: 2.5 mg/kg enrofloxacin, treatment on three consecutive days, 12 pigs; Group T3: 0.9% saline treatment, 11 animals at Day 0, 4 pigs from Day 0 + 4 h onwards, 3 pigs from Day 2 onwards; Day 0 = time of intention to first treatment, h = hours, Day 1 = 24 h after first treatment, Day 2–6 = 48–144 h after first treatment, dotted line = marking the threshold for physiological body temperature of 40.0 °C

score > 1. The depression score was 0 for all animals in groups T1 and T2 at 24 h after first treatment and had returned to normal for the pigs in group T3 on day 4 (Fig. 1).

The rectal temperature returned to < 40.3 °C eight hours after treatment initiation in groups T1 and T2 and on day two in all remaining pigs of group T3. There was a small increase in temperature for less than 24 h on day three after the first treatment in group T1 and on day five after the first treatment in group T2 (Fig. 1). Regarding the course of disease, the differences were statistically significant between groups T1 and T3 as well as between groups T2 and T3 ($p < 0.0001$).

Of the ITT population, 10 pigs (90.9%) belonging to group T1, 10 pigs (83.3%) belonging to group T2 and 1 pig (9.1%) belonging to group T3 were considered cured on day 6 (Table 3). The difference was statistically significant between T1 and T3 and between T2 and T3 ($p < 0.001$).

The average daily weight gain (kg per day) also differed significantly ($p < 0.05$) between the groups T1 and T3 and between the groups T2 and T3 (Table 4).

Lung lesion score (LLS)

The LLS was the primary efficacy criterion. As two pigs were treated despite not fulfilling all inclusion criteria only 32 pigs were included in this analysis (see Clinical data; Table 4). After log transformation of the data, a statistically significant superiority of T1 and T2 compared to T3 was proven ($p < 0.0001$; Table 4).

Bacteriological examination

For the assessment of the bacteriological cure, the whole ITT population of 34 animals was included (Table 4). In group T1 A. pleuropneumoniae was re-isolated from the lungs from none (0.0%) of the pigs, in group T2 from one pig (8.3%) and from all pigs (100.0%) in group T3. Using the Fisher's exact test, a statistically significant difference was confirmed between groups T1 and T3 and also between groups T2 and T3 ($p < 0.001$). There was no statistically significant difference between groups T1 and T2.

Safety criteria

One animal of group T3 was found dead 24 h after treatment initiation. As this was the group treated with 0.9% NaCl-solution, the death was considered to be due to disease progression and not as a consequence of treatment.

No injection site reactions were observed in any of the treatment groups.

Discussion

The results of this study show that treatment with marbofloxacin and enrofloxacin was significantly superior to the mock-treatment of 0.9% saline solution. Enrofloxacin was chosen as reference product for the positive controls because like marbofloxacin, it belongs to the second generation fluoroquinolones and has similar pharmacokinetic properties. Additionally, the selected product Baytril®- Das Original 50 mg/ml (Bayer Vital GmnH, Germany) is already registered for the treatment of A. pleuropneumoniae infection in swine. The significant reduction of the need to euthanize pigs due to the severity of symptoms confirms the importance of antibiotic treatment to treat and save infected pigs after the onset of clinical signs for animal welfare reasons. Both antibiotic treatment regimens (T1 and T2) induced a faster return to a normal rectal temperature as well as a faster recovery of the general condition and respiratory parameters. The observed minor fluctuation in body temperature observed in animals in groups T1 and T2 after treatment could probably be linked to changes in activity behavior of the pigs [38] but an hypothesis of relapse, even though less probable because of the absence of other clinical signs, could not be totally excluded. If the treatment was insufficient for example due to a short treatment period a relapse of infection and inflammation might occur accompanied by a repeated increase in body temperature. As the study was terminated on day seven post inoculation no definitive statement can be made if the increase would have led to a relapse of clinical disease or if it was only a short-term fluctuation.

Although there was a somewhat faster improvement of general condition, respiratory parameters and rectal temperature, there were no statistically significant differences between the marbofloxacin and enrofloxacin-treated groups. This also applies to the clinical cure, the lung lesion score and the bacteriological examination. Lung lesions were less prominent in the marbofloxacin-treated pigs. Isolation of A. pleuropneumoniae from the lung tissue was possible in a greater number of animals from the enrofloxacin-treated than from the marbofloxacin-treated animals although the difference was only one pig and is therefore not significant.

Comparing the results of this study with previous studies that also assessed the influence of fluoroquinolones on A. pleuropneumoniae infection, these results are comparable with the results from Grandemange et al. [39] who also tested the efficacy and safety of marbofloxacin and enrofloxacin for the treatment of porcine pleuropneumonia. The outcome of the Grandemange study also concluded that both antibiotics were equally effective. However, comparison of efficacy results between different studies should be made with care. It should be taken into account that small setup-related differences e.g. in applied infection dose, environmental conditions, used serotype or dosage may significantly influence the development of disease [4–6] and therefore the study results. Most published studies evaluating the efficacy of marbofloxacin on *A. pleuropneumoniae* infection are conducted either as field [33, 40] or in-vitro studies [41–44]. An advantage of experimental infections under standardized conditions is that confounding environmental factors, that are often discussed as reasons for failure or reduced efficacy in field studies, can be eliminated. Studies that evaluate the efficacy of marbofloxacin and enrofloxacin on porcine pleuropneumonia under experimental conditions [45–47] show cure rates of 80–100%. For the one-shot high dose marbofloxacin treatment of porcine pleuropneumonia an experimental counterpart eliminating the environmental factors has not been conducted before. Other studies evaluating the efficacy of marbofloxacin to treat porcine pleuropneumonia investigated the efficacy of dosages between 1.5 mg/kg and 5 mg/kg bodyweight, administered on four consecutive days [47]. Nevertheless the results are in accordance with the results of this study regardless of the fact that fluoroquinolones develop their main bactericidal activity in a concentration-dependent manner [31, 32].

Another fact is, that especially in field studies, where the exact time of infection of the individual animal cannot be determined; the efficacy of antibiotic treatment can be reduced due to the biofilm formation within the porcine lungs if treatment is initiated too late. It has been demonstrated that *A. pleuropneumoniae* takes active part in the biofilm formation [48]. Biofilms are a biopolymer matrix attached to the biotic surfaces produced by the local microflora. Bacteria, such as *A. pleuropneumoniae*, are able use such biofilms to shield themselves from the immune system or antimicrobial treatment due to a developing gradient of diffusion [49]. Biofilm formation starts a few hours after infection and can seriously affect the efficacy of administered antibiotics. Due to the acute infection in this study, the fact that the pigs were tested negative for *A. pleuropneumoniae* prior to inoculation and the early onset of treatment, it is unlikely that a protective biofilm matrix influenced the efficacy of either of the antibiotics.

In this study *A. pleuropneumoniae* could not be re-isolated from lung tissue of any of the marbofloxacin-treated animals, indicating that the bacterial cure of the lung tissue was 100%. Other related studies have already shown that enrofloxacin is also capable of eliminating *A. pleuropneumoniae* from lung tissue after controlled experimental infection [45, 46]. A main difference between these presented results and previous studies concluding that an antibiotic treatment (e.g. tulathromycin, tilmicosin) is unable to completely eliminate *A. pleuropneumoniae* from colonized pigs is that other studies used PCR protocols for the pathogen detection and also tested the tonsils of the infected pigs after treatment [18, 50]. Tonsils and evolved lung sequesters are the

main locations described where *A. pleuropneumoniae* can survive despite a systemic antibiosis of the host [8, 51]. The PCR technique may also detect dead DNA, while culture depends on viability of the bacteria investigated [52]. Therefore conclusions regarding superiority or inferiority of fluoroquinolones for the elimination of *A. pleuropneumoniae* from infected pigs cannot be drawn based on the results of this study. Previous studies have demonstrated that marbofloxacin achieves a good penetration of tonsillar tissue and may reach sufficient concentration levels to remove *A. pleuropneumoniae* [53]. Nevertheless, no prediction of total clearance from animals can be made based upon the lack of isolation of bacteria from the lung tissue. Regarding the limitations of this study it should be mentioned that it only demonstrated the basic potential of this treatment procedure. A direct transfer of the results to field conditions cannot be made due to the diversity of the already mentioned environmental confounders and interactions with different microflora settings on different farms and within different animals.

Although the results of this study state a good efficacy and safety for the treatment of porcine pleuropneumonia with fluoroquinolones, the high importance of fluoroquinolones for use in human medicine should be stressed. It is therefore essential to limit the administration of fluoroquinolones to specific identified cases in order to maintain their efficacy and the low level of resistance which are equally important for their further use within the field of veterinary and human infectious diseases. Other measures such as improvement of husbandry practices and vaccination that have a major impact on the spreading of *A. pleuropneumoniae* infection [4] should be the method of choice when it comes to strategic containment of *A. pleuropneumoniae* leaving the use of fluoroquinolones for the treatment of clinical conditions that do not respond to other classes of antimicrobials.

Conclusions

The one-shot 8 mg/kg marbofloxacin treatment was proven to be efficacious and safe for the treatment of porcine pleuropneumonia caused by an experimental aerosol inoculation, as confirmed by clinical, pathomorphological and bacteriological examination. A superiority of the marbofloxacin treatment compared to the 2.5 mg/kg enrofloxacin treatment administered on three consecutive days was not demonstrated. Nevertheless, the one-shot marbofloxacin treatment demonstrated the same efficacy as the three-shot enrofloxacin treatment while reducing the stress to the animals and the risk for administration errors due to the single administration. This study also demonstrated the importance of antibiotic treatment to reduce mortality during the acute phase of the disease compared to a mock-treated group.

Abbreviations

A. pleuropneumoniae: *Actinobacillus pleuropneumoniae*; D6: Day six after first treatment; IM: Intramuscular; ITT: Intention-to-treat population; kg: kilogram; LLS: Lung lesion score; m: mean; mg: milligram; MIC: Minimal inhibitory concentration; p.inf.: Post infection; SD: Standard deviation

Acknowledgements

The authors would like to thank M. Homuth (IVD GmbH, Hannover, Germany) for conducting the serological examinations and P. Klein for the statistical analyses (dsh statistical services, Pfaffenhofen, Germany).

Funding

This study was financially supported by Vetoquinol SA as part of the work required for approval by the Agencies of European Countries for marketing authorization of Forcyl® for use in swine.

Authors' contributions

All authors contributed to the study design, interpretation of the data and drafting of the manuscript. BB and KH managed and monitored the study, DH was the principal investigator, JR performed the microbiological analyses.

Competing interests

The authors declare that they have no competing interests.

Author details

[1]Clinic for Swine, Small Ruminants, forensic Medicine and Ambulatory Service, University of Veterinary Medicine Hannover, Foundation, Bischofsholer Damm 15, D-30173 Hannover, Germany. [2]Institute for Microbiology, University of Veterinary Medicine Hannover, Foundation, Bischofsholer Damm 15, D-30173 Hannover, Germany. [3]Klifovet AG, Geyerspergerstr. 27, D-80689 Munich, Germany. [4]Vetoquinol SA, Research and Development Centre, B.P. 189, Cedex 70204 Lure, France.

References

1. Gottschalk M. Actinobacillus pleuropneumoniae is a current and continuing pathogen. Albéitar. 2012;159:4–5.
2. Von Altrock A. Occurrence of bacterial infectious agents in pathologically/anatomically altered lungs of pigs and compilation of resistance spectra. Berl Munch Tierarztl Wochenschr. 1998;111(5):164–72.
3. Rycroft AN, Garside LH. Actinobacillus species and their role in animal disease. Vet J. 2000;159(1):18–36.
4. Tobias T. Actinobacillus pleuropneumoniae transmission and clinical outbreaks. Utrecht: Utrecht University; 2014.
5. Hoeltig D, Hennig-Pauka I, Thies K, Rehm T, Beyerbach M, Strutzberg-Minder K, Gerlach GF, Waldmann K-H. A novel respiratory health score (RHS) supports a role of acute lung damage and pig breed in the course of an Actinobacillus pleuropneumoniae infection. BMC Vet Res. 2009;5(1):14.
6. Jacobsen M, Nielsen J, Nielsen R. Comparison of virulence of different Actinobacillus pleuropneumoniae serotypes and biotypes using an aerosol infection model. Vet Microbiol. 1996;49:159–68.
7. Gottschalk M. Actinobacillus pleuropneumoniae: an old but still relevant swine pathogen in the XXI century. In: Proc 22nd international pig veterinary society congress: 2012; 2012. p. 26–31.
8. Gottschalk M. Actinobacillosis. In: Straw BE, Zimmerman JJ, D'Allaire S, Taylor, editors. Disease of Swine. 10th ed. Oxford: Wiley-Blackwell; 2012. p. 653–69.
9. Brackmann J, Beckmann K, Lücken C, Baier S. Zur Verbreitung und Diagnostik von Actinobacillus pleuropneumoniae. Prakt Tierarzt. 2015;96:372–81.
10. Done S, White M. Porcine respiratory disease and complexes: the story to date. In Pract. 2003;25(7):410–7.
11. Hoy S, Mehlhorn G, Eulenberger K, Erwerth W, Johannsen U, Dorn W, Hörügel K. Zum Einfluß entzündlicher Lungenveränderungen auf ausgewählte Parameter der Schlachtleistung beim Schwein. Mh. Vet Med. 1985;40:584–7.
12. Hoy S, Mehlhorn G, Eulenberger K, Erwerth W, Johannsen U, Dorn W, Hörügel K. Zusammenhang zwischen entzündlichen Lungenveränderungen und der Lebendmasseentwicklung beim Schwein. Mh. *Vet Med*. 1985;40:579–84.
13. Mateusen B, Maes D, Hoflack G, De Vliegher S, Verdonck M, de Kruif A. Efficacy of tilmicosin phosphate in feed for the treatment of a clinical outbreak of Actinobacillus pleuropneumoniae infection in growing-finishing pigs. In: Proceedings 16th IPVS Congress Melbourne Australia 2000; 2000. p. 130.
14. Mengelers M, Kuiper H, Pijpers A, Verheijden J, Van Miert A. Prevention of pleuropneumonia in pigs by in-feed medication with sulphadimethoxine and sulphamethoxazole in combination with trimethoprim. Vet Q. 2000; 22(3):157–62.
15. Tumamao J, Bowles R, Hvd B, Klaasen H, Fenwick B, Storie G, Blackall P. Comparison of the efficacy of a subunit and a live streptomycin-dependent porcine pleuropneumonia vaccine. Austr Vet J. 2004;82(6):370–4.
16. Higgins R, Lariviere S, Mittal K, Martineau G, Rousseau P, Cameron J. Evaluation of a killed vaccine against porcine pleuropneumonia due to Haemophilus pleuropneumoniae. Can Vet J. 1985;26(2):86.
17. Velthuis A, De Jong M, Kamp E, Stockhofe N, Verheijden J. Design and analysis of an Actinobacillus pleuropneumoniae transmission experiment. Prev Vet Med. 2003;60(1):53–68.
18. Angen Ø, Andreasen M, Nielsen E, Stockmarr A, Baekbo P. Effect of tulathromycin on the carrier status of Actinobacillus pleuropneumoniae serotype 2 in the tonsils of pigs. Vet Rec. 2008;163(15):445–7.
19. Bossé JT, Li Y, Rogers J, Crespo RF, Li Y, Chaudhuri RR, Holden MT, Maskell DJ, Tucker AW, Wren BW. Whole genome sequencing for surveillance of antimicrobial resistance in Actinobacillus pleuropneumoniae. Front Microbiol. 2017;8
20. White DG, Zhao S, Simjee S, Wagner DD, McDermott PF. Antimicrobial resistance of foodborne pathogens. Microbes Infect. 2002;4(4):405–12.
21. Bossé JT, Li Y, Atherton TG, Walker S, Williamson SM, Rogers J, Chaudhuri RR, Weinert LA, Holden MT, Maskell DJ. Characterisation of a mobilisable plasmid conferring florfenicol and chloramphenicol resistance in Actinobacillus pleuropneumoniae. Vet Microbiol. 2015;178(3):279–82.
22. Dayao D, Gibson J, Blackall P, Turni C. Antimicrobial resistance genes in Actinobacillus pleuropneumoniae, Haemophilus parasuis and Pasteurella multocida isolated from Australian pigs. Austr Vet J. 2016;94(7):227–31.
23. Dayao DAE, Gibson JS, Blackall PJ, Turni C. Antimicrobial resistance in bacteria associated with porcine respiratory disease in Australia. Vet Microbiol. 2014;171(1):232–5.
24. Sweeney MT, Lindeman C, Johansen L, Mullins L, Murray R, Senn MK, Bade D, Machin C, Kotarski SF, Tiwari R. Antimicrobial susceptibility of Actinobacillus pleuropneumoniae, *Pasteurella multocida*, Streptococcus suis, and Bordetella bronchiseptica isolated from pigs in the United States and Canada, 2011 to 2015. J Swine Health Prod. 2017;25(3):106–20.
25. WHO Advisory group on integrated surveillance of antimicrobial resistance (AGISAR). Critically important antimicrobials for human medicine -5th rev. Geneva: World Health Organization; 2017. Licence: CC BY-NC-SA 3.0 IGO
26. Anthony F, Acar J, Franklin A, Gupta R, Nicholls T, Tamura Y, Thompson S, Threlfall E, Vose D, Van Vuuren M. Antimicrobial resistance: responsible and prudent use of antimicrobial agents in veterinary medicine. Rev Sci Tech. 2001;20(3):829–37.
27. Teale C, Moulin G. Prudent use guidelines: a review of existing veterinary guidelines. Rev Scienti Techniq OIE. 2012;31(1):343.
28. Ungemach FR, Müller-Bahrdt D, Abraham G. Guidelines for prudent use of antimicrobials and their implications on antibiotic usage in veterinary medicine. Int J Med Microbiol. 2006;296:33–8.
29. Weese JS: Prudent use of antimicrobials. Antimicrobial Therapy in Veterinary Medicine, Prescott JF, Baggot JD, Walker RD 2006: 437–448.

30. Friendship R. Antimicrobial drug use in swine. In: Prescott JF, Baggot JD, Walker RD, editors. Antimicrobial therapy in veterinary medicine; 2000. p. 602–16.

31. Ahmad I, Huang L, Hao H, Sanders P, Yuan Z. Application of PK/PD modeling in veterinary field: dose optimization and drug resistance prediction. Biomed Res Int. 2016;2016

32. Martinez M, McDermott P, Walker R. Pharmacology of the fluoroquinolones: a perspective for the use in domestic animals. Vet J. 2006;172(1):10–28.

33. Thomas E, Grandemange E, Pommier P, Wessel-Robert S, Davot J. Field evaluation of efficacy and tolerance of a 2% marbofloxacin injectable solution for the treatment of respiratory disease in fattening pigs. Vet Q. 2000;22(3):131–5.

34. Wayne P. CLSI. Performance Standards for Antimicrobial Disk and Dilution Susceptibility Tests for Bacteria Isolated from Animals. In: CLSI Supplement VET01S, Clinical and Laboratory Standards Institute. 3rd ed; 2015. Table 21.

35. Jacobsen MJ, Nielsen JP. Development and evaluation of a selective and indicative medium for isolation of Actinobacillus pleuropneumoniae from tonsils. Vet Microbiol. 1995;47(1–2):191–7.

36. Frey J. Detection, identification, and subtyping of Actinobacillus pleuropneumoniae. PCR Detect Microb Pathogens. 2003:87–95.

37. Hannan P, Bhogal B, Fish J. Tylosin tartrate and tiamutilin effects on experimental piglet pneumonia induced with pneumonic pig lung homogenate containing mycoplasmas, bacteria and viruses. Res Vet Sci. 1982;33:76–88.

38. Ingram D, Legge K. Variations in deep body temperature in the young unrestrained pig over the 24 hour period. J Physiol. 1970;210(4):989–98.

39. Grandemange E, Perrin P-A, Cvejic D, Haas M, Rowan T, Hellmann K. Randomised controlled field study to evaluate the efficacy and clinical safety of a single 8 mg/kg injectable dose of marbofloxacin compared with one or two doses of 7.5 mg/kg injectable enrofloxacine for the treatment of Actinobacillus pleuropneumoniae infections in growing-fattening pigs in Europe. Porcine Health Mang. 2017;3(1):10.

40. Sala V, Gusmara C, Invernizzi F, Gazza C. Control of sow to litter spreading of APP by injectable marbofloxacine (Marbocyl® 10%). In: Atti della Società Italiana di Patologia ed Allevamento dei Suini, XXXV Meeting Annuale, Modena, Italia, 12–13 Marzo 2009: Società Italiana di Patologia ed Allevamento dei Suini (SIPAS); 2009, 2009. p. 468–76.

41. Dorey L, Hobson S, Lees P. Factors influencing the potency of marbofloxacin for pig pneumonia pathogens Actinobacillus pleuropneumoniae and Pasteurella multocida. Res Vet Sci. 2017;111:93–8.

42. Nadeau M, Lariviere S, Higgins R, Martineau G. Minimal inhibitory concentrations of antimicrobial agents against Actinobacillus pleuropneumoniae. Can J Vet Res. 1988;52(3):315.

43. Rose M, Menge M, Bohland C, Zschiesche E, Wilhelm C, Kilp S, Metz W, Allan M, Röpke R, Nürnberger M. Pharmacokinetics of tildipirosin in porcine plasma, lung tissue, and bronchial fluid and effects of test conditions on in vitro activity against reference strains and field isolates of Actinobacillus pleuropneumoniae. J Vet Phar Ther. 2013;36(2):140–53.

44. Vilalta C, Giboin H, Schneider M, El Garch F, Fraile L. Pharmacokinetic/pharmacodynamic evaluation of marbofloxacin in the treatment of Haemophilus parasuis and Actinobacillus pleuropneumoniae infections in nursery and fattener pigs using Monte Carlo simulations. J Vet Phar Ther. 2014;37(6):542–9.

45. Herradora L, Martínez-Gamba R. Effect of oral enrofloxacine and florfenicol on pigs experimentally infected with Actinobacillus pleuropneumoniae serotype 1. Transbound Emerg Dis. 2003;50(5):259–63.

46. Wallgren P, Segall T, Pedersen MA, Gunnarsson A. Experimental infections with Actinobacillus pleuropneumoniae in pigs-I. Comparison of five different parenteral antibiotic treatments. Zentralblatt fur Veterinarmedizin Reihe B J Vet Med Ser B. 1999; 46(4):249–60.

47. Zou M, Zeng Z. Efficacy of marbofloxacin against experimentally induced Actinobacillus pleuropneumoniae in swine. Southwest China J Agric Sci. 2012;25(6):2333–7.

48. Li Y, Cao S, Zhang L, GW Lau Y, Wen RW, Zhao Q, Huang X, Yan Q, Huang Y, Wen X. A TolC-like protein of Actinobacillus pleuropneumoniae is involved in antibiotic resistance and biofilm formation. Front Microbiol. 2016;7:1618.

49. Hoiby N, Bjarnsholt T, Givskov M, Molin S, Ciofu O. Antibiotic resistance of bacterial biofilms. Int J Antimicrob Agents. 2010;35:322–32.

50. Fittipaldi N, Klopfenstein C, Gottschalk M, Broes A, Paradis M, Dick C. Assessment of the efficacy of tilmicosin phosphate to eliminate Actinobacillus pleuropneumoniae from carrier pigs. Can J Vet Res. 2005; 69(2):146.

51. Vigre H, Angen Ø, Barfod K, Lavritsen DT, Sørensen V. Transmission of Actinobacillus pleuropneumoniae in pigs under field-like conditions: emphasis on tonsillar colonisation and passively acquired colostral antibodies. Vet Microbiol. 2002;89(2):151–9.

52. Gram T, Ahrens P, Nielsen J. Evaluation of a PCR for detection of Actinobacillus pleuropneumoniae in mixed bacterial cultures from tonsils. Vet Microbiol. 1996;51(1–2):95–104.

53. Vilalta C, Schneider M, LÓPEZ-JIMENEZ R, Caballero J, Gottschalk M, Fraile L. Marbofloxacin reaches high concentration in pig tonsils in a dose-dependent fashion. J Vet Phar Ther. 2011;34(1):95.

20

Diarrhoea in neonatal piglets: a case control study on microbiological findings

Hanne Kongsted[1,2]* ⓘ, Karl Pedersen[3], Charlotte Kristiane Hjulsager[3], Lars Erik Larsen[3], Ken Steen Pedersen[2], Sven Erik Jorsal[3] and Poul Bækbo[2]

Abstract

Background: Many factors can influence the occurrence of neonatal diarrhoea in piglets. Currently, well-known pathogens such as enterotoxigenic *Escherichia coli* and *Clostridium perfringens* type C appear to play a minor role in development of disease. Other infectious pathogens may be involved. In this study, we aimed to investigate the presence of selected infectious pathogens in neonatal piglets with clinical and pathological signs of enteric disease. The association between rotavirus A, Enterococcus hirae, Clostridium difficile and *Clostridium perfringens* type A/C and diarrhoea was investigated in a case control study on piglet level. The possible role of *E. coli* virulence factors was investigated in a multistep-procedure using herd-pools of E.coli isolates to screen for their presence.

Results: Rotavirus A was detected more often in cases (25%) than in controls (6%) ($P < 0.001$). The detection rate of *Enterococcus hirae, Clostridium difficile* and *C. perfringens* type A positive for beta2 genes was the same in the two groups of piglets. *C. perfringens* type C was not detected in the study. Investigations on *E. coli* virulence factors showed a high prevalence of EAST1 toxin genes (55% of tested case piglets were positive) and AIDA-1 adhesin genes (63% of toxin positive case piglets were positive) in case piglets.

Conclusions: Detection of rotavirus A was statistically significantly associated with neonatal piglet diarrhoea. An aetiologic role of *E. coli* carrying virulence factors EAST1 and AIDA-1 needs further investigation as the study points out these two factors as possible causative factors in neonatal diarrhoea.
Detection of *E.hirae, C.difficile* and *C. perfringens* type A carrying beta 2 genes was not associated with neonatal piglet diarrhoea. However, the study suggested that massive overgrowth by *E. hirae* could be part of the pathogenesis in some cases of neonatal diarrhoea.

Keywords: Piglets, Neonatal diarrhoea, Rotavirus a, *E. coli* virulence factors, EAST1, AIDA-1, *C. difficile, C. perfringens* type a, Beta 2, *Enterococcus hirae*

Background

Many sow herds experience diarrhoea in piglets within the first week of life (neonatal diarrhoea), and it is an ongoing challenge to diagnose the underlying cause of symptoms in individual herds. In many cases, the pattern of disease indicates an infectious aetiology, but no causative agents are identified by traditional laboratory investigations. Previous examinations of neonatal diarrhoea in Danish and Swedish herds suggested that

Enterococcus spp., rotavirus A and *E. coli* carrying EAST1 virulence genes might be of significance [1–3]. Other studies suggest that *Clostridium difficile* (*C. difficile*) and *C. perfringens* type A containing beta2 toxin gene (CPA cpb2) may be relevant to investigate further in relation to neonatal diarrhoea [4–6].

This study intended to study potential aetiologies of neonatal diarrhoea in a large number of herds throughout Denmark, focusing on specific agents previously suggested to be relevant in a North European setting. We limited our detection of agents to include rotavirus A, toxigenic *E.coli* (*E.coli* carrying genes for LT, STa, STb or EAST1), CPA cpb2, *C. perfringens* type C (CPC), *C. difficile* and *E. hirae*. Rotavirus C was not included due to earlier studies indicating a very low prevalence

* Correspondence: hanne.kongsted@anis.au.dk
[1]Department of Animal Science, Aarhus University, Blichers Allé 20, DK-8830 Tjele, Denmark
[2]SEGES Danish Pig Research Centre, Axeltorv 3, DK-1609 Copenhagen V, Denmark
Full list of author information is available at the end of the article

and no association with neonatal diarrhoea in Danish and Swedish herds [1, 7, 8]. As no PED or TGE outbreaks have been described in Denmark, coronaviruses were not investigated. In order to obtain a clear definition of a diarrhoeic case vs. a non-diarrhoeic control we used a combination of clinical and pathological examinations.

Methods
Enrolment of piglets
The study was performed as a case control study involving diarrhoeic and non-diarrhoeic piglets from commercial production herds. Piglets from 60 herds were selected by 23 different local practitioners (1–8 herds per practitioner) and enrolled from October 2013 to October 2014. Herd owners were asked to fill in questionnaires on vaccination schemes.

Within each herd, the local practitioners were asked to select four diarrhoeic (but otherwise apparently healthy) and two non-diarrhoeic and otherwise apparently healthy 1–5 days old piglets from different litters. Antibiotic treatment against diarrhoea was prohibited in the selected piglets, but metaphylactic antibiotic treatment on the day of birth was allowed.

Necropsy
Piglets were euthanized by a stroke to the head and marked as diarrhoeic or non-diarrhoeic. They were packaged with cooling elements and shipped by mail to Laboratory for Pig Diseases, SEGES Pig Research Centre for necropsy on the following day. This procedure is equivalent to routine laboratory diagnostics in Denmark. Histological examination of intestinal epithelium was not an option under this setup because it requires fresh material sampled immediately after euthanasia. Necropsies were performed by experienced pathologists using a standardized scheme. The diagnosis enteritis was based upon the appearance of intestinal walls ant the consistency of colon content.

From each piglet, a section of mid-jejunum was cultured for E. coli. Other intestinal segments and intestinal contents were evacuated and stored at – 80 °C until further use.

Laboratory analyses
E. coli culture and PCR
Intestinal contents were streaked onto Columbia agar plates (Oxoid) with 5% calf blood and incubated aerobically at 37 °C for 24 h. For verification of the presence of E. coli colonies, parallel culturing on Drigalski (in house selective and indicative medium for coliforms) was performed. When E. coli colonies were present, two colonies per piglet were mixed in a herd pool (containing up to twelve colonies in total, from the six piglets pr. herd) and frozen at – 80 °C in Luria-Bertani broth with 15% glycerol for subsequent PCR analyses. If present, β-haemolytic colonies were selected. Otherwise, two typical non-haemolytic colonies were selected. Subcultures of all selected colonies were frozen individually using the same procedure.

PCR-analyses were performed stepwise. All herd pools ($n = 60$) were tested for the presence of heat-labile enterotoxin (LT), heat-stable toxin a (STa) and b (STb) and enteroaggregative Escherichia coli heat-stable enterotoxin1 (EAST1). LT, STa, and STb were detected by real-time PCR [8] in a Rotor-Gene Q real-time PCR machine (QIAGEN). Samples with Ct < 30 were considered positive. Detection of EAST1 was carried out by conventional PCR and subsequent separation by agarose gel electrophoresis. We used the method described by Zhang et al. [9] with the exception that AmpliTaq Gold Polymerase (ThermoFisher Scientific) was used and amplification was conducted in a total volume of 50 μl including 5 μl template in a TRIO thermocycler (Biometra GmbH, Germany). Herd-pools that were positive for LT, STa, STb or EAST1 were tested for the fimbrial adhesins F4, F5, F6, F18 and F41 (by real-time PCR as described for LT, STa and Stb) and adhesin involved in diffuse adherence-1 (AIDA-1) (by conventional PCR as described for EAST1). The stepwise procedure used for herd-pool testing is shown in Fig. 1.

Isolates from herd pools being positive for minimum one toxin gene and one adhesin gene were tested for STb and EAST1 genes (the most prevalent toxin genes in the herd pools). Subsequently, piglets that were positive for EAST-1 and/ or STb genes were tested for F41 and AIDA-1 genes (the most prevalent adhesin genes in the herd pools). For each virulence factor, we tested two isolates per piglet and considered a piglet positive if at least one of the two tested isolates was positive for the virulence factor in question.

E. hirae culture and identification by MALDI-TOF
A section of distal jejunum was used for culturing of E. hirae. Intestinal contents were plated on Slanetz-Bartley agar (Oxoid) and incubated aerobically at 37 °C for 48 h. Dominant colony types (1–3 colony types per specimen), were subcultured on blood agar and identified to species-level using MALDI-TOF (Bruker Daltronics, Bremen, Germany). Growth of E. hirae was semi quantitatively assessed. In the analyses we evaluated 1) Presence of E. hirae and 2) Massive growth of E. hirae (pure or massive growth).

PCR on intestinal contents
Jejunal contents were used for detection of rotavirus A, C. difficile and C. perfringens. Samples were prepared as a 10% suspension in PBS, beated for 20 s at 15 Hz, and centrifuged at 10.000 rpm for 90 s. Nucleic acids were

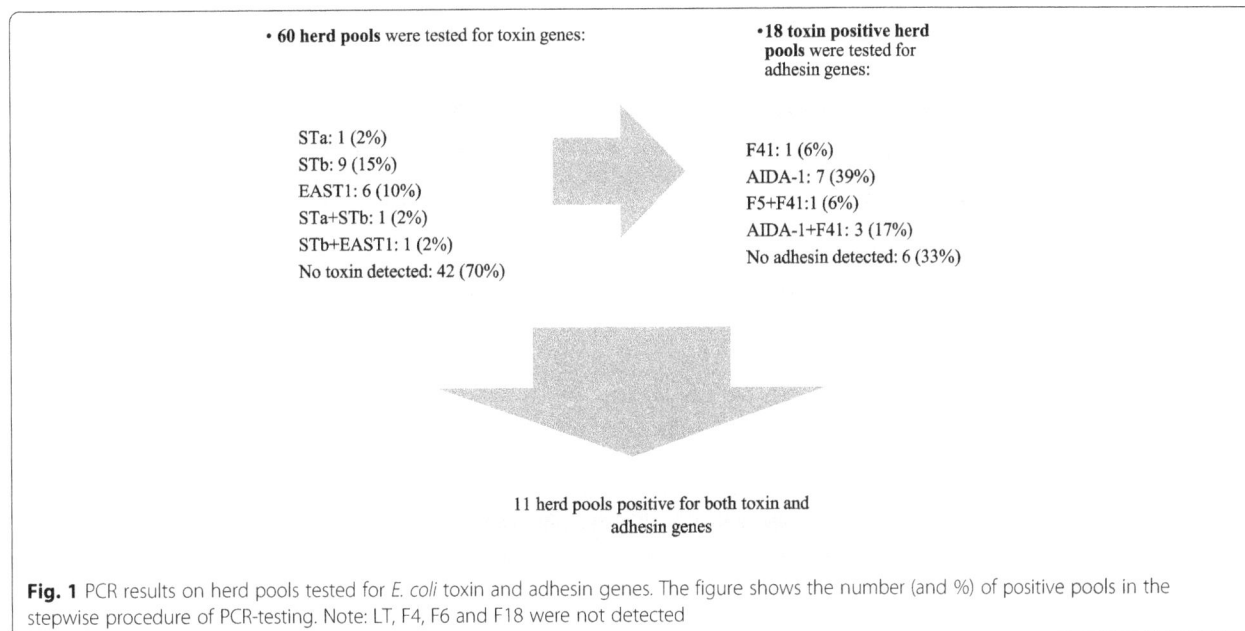

Fig. 1 PCR results on herd pools tested for *E. coli* toxin and adhesin genes. The figure shows the number (and %) of positive pools in the stepwise procedure of PCR-testing. Note: LT, F4, F6 and F18 were not detected

extracted from 200 μl supernatant with the QIAsymphony DSP Virus/Pathogen Mini Kit (QIAGEN, Denmark), protocol "Complex 200 V6 DSP" without carrier, automated on the QIAsymphony (QIAGEN) extraction robot. Nucleic acid extracts were stored at − 80 °C until analysis.

Previously published RT-qPCR assay primers and probe targeting the NSP3 gene and designed to detect all rotavirus A genotypes from humans and animals, were used [10]. Each PCR reaction contained 2 μl template, 1 x RT-PCR Buffer and 1 x RT-PCR Enzyme Mix (AgPath-ID™ OneStep RT-PCR Kit, ThermoFisher Scientific), 400 nM of each primer and 120 nM probe in a total volume of 15 μl. PCR was performed on Rotor-Gene Q real-time PCR machine with cycling conditions: 10 min at 45 °C, 10 min at 95 °C, 48 cycles of 15 s at 95 °C, 45 s at 60 °C. Samples with Ct < 33 were considered positive.

Detection of *C. difficile* was carried out by the PCR method described by Penders et al. [11] with the exception that detection was carried out on a Rotor-Gene Q real-time PCR machine. Purified DNA from reference strain CCUG 4938 served as positive control in the PCR. Samples with Ct < 37 were considered positive. Alfa-, beta- and beta2 toxin genes related to *C. perfringens* were detected by PCR using primers and probes described previously [12]. Primers and probes were multiplexed on Rotor-Gene Q with FAM-BHQ1 fluorophore pair for the alfa-toxin gene probe, HEX-BHQ1 for the beta-toxin gene probe and Cy5-BHQ2 for the beta2-toxin gene probe. PCR reactions contained 1× JumpStart™ *Taq* ReadyMix™ (SIGMA-Aldrich), 3.5 mM MgCl$_2$, 300 nM of each primer, 400 nM of each probe

and 3 μl template in a total volume of 25 μl. Results for alfa-toxin, beta-toxin and beta2-toxin were detected in the green, yellow and red channels, respectively. Cut-off was Ct = 37. Only samples with positive results for alfa toxin genes were considered *C. perfringens* positive.

Case/control definition and statistical evaluation

A case piglet was defined as a piglet selected as diarrhoeic in the herd and given the diagnosis enteritis at necropsy. A control piglet was defined as a piglet selected as non-diarrhoeic in the herd and found healthy at necropsy. Fisher's exact test (significance level = 0.05) was used to test statistical significant differences between microbiological findings in cases vs. controls.

Results
Piglets selected in the herds and herd vaccination protocols

In total, 230 piglets selected as diarrhoeic and 125 piglets selected as non-diarrhoeic were submitted from 60 herds in the study (not all herds followed the instructions on submitting four diarrhoeic and 2 non-diarrhoeic piglets). Fourtynine (82%) of the participating herds returned the questionnaires on vaccination routines. Almost all (94–98%) of these herds vaccinated breeding stock against enterotoxigenic *E. coli* (ETEC) and *C. perfringens* type C (mainly by using polyvalent vaccines containing *E. coli* F4, F5, F6 and *C. perfringens* betatoxoid antigens). Twenty-seven % of the herds returning questionnaires vaccinated breeding stock against *C. perfringens* type A.

Necropsy and inclusion as cases and controls

Extra-intestinal diagnoses were scarce. Pneumonia, arthritis, trauma from castration and unspecific findings were registered in 2, 3, 3, 9 piglets, respectively. Diagnoses at necropsy were not consistently in agreement with the clinical diagnoses in the herds. Thus, 11% of piglets with diarrhoea and 8% of the piglets selected as healthy in the herds were diagnosed with starvation as the only diagnosis at necropsy. Also, 13% of the piglets selected as diarrhoeic were diagnosed as healthy and 9% of the piglets selected as healthy were diagnosed with enteritis at necropsy (Table 1).

Altogether, 171 (74%) of the diarrhoeic piglets were diagnosed with enteritis and 97 (78%) of the non-diarrhoeic piglets were diagnosed as healthy at necropsy. These two groups of piglets served as cases and controls in the study. Descriptive information on necropsy findings in case and control piglets is given in Additional file 1.

Laboratory analyses

E. coli As described, detection of *E. coli* virulence factors was performed stepwise, initially testing herd pools of *E. coli* isolates from all 60 herds submitting piglets for the study. Toxin genes were detected in 30% of herd pools with STb being the most common toxin gene. Figure 1 summarizes the stepwise testing procedure and PCR results on pool level. In total, eleven herd pools (18%) were positive for both toxin and adhesin genes.

Fourty-five piglets from these eleven herds were selected as either cases ($n = 29$) or controls ($n = 16$) and thus tested individually. More case (55%) than control piglets (19%) tested positive for *E. coli* toxin genes STb and/or EAST-1 ($P = 0.03$). Sixty-three percent of toxin gene positive piglets were positive for the adhesion gene AIDA-1, whereas F41 was not detected in any (Table 2).

C. perfringens, C. difficile, E. hirae and rotavirus a

CPA cpb 2 and *C. difficile* were frequently detected in both case and control piglets. Thus, more than half of the piglets in both groups were *C. difficile* positive by PCR and close to 100% of piglets in both groups were positive for CPA cpb2. None of the 268 piglets tested positive for *C. perfringens* type C (=beta toxin genes). Approximately 40% of piglets in both groups were positive for *E. hirae* by culture, but only 14% (16% of case

piglets vs. 9% of control piglets ($P = 0.1$)) exhibited abundant or massive growth of this bacterial species on agar plates.

A low prevalence of Rotavirus A was detected (18% of piglets were positive by PCR), however, Rotavirus A was the only agent statistically significantly associated with case piglets ($P = 0.001$). Results on the detection of *C. difficile*, CPA cpb2, *E. hirae* and rotavirus A are presented in Table 3. Several other Streptococcus and Enterococcus species were also commonly found, most commonly *E. faecalis*, *E. faecium*, *E. durans*, *S gallolyticus* or *S. bovis*.

Discussion

The object of this study was to investigate potential microbiological aetiologies of diarrhoea in a large number of herds throughout Denmark in order to elucidate the potential significance of specific agents.

Studies using fluorescence in situ hybridization (FISH) and multiplex qPCR ("Gut Microbiotassay") methods previously suggested a potential significance of Enterococcus spp. and non-ETEC *E. coli* in Danish cases of neonatal diarrhoea [13, 14]. Furthermore, the study by Hermann-Bank et al. showed a disturbed bacterial composition of the gut flora in diarrhoeic piglets. These studies have served as an inspiration when choosing the focus of the current study. However, we chose not to include FISH and "Gut Microbiotassay" analyses in the present study, as we wanted to work under standard diagnostic conditions. We used piglets euthanized the day before necropsy and limited ourselves from using these methods.

Diarrhoeic cases and healthy controls were defined using a combination of clinical and pathological diagnostics. This approach reduced the number of clinically evaluated piglets from 355 initially submitted to 268 piglets finally included as cases and controls based on necropsy findings. The fact that 24% of piglets selected as diarrhoeic cases in the herds were either diagnosed with starvation or as being healthy at necropsy shows that diarrhoeic symptoms do not always reflect an enteric pathological condition. Furthermore, 9% of the piglets selected as healthy controls were diagnosed with enteritis at necropsy emphasizing that it is challenging to select the correct piglets for laboratory confirmation. Further, this might explain a part of the difficulties

Table 1 Diagnoses assigned at necropsy in 230 piglets selected as diarrhoeic and 125 piglets selected as non-diarrhoeic by the veterinary practitioners in the herds prior to euthanazia. Single piglets were given one to two diagnoses at necropsy

	Enteritis	Starvation	Arthritis	Pneumonia	Trauma from castration	Healthy	Unspecific
Diarrhoeic	171 (74%)	31 (13%)[a]	2 (1%)	1 (0.5%)	2 (1%)	30 (13%)	4 (2%)
Non-diarrhoeic	11 (9%)	11 (9%)[b]	1 (1%)	1 (1%)	1 (1%)	97 (78%)	5 (4%)

[a]26 (11%) had starvation as the only diagnosis. [b]10 (8%) had starvation as the only diagnosis

Table 2 *E. coli* virulence factors detected in case and control piglets (only isolates from herd-pools with positive results for both toxin(s) and adhesin(s) were individually tested)

Piglets tested for EAST-1 and STb genes (n = 45)	Case piglets (n = 29)	Control piglets (n = 16)	P-value*
EAST-1	6 (21%)	1 (6%)	0.4
EAST-1 + STb	10 (34%)	2 (13%)	0.2
Toxin detected	16 (55%)	3 (19%)	0.03
Piglets tested for F41 and AIDA-1 genes (n = 19)	Case piglets (n = 16)	Control piglets (n = 3)	
AIDA-1[#]	10 (63%)	2 (67%)	1
F41	0 (0%)	0 (0%)	1

*Two-sided Fisher's exact test. [#]All piglets that were positive for AIDA-1 were positive for both EAST-1 and STb

reported in relation to diagnosing causes of neonatal diarrhoea in other studies [3, 15].

Out of several infectious agents investigated, only rotavirus A was statistically significantly associated with being a case. Rotavirus A is by many considered ubiquitous in suckling piglets, but previous Danish studies have shown that the prevalence within the first week of life can be very low [16]. Studies focusing on the possible viral aetiology of the newly described phenomenon New Neonatal Porcine Diarrhoea Syndrome (NNPDS) conclude that viruses do not seem to pose a significant contribution to diarrhoeal symptoms in affected herds [7, 16]. However, these herds (four in Denmark and ten in Sweden) were selected as representative for a new type of diarrhoea not caused by known agents, including rotavirus A [1]. In the present study, we did not focus on NNPDS and did not exclude any herds due to presence of rotavirus A. Instead, we included a large number (60) of different herds in order to get a broader picture of diarrhoeal aetiologies in neonatal pigs. Interestingly, our findings support a recent study in two Danish herds. In that study, examining samples from 132 neonatal piglets, 89% of diarrhoeic piglets vs. 48% of non-diarrhoeic piglets were rotavirus A positive by PCR [2]. Taken together, these results suggest that rotavirus A has an important clinical significance in neonatal piglets, although the prevalence of case herds may be rather low as indicated by the low prevalence (18%) shown in this study.

Piglets in the study seemed to be protected against ETEC and *C. perfringens* type C by sow vaccination. The low herd-pool prevalence of *E. coli* fimbrial genes, including the previously clinically important F4 gene that was not detected at all, and the fact that *C. perfringens* type C was not detected at all probably reflects a successful vaccination scheme. Also, antibiotics used as metaphylaxis in some of the herds and the Danish breeding programme for F4 resistant pigs [17] could have an influence on the absence of F4 positive *E. coli*. STb was the only ETEC-associated toxin gene detected at a relatively high prevalence (19% of herd pools were positive). Whether a result of vaccination or not, *E. coli* results in this study support laboratory surveillance data indicating that ETEC are no longer dominant agents in neonatal diarrhoea [5, 18]. Also *C. perfringens* type C is an extremely rare agent detected in routine diagnostics in Denmark.

PCR results from *E. coli* herd pools in this study suggested that the toxin gene EAST1 and the adhesion gene AIDA-1 could be relevant to investigate further, as both these virulence factors were moderately prevalent. Few studies have evaluated the possible role of EAST1 and AIDA-1 in neonatal diarrhoea. A Danish study found that 48% of diarrhoeic vs. 18% of non-diarrhoeic neonatal piglets were positive for EAST1. In one of the investigated herds in this study, ten out of ten diarrhoeic piglets were positive for EAST1 [1].Vu-Khac et al.

Table 3 Comparative results on *E. hirae* culture and PCR detection of rotavirus A, *C. difficile* and *C. perfringens* type A carrying beta2 genes (CpA-cpb2) in case vs. control piglets

	Case piglets (n = 171)	Control piglets (n = 97)	P-value*
C. difficile	111 (65%)	55 (57%)	0.2
CpA cpb2	157 (96%)	90 (97%)	1
E. hirae present	76 (44%)	42 (43%)	0.9
Massive growth of *E. hirae*	28 (16%)	9 (9%)	0.1
Rotavirus A	42 (25%)	6 (6%)	< 0.001

*Two-sided Fisher's exact test

detected EAST1 genes in 65% of *E. coli* isolates from diarrhoeic piglets vs. 27% of isolates from non-diarrhoeic ones [19]. Other studies did not find any association between the detection of EAST1 and diarrhoea [20–22]. Previous studies on AIDA-1 found a quite low prevalence (3–17%) in isolates from diarrhoeic suckling piglets [20, 21, 23–25]. Two of these studies included non-diarrhoeic specimens and did not detect AIDA-1 in any of those [20, 21]. The current study provides limited information on the piglet level, as only 45 piglets from toxin and adhesin positive pools were individually tested as cases and controls. However, EAST1 being present in 55% of individually tested case piglets with the majority being positive for AIDA-1 also, supports relevance of further investigation of the role of these virulence factors in neonatal diarrhoea.

E. hirae is part of the normal intestinal flora of pigs [26], but Swedish and Danish studies have suggested a possible relation to neonatal diarrhoea [3, 13]. The Swedish study examined 29 piglets and found that 100% of diarrhoeic piglets vs. none of the non-diarrhoeic control piglets exhibited enteroadherent enterococci in the small intestine when examined by fluorescence in situ hybridisation. The Danish study examined 101 piglets and found that 37% of diarrhoeic vs. 14% of non-diarrhoeic specimens had enteroadherent enterococci in the small intestine. The present study did not find any association between the detection of *E. hirae* in intestinal contents and diarrhoea, but the results indicated that a massive growth of *E. hirae* might have clinical impact. The massive growth seen in some of the piglets in this study may, however, merely be a reflection of a disturbed microbiota.

It has been established that *C. difficile* can cause enteritis in neonatal piglets [27–29], but epidemiologic studies do not support the idea of *C. difficile* being a primary diarrhoeic pathogen in pigs [4, 13, 30–32]. In accordance with this, the detection of *C. difficile* was not associated with being a case in this study. However, it may be that histopathological examination is essential in the diagnostics on *C. difficile* related diarrhoea, and that studies merely detecting the agent or its toxins give misleading results.

Many studies have found that CPA cpb2 does not seem to be associated with neonatal diarrhoea [6, 32–34], which is supported by this study. For many years, *C. perfringens* type A has been a suspected pathogen in neonatal diarrhoea, but no studies have convincingly supported this claim. One study demonstrated a (minor) cytotoxic effect of supernatant from porcine CPA cpb2, but also showed that the cytotoxic effect was not related to beta2 toxin [35]. Thus, that study suggests that the potential role of *C. perfringens* type A in neonatal diarrhoea is not due to its ability to produce beta2 toxin. Investigations into the diarrhoea-causing capability of other toxins produced by *C. perfringens* type A may be relevant.

Conclusions

Rotavirus A was the only agent in the study statistically significantly associated with diarrhoea, and probably plays an important role in the development of neonatal diarrhoea in some herds. The study stresses that rotavirus A is not ubiquitous in neonatal piglets. The detection of this virus in cases of neonatal diarrhoea can therefore be a useful method to support decisions on vaccination regimes.

The possible role of the *E. coli* virulence factors EAST1 and AIDA-1 needs further investigation as our results suggested these factors to be more relevant in relation to neonatal diarrhoea in today's pig herds than the classical ETEC virulence factors.

CPC was not detected in any of 60 herds in the study and seems to be well controlled by vaccination as well as classical ETEC. Detection of *E.hirae*, *C.difficile* and CPA cpb2 was not related to diarrhoeal status. However, results in a small subset of piglets show that massive overgrowth by *E. hirae* could be part of the pathogenesis in some cases of neonatal diarrhoea.

Acknowledgements

We would like to thank herd-owner and field veterinarians for the submission of piglets. We are also very thankful to laboratory staff at Laboratory for Pig Diseases, SEGES Danish Pig Research Centre and National Veterinary Institute, Technical University of Denmark.

Funding

The study was supported by The Danish Ministry of Food, Agriculture and Fisheries and The Pig Levy Fond.

Authors' contributions

All authors contributed to the design of the study. Inclusion of piglets was carried out by KSP. CKJ and LEL performed the PCR analyses. KP performed the culturing of *Enterococcus spp.* Descriptive and statistical evaluations were carried out by HK. All authors contributed to drafts and proofreading of the manuscript. All authors read and approved the final manuscript.

Competing interests

The authors declare that they have no competing interests.

Author details
[1]Department of Animal Science, Aarhus University, Blichers Allé 20, DK-8830 Tjele, Denmark. [2]SEGES Danish Pig Research Centre, Axeltorv 3, DK-1609 Copenhagen V, Denmark. [3]National Veterinary Institute, Technical University of Denmark, Kemitorvet, 2800 Kgs. Lyngby, Denmark.

References
1. Kongsted H. New neonatal porcine Diarrhoea syndrome - a study on its aetiology, epidemiology and clinical manifestations. Copenhagen: SL Grafik; 2014. 978-87-7611-772-6
2. Rasmussen M, Moeller C, Hjulsager CK, Kongsted H, Hansen C, Larsen LE. Rotavirus type A associated diarrhoea in neonatal piglets: Importance and biodynamics. Proceedings of the 9th European Symposium of Porcine Health Management VVD-046. Prague; 2017. http://orbit.dtu.dk/files/140539459/ESPHM2017_Proceedings_Rotavirus.pdf.
3. Larsson J, Lindberg R, Aspan A, Grandon R, Westergren E, Jacobson M. Neonatal piglet Diarrhoea associated with Enteroadherent enterococcus hirae. J Comp Pathol. 2014;151:137–47.
4. Silva ROS, Salvarani FM, Cruz Junior ECC, Pires PS, Santos RLR, Antunes de Assis R, Guedes RMC, Lobato FCF. Detection of enterotoxin a and cytotoxin B, and isolation of Clostridium difficile in piglets in Minas Gerais, Brazil. Cienc Rural. 2011;41(8):1430–5.
5. Chan G, Farzan A, DeLay J, McEwen B, Prescott JF, Friendship RM. A retrospective study on the etiological diagnoses of diarrhea in neonatal piglets in Ontario, Canada between 2001 and 2010. Can J Vet Res. 2013;77(4):254–60.
6. Cruz EC Jr, Salvarani FM, Silva ROS, Silva MX, Lobato FCF, Guedes RMC. A surveillance of enteropathogens in piglets from birth to seven days of age in Brazil. Pesquisa Vet Brasil. 2013;33(8):963–9.
7. Karlsson OE, Larsson J, Hayer J, Berg M, Jacobson M. The intestinal eukaryotic Virome in healthy and Diarrhoeic neonatal piglets. PLoS One. 2016; https://doi.org/10.1371/journal.pone.0151481.
8. Frydendahl K, Imberechts H, Lehmann S. Automated 5' nuclease assay for detection of virulence factors in porcine Escherichia coli. Mol Cell Probes. 2001;15(3):151–60.
9. Zhang WP, Zhao MJ, Ruesch L, Omot A, Francis D. Prevalence of virulence genes in Escherichia coli strains recently isolated from young pigs with diarrhea in the US. Vet Microbiol. 2007;123(1/3):145–52.
10. Pang XL, Lee B, Boroumand N, Leblanc B, Preiksaitis JK, Yu Ip CC. Increased detection of rotavirus using a real time reverse transcription-polymerase chain reaction (RT-PCR) assay in stool specimens from children with diarrhea. J Med Virol. 2004;72(3):496–501.
11. Penders J, Vink C, Driessen C, London N, Thijs C, Stobberingh EE. Quantification of Bifidobacterium spp., Escherichia coli and Clostridium difficile in faecal samples of breast-fed and formula-fed infants by real-time PCR. FEMS Microbiol Lett. 2005;243(1):141–7.
12. Albini S, Brodard I, Jaussi A, Wollschlaeger N, Frey J, Miserez R, Abril C. Real-time multiplex PCR assays for reliable detection of Clostridium perfringens toxin genes in animal isolates. Vet Microbiol. 2008;127(1–2):179–85.
13. Jonach B, Boye M, Stockmarr A, Jensen T. Fluorescence in situ hybridization investigation of potentially pathogenic bacteria involved in neonatal porcine diarrhea. BMC Vet Res. 2014;10(1):68.
14. Hermann-Bank ML, Skovgaard K, Stockmarr A, Strube ML, Larsen N, Kongsted H, Ingerslev HC, Mølbak L, Boye M. Characterization of the bacterial gut microbiota of piglets suffering from new neonatal porcine diarrhoea. BMC Vet Res. 2015;11:139.
15. Kongsted H, Jonach B, Haugegaard S, Angen O, Jorsal SE, Kokotovic B, Larsen LE, Jensen TK, Nielsen JP. Microbiological, pathological and histological findings in four Danish pig herds affected by a new neonatal diarrhoea syndrome. BMC Vet Res. 2013;9:206.
16. Goecke NB, Hjulsager CK, Kongsted H, Boye M, Rasmussen S, Granberg F, Fischer TK, Midgley SE, Rasmussen LD, Angen Ø, Nielsen JP, Jorsal SE, Larsen LE. No evidence of enteric viral involvement in the new neonatal porcine diarrhoea syndrome in Danish pigs. BMC Vet Res. 2017;13(1):315.
17. Anonymous. The National Committee for pig production. Annu Rep. 2004; 2004(6):10–1.
18. Svensmark B. New neonatal Diarrhoea syndrome in Denmark. Proceedings of the 1st ESPHM: 27–28/8–2011; Faculty of Life Sciences. Copenhagen: Denmark; 2009. p. 27.
19. Vu-Khac H, Holoda E, Pilipcinec E, Blanco M, Blanco JE, Dahbi G, Mora A, Lopez C, Gonzalez EA, Blanco J. Serotypes, virulence genes, intimin types and PFGE profiles of Escherichia coli isolated from piglets with diarrhoea in Slovakia. Vet J. 2007;174(1):176–87.
20. Chapman TA, Wu X, Barchia I, Bettelheim KA, Driesen S, Trott D, Wilson M, Chin JJC. Comparison of virulence gene profiles of Escherichia coli strains isolated from healthy and diarrheic swine. Appl Environ Microbiol. 2006;72(7):4782–95.
21. Ngeleka M, Pritchard J, Appleyard G, Middleton DM, Fairbrother JM. Isolation and association of Escherichia coli AIDA-I/STb, rather than EAST1 pathotype, with diarrhea in piglets and antibiotic sensitivity of isolates. J Vet Diagn Investig. 2003;15(3):242–52.
22. Zajacova ZS, Konstantinova L, Alexa P. Detection of virulence factors of Escherichia coli focused on prevalence of EAST1 toxin in stool of diarrheic and non-diarrheic piglets and presence of adhesion involving virulence factors in astA positive strains. Vet Microbiol. 2012;154(3/4):369–75.
23. Byun JW, Jung BY, Kim HY, Fairbrother JM, Lee MH, Lee WK. O-serogroups, virulence genes of pathogenic Escherichia coli and pulsed-field gel electrophoresis (PFGE) patterns of O149 isolates from diarrhoeic piglets in Korea. Vet Med. 2013;58(9):468–76.
24. Liu W, Yuan C, Meng X, Du Y, Gao R, Tang J, Shi D. Frequency of virulence factors in Escherichia coli isolated from suckling pigs with diarrhoea in China. Vet J. 2014;199(2):286–9.
25. Ha SK, Choi C, Jung K, Kim J, Han DU, Ha Y, Lee SD, Kim SH, Chae C. Genotypic prevalence of the adhesin involved in diffuse adherence in Escherichia coli isolates in pre-weaned pigs with diarrhoea in Korea. J Vet Med Series B. 2004;51(4):166–8.
26. Fisher K, Phillips C. The ecology, epidemiology and virulence of enterococcus. Microbio. 2009;155(6):1749–57.
27. Steele J, Feng H, Parry N, Tzipori S. Piglet models of acute or chronic Clostridium difficile illness. J Infect Dis. 2010;201(3):428–34.
28. Arruda PHE, Madson DM, Ramirez A, Rowe E, Lizer JT, Songer JG. Effect of age, dose and antibiotic therapy on the development of Clostridium difficile infection in neonatal piglets. Anaerobe. 2013;22:104–10.
29. McElroy MC, Hill M, Moloney G, MacAogain M, McGettrick S. Typhlocolitis associated with Clostridium difficile ribotypes 078 and 110 in neonatal piglets from a commercial Irish pig herd. Ir Vet J. 2016;69:10.
30. Yaeger MJ, Kinyon JM, Glenn Songer J. A prospective, case control study evaluating the association between Clostridium difficile toxins in the colon of neonatal swine and gross and microscopic lesions. J Vet Diagn Investig. 2007;19(1):52–9.
31. Alvarez-Perez S, Alba P, Blanco JL, Garcia ME. Detection of toxigenic Clostridium difficile in pig feces by PCR. Vet Med. 2009;54(8):360–6.
32. Larsson J, Aspan A, Lindberg R, Grandon R, Baverud V, Fall N, Jacobson M. Pathological and bacteriological characterization of neonatal porcine diarrhoea of uncertain aetiology. J Med Microbiol. 2015;64(8):916–26.
33. Farzan A, Kircanski J, DeLay J, Soltes G, Songer JG, Friendship R, Prescott JF. An investigation into the association between cpb2-encoding Clostridium perfringens type a and diarrhea in neonatal piglets. Can J Vet Res. 2013;77(1):45–53.
34. Bueschel DM, Jost BH, Billington SJ, Trinh HT, Songer JG. Prevalence of cpb2, encoding beta2 toxin, in Clostridium perfringens field isolates: correlation of genotype with phenotype. Vet Microbiol. 2003;94(2):121–9.
35. Allaart JG, AJAM v A, Vernooij JCM, Gröne A. Beta2 toxin is not involved in in vitro cell cytotoxicity caused by human and porcine cpb2-harbouring Clostridium perfringens. Vet Microbiol. 2014;171(1/2):132–8.

21

Initial vaccination and revaccination with Type I PRRS 94881 MLV reduces viral load and infection with porcine reproductive and respiratory syndrome virus

Jeremy Kroll[1]*, Michael Piontkowski[2], Christian Kraft[3], Teresa Coll[3] and Oliver Gomez-Duran[4]

Abstract

Background: Porcine reproductive and respiratory syndrome (PRRS) causes respiratory distress in pigs, reproductive failure in breeding-age gilts and sows, and can have devastating economic consequences in domestic herds. Several PRRS vaccines are available commercially. This study compared the effectiveness of single-vaccination and revaccination schedules using the PRRS 94881 Type I modified live virus (MLV) vaccine ReproCyc® PRRS EU with no vaccination (challenge control) in protecting against a PRRS virus (PRRSV) challenge in non-pregnant gilts.

Results: Data were available from 48 gilts across three groups: a challenge control group ($n = 16$), which received no vaccination; a revaccination group ($n = 16$), which received ReproCyc® PRRS EU on Days 0 and 56; and a single vaccination group ($n = 16$), which received ReproCyc® PRRS EU on Day 56. All gilts were PRRSV RNA-negative (based on reverse transcription and quantitative polymerase chain reaction [RT-qPCR]) and PRRSV seronegative (based on enzyme-linked immunosorbent assay [ELISA]) at Day 0. All gilts were challenged with PRRSV strain 190136 on Day 91. Viral RNA loads in both vaccination groups were significantly reduced compared with the challenge control group on Days 98 ($P < 0.0001$) and 101 ($P < 0.0001$), indicating that vaccinated gilts were better able to respond to challenge than unvaccinated gilts. At all timepoints following challenge, mean viral RNA load and the percentage of PRRSV RNA-positive gilts were numerically higher in the single-vaccination group than in the revaccination group; these differences were statistically significant on Day 101 ($P = 0.0434$). Furthermore, viremia levels after challenge were significantly lower in the revaccination group than in the single-vaccination group based on median area under the curve (AUC) values for viral RNA load from Day 91 to Day 112, suggesting that revaccinated gilts had better protection from viral infection than gilts who received a single vaccination. Protection from viremia did not correlate with the proportion of seropositive gilts on Day 91. In the single-vaccination group, 94% of pigs were seropositive on Day 91 compared with 56% in the revaccination group. Vaccination was well tolerated and no safety concerns were identified.

Conclusions: Both single-vaccination and revaccination with ReproCyc® PRRS EU were effective in reducing PRRSV viremia post-challenge. These findings have important implications for herd management as both the single-vaccination and revaccination schedules protect against PRRSV challenge, with revaccination appearing to provide better protection from viremia than single vaccination.

Keywords: Porcine reproductive respiratory syndrome (PRRS), Viral RNA load, Revaccination, PRRS 94881 MLV

* Correspondence: jeremy.kroll@boehringer-ingelheim.com
[1]Department of Research and Development, Boehringer Ingelheim Animal Health Inc, 2412 South Loop Drive, Ames, IA 50010, USA
Full list of author information is available at the end of the article

Background

Porcine reproductive and respiratory syndrome (PRRS) is a viral disease that causes respiratory distress, reproductive failure and increases mortality in pigs [1–3]. PRRS was initially reported in North America in the late 1980s and in Europe in the 1990s and has since spread rapidly [3, 4]. It is now known to affect swine worldwide [3] and is responsible for devastating economic losses in domestic herds [2, 5].

PRRS is caused by the PRRS virus (PRRSV), a positive strand RNA virus belonging to the *Arteriviridae* family [2, 3]. Historically, PRRSV has been divided into two main genotypes: a Type I European (EU) genotype and a Type II North American (NA) genotype, which are antigenically different [3] and are now considered to be different species [6]. A variant of the NA genotype designated as highly pathogenic PRRSV recently emerged in Asia and has been shown to cause severe disease [3].

PRRSV is transmitted through direct contact with body fluids such as saliva, urine, milk and semen (naturally and through artificial insemination), and through indirect means such as contamination via needles, fomites, farm personnel, vehicles, insect vectors, and airborne mechanisms including aerosolization [3, 4, 7–9]. The virus can therefore spread quickly through a herd, especially if the animals are kept in close proximity, and may also spread to nearby herds [3].

Although infection can be asymptomatic, clinical features occur due to acute viremia in adult or weaned pigs and transmission of the virus across the placenta to developing fetuses. Concomitant infection with other pathogenic microorganisms may also occur. Clinical features typically include systemic effects (such as loss of appetite, weight loss, fever, diarrhea, and lethargy), and effects on the respiratory system (e.g. labored breathing and respiratory distress) and on reproduction (e.g. premature farrowing and abortion, still birth, pre-weaning death, mummified fetuses, and variable size and weak-born piglets) [3, 10]. The severity of disease depends on many factors, including the strain of virus, immune status of the animal, the age of the infected animal and herd husbandry [3, 9]. Effective PRRSV prevention and control strategies such as pig flow, gilt acclimation and herd management are therefore essential, especially as pigs are still contagious for a period following recovery from clinical disease [11–13].

Vaccines against PRRS are available but are usually used to reduce clinical signs and control disease rather than to prevent infection due to the difficulty in protecting from heterologous PRRSV strains [5]. At least 20 different vaccines are commercially available worldwide, comprising modified live viruses (MLVs) and killed PRRS viruses [5, 14]. Of these, MLV vaccines are considered most effective in protecting pigs from circulating PRRSV, provided the MLV is antigenically similar to the circulating strain [14].

PRRS MLV vaccines have been shown to significantly reduce fetal infection, to improve pig health and reproductive performance, and to enhance the body weight and survival rate at weaning of piglets born to vaccinated gilts compared with piglets born to non-vaccinated gilts [5, 15, 16]. In growing pigs, PRRS MLV vaccines can reduce viremia, and improve respiratory signs and growth performance [17, 18].

Despite these positive results, questions over the efficacy and safety of current PRRS MLV vaccines have been raised, including concerns over virus genotype-specific protection, interference with other swine vaccines, and reversion to virulence [5]. In addition, there is disagreement within the swine health field on the most appropriate vaccination schedule; it is unclear whether multiple injections (repeated at 8-weekly intervals) are better than a single injection at limiting clinical signs and providing immunity against subsequent infection. There are continuing efforts to develop new PRRS vaccines that are safe, highly immunogenic, and confer broad protection across PRRSV strains [19, 20].

ReproCyc® PRRS EU is a PRRS MLV which has previously been shown to be safe and efficacious in several clinical trials [21–24]. This study evaluated whether revaccination with ReproCyc® PRRS EU using a two-dose vaccination scheme would result in protection from viremia equivalent to or greater than with a single-dose vaccination.

Results

Data were available from 48 non-pregnant gilts across three groups: a challenge control group ($n = 16$), which received no vaccination; a revaccination group ($n = 16$), which received ReproCyc® PRRS EU on Days 0 and 56; and a single-vaccination group ($n = 16$), which received ReproCyc® PRRS EU on Day 56 only. All gilts were PRRSV RNA-negative (as determined by reverse transcription and quantitative polymerase chain reaction [RT-qPCR]) and PRRSV seronegative (as determined by enzyme-linked immunosorbent assay [ELISA]) at the start of the study.

Viremia and viral RNA load

The percentage of gilts that were positive for PRRSV RNA from day of challenge (Day 91) to Day 112 based on RT-qPCR is shown in Fig. 1. After the challenge on Day 91, all gilts tested positive for PRRSV RNA by Day 94. The percentage of PRRSV RNA-positive gilts then declined sharply in both the revaccination and single-vaccination groups, and by Day 98 both vaccination groups had significantly lower percentages of PRRSV RNA-positive gilts than the challenge control group ($P < 0.0001$). After Day 101

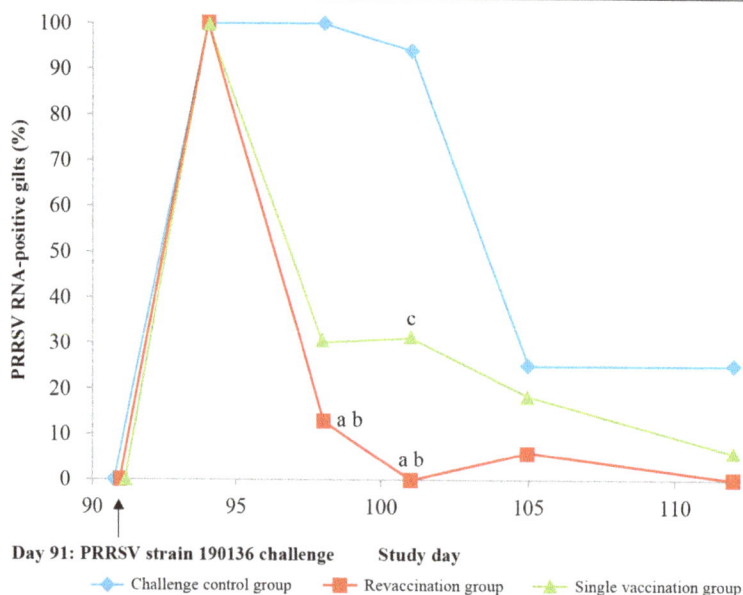

Fig. 1 Percentage of PRRSV RNA-positive gilts after challenge with PRRSV strain 190,136. Viral load was assessed using RT-qPCR. All gilts were challenged with PRRSV strain 190136 on Day 91. Prior to challenge (Day 0–91), 0% of gilts were PRRSV RNA-positive. On Day 94, 100% tested positive for PRRSV RNA. The percentage of PRRSV RNA-positive gilts then declined sharply in both the revaccination and single-vaccination groups. By Day 98 both vaccination groups had significantly lower percentages of PRRSV RNA-positive gilts than the challenge control group ($P < 0.0001$). Challenge control group ($n = 16$); Revaccination group ($n = 16$); Single-vaccination group ($n = 16$). [a]$P < 0.0001$ for challenge control vs revaccination group; [b]$P < 0.001$ for challenge control vs single-vaccination group; [c]$P < 0.05$ for revaccination group vs single-vaccination group

(10 days after challenge), the percentage of PRRSV RNA-positive gilts in the challenge control group fell considerably and there were no significant differences in the percentages of PRRSV RNA-positive gilts between the vaccine groups and the challenge control group by Day 105.

At all timepoints following challenge, the percentage of PRRSV RNA-positive gilts was numerically higher in the single-vaccination group than in the revaccination group, and this difference was statistically significant on Day 101 ($P = 0.0434$).

Serum PRRS viral RNA load based on RT-qPCR was baseline in all groups from study initiation to Day 91, indicating that vaccinated gilts were free of PRRSV up until the point of challenge on Day 91 (Fig. 2). Viral RNA load increased sharply between challenge and Day 94 in all groups. However, the revaccination group had significantly lower median viral RNA loads compared with the challenge control group on Day 94 ($P = 0.0007$). The duration of viremia post-challenge was shorter in the revaccination and single-vaccination groups compared with the challenge control group. On Day 98, all challenge control gilts were still viremic whereas only two revaccinated gilts and five single-vaccinated gilts were PRRSV RNA-positive. The viral RNA loads of both vaccination groups were significantly reduced compared with the challenge control group on Day 98 ($P < 0.0001$ for both) and Day 101 ($P < 0.0001$ for both).

As with the percentage of PRRSV RNA-positive gilts, mean viral RNA load at all timepoints following challenge was numerically higher in the single-vaccination group than in the revaccination group, and this difference was statistically significant on Day 101 ($P = 0.0434$).

The median AUC values for viral RNA load from Day 91 to Day 112 (AUC_{91-112}) are shown in Table 1. Median AUC_{91-112} values were significantly lower for both vaccination groups compared with the challenge control group (both $P < 0.0001$) and the median AUC_{91-112} for the revaccination group was significantly lower than for the single-vaccination group ($P = 0.0029$).

Gilt PRRS serology

PRRS serology results from Day 0 to Day 91 are shown in Table 2. All gilts were PRRSV seronegative at the start of the study, as indicated by ELISA. As expected, all challenge control gilts were PRRSV seronegative up to Day 91 (day of challenge). Gilts in the revaccination group were all seronegative on Day 0 (day of first vaccination), 25% were PRRS seropositive at Day 14, and 69% were seropositive at Day 56 (day of second vaccination), consistent with a serological response to the first vaccination. The proportion of seropositive gilts did not increase further following the second vaccination. In the single-vaccination group, all gilts were PRRSV seronegative up to Day 56 (day of vaccination) and 69% were PRRSV seropositive by Day 70, consistent

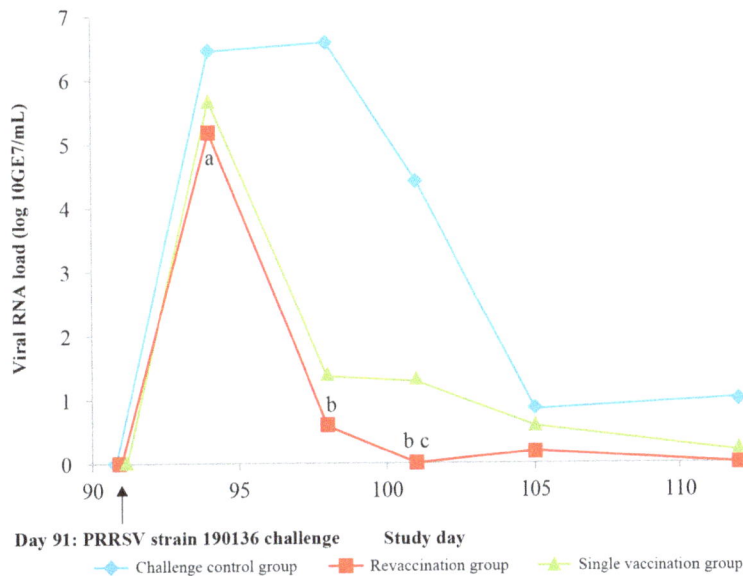

Fig. 2 PRRSV viral RNA load in gilts after challenge with PRRSV strain 190136. Serum PRRS viral RNA load was assessed using RT-qPCR. Viral RNA load was baseline in all groups from Day 0–91. All gilts were challenged with PRRSV strain 190,136 on Day 91. The viral RNA loads of both vaccination groups were significantly reduced compared with the challenge control group on Days 98 ($P < 0.0001$) and Day 101 ($P < 0.0001$). Challenge control group ($n = 16$); Revaccination group ($n = 16$); Single-vaccination group ($n = 16$). [a]$P < 0.001$ for challenge control vs revaccination group; [b]$P < 0.0001$ for challenge control vs revaccination or single-vaccination group; [c]$P < 0.05$ for revaccination group vs single-vaccination group

with a serological response to vaccination. From Day 77, a numerically higher percentage of gilts in the single-vaccination group (94%) were seropositive compared with the revaccination group (69%), and this difference was statistically significant at Day 91 (94% vs 56%, respectively; $P = 0.0373$).

Clinical signs

Three of the 16 gilts (19%) in both the challenge control and revaccination groups, and two of 16 gilts (13%) in the single-vaccination group, exhibited abnormal clinical signs such as skin lesions, lameness, and thinness. In three challenge control gilts, these abnormal clinical observations were exhibited before challenge on Day 91, and one of the single-vaccination gilts also exhibited clinical signs before

Table 1 AUC median values from Day 91 to Day 112 in gilt groups, after challenge with PRRSV strain 190136

Group	Median AUC from Day 91–112 (min, max)	P-value (vs challenge control)	P-value (vs revaccination)
Challenge control	65.4 (61.0, 79.2)	N/A	< 0.0001
Revaccination	20.2 (19.2, 22.9)	< 0.0001	N/A
Single vaccination	34.9 (24.5, 41.4)	< 0.0001	0.0029

Challenge control group ($n = 16$); Revaccination group ($n = 16$); Single vaccination group ($n = 16$)
Viral RNA load and AUC were assessed using RT-qPCR
AUC area under the curve, *N/A* not applicable, *PRRSV* Porcine reproductive and respiratory syndrome virus, *RT-qPCR* reverse transcription quantitative polymerase chain reaction

receiving a vaccination on Day 56, all clinical signs were recorded before challenge. These clinical signs were determined by the study investigator as not interfering with animal welfare and to be unrelated to PRRS or study medication.

Discussion

The study aimed to determine if a revaccination schedule with ReproCyc® PRRS EU has a vaccine efficacy at least equivalent (quantitatively and qualitatively) to that seen with a single-vaccination scheme. All gilts entering the study were free from PRRSV as demonstrated by the absence of PRRSV RNA in their serum followed by PRRS seronegative ELISA test results on Day 0. In addition, RT-qPCR and serology results indicated all gilts were free from PRRSV from Day 0 to Day 91.. These data confirm that no extraneous PRRSV exposure or cross-contamination among treatment and control groups occurred up to the point of challenge on Day 91, validating subsequent findings of this study. Viremia in adult animals is usually short-lasting; therefore, the lack of observed vaccine-induced viremia prior to challenge may be due to resolution of viremia before the initial blood samples were taken 14 days post-vaccination.

The study found that both single vaccination and revaccination with ReproCyc® PRRS EU significantly reduced PRRSV viremia post-challenge compared with non-vaccinated challenged controls. However, the revaccination group had a significantly lower viral RNA load and

Table 2 Percentage of gilts who were seropositive for PRRSV based on ELISA

Day	Group	% seropositive (95% CI)	P-value (vs challenge control)	P-value (vs revaccination)
0	Challenge control	0	–	–
	Revaccination	0	–	–
	Single vaccination	0	–	–
14	Challenge control	0 (0.0, 20.6)	N/A	
	Revaccination	25 (7.3, 52.4)	0.101	N/A
	Single vaccination	0 (0.0, 20.6)	ND	0.101
21	Challenge control	0 (0.0, 20.6)	N/A	
	Revaccination	56 (29.9, 80.2)	0.0008	N/A
	Single vaccination	0 (0.0, 20.6)	ND	0.0008
56	Challenge control	0 (0.0, 20.6)	N/A	
	Revaccination	69 (41.3, 89.0)	0.0001	N/A
	Single vaccination	0 (0.0, 20.6)	ND	0.0001
70	Challenge control	0 (0.0, 20.6)	N/A	
	Revaccination	69 (41.3, 89.0)	0.0001	N/A
	Single vaccination	69 (41.3, 89.0)	0.0001	1.0000
77	Challenge control	0 (0.0, 20.6)	N/A	
	Revaccination	69 (41.3, 89.0)	0.0001	N/A
	Single vaccination	94 (69.8, 99.8)	< 0.0001	0.172
91	Challenge control	0 (0.0, 20.6)	N/A	
	Revaccination	56 (29.9, 80.2)	0.0008	N/A
	Single vaccination	94 (69.8, 99.8)	< 0.0001	0.0373

Challenge control group ($n = 16$); Revaccination group ($n = 16$); Single-vaccination group ($n = 16$)
PRRS serology was assessed using ELISA
CI confidence interval, ELISA enzyme-linked immunosorbent assay, N/A not applicable, ND not determined, PRRSV Porcine reproductive and respiratory syndrome virus

fewer PRRSV RNA-positive gilts on Day 101 compared with the single vaccination group. Furthermore, at all time-points following challenge, both the mean viral RNA loads and the percentage of PRRSV RNA-positive gilts were numerically higher in the single-vaccination group than in the revaccination group. In addition, the revaccination group had a significantly lower viremia AUC_{91-112} compared with the single-vaccination group.

These findings suggest that previous vaccination with ReproCyc® PRRS EU increases the effectiveness of subsequent vaccination with the same product, and revaccination may be slightly more effective against PRRSV post-challenge than a single-vaccination schedule. Although there was no correlation between the PRRS seroconversion and viremia reductions across the vaccination schemes, the consistently greater reduction in viremia observed with revaccination compared with single vaccination suggests an element of protective immunity provided by the revaccination schedule, possibly linked to the presence of memory T cells.

Seroconversion of gilts was not complete in either the single-vaccination or revaccination group. Furthermore, the seroconversion rate was particularly low in the

revaccination group (56% seropositive on Day 91) and did not increase following the second vaccination, despite the greater reduction in viremia observed with revaccination compared with single vaccination. The authors do not have an explanation for this unexpected finding, which differs from other studies that have shown consistent seroconversion following vaccination [25, 26]. These observations suggest that seroconversion is not an indicative measure of protection in adult animals. Some animals did not test positive by either RT-qPCR or ELISA and showed the same level of protection upon challenge compared with animals that had seroconverted. Incomplete seroconversion alongside full protection from PRRS has already been observed in other studies [27] and most likely reflects variability in immune responses between animals.

Previous studies demonstrated that a single-dose of ReproCyc® PRRS EU was successful in protecting piglets [22, 24], bred gilts [21], and farrowing gilts [23] from PRRS. Vaccinating gilts helps prevent viral shedding and reduces both horizontal (sow to sow) and vertical PRRSV transmission (sow to piglet). This study suggests that a single shot of vaccination is sufficient to protect gilts based on reduced viremia, and thereby likely to reduce the risk of transmission as well. It also showed that revaccinating non-pregnant gilts reduced challenge-induced viremia compared with single vaccination; this effect could reduce shedding, thus decreasing airborne levels of PRRSV, preventing infection of pregnant gilts and consequently reducing transmission of PRRSV to unborn piglets. Given the duration of immunity defined in other studies [28], we estimate that a revaccination schedule of every 3 to 4 months would be sufficient to avoid gaps in protection from PRRS.

Due to the wide heterology of PRRSV field strains [29] the level of protection provided by a single vaccine strain may differ from farm to farm. Although genetic distance in the ORF5 gene locus is not a stoichiometric indicator of the likelihood of protection, the protection demonstrated in this study with the chosen genetic distance of less than 87% homology between the vaccine and challenge should provide a good level of assurance that the vaccine could protect against heterologous PRRSV strains. As in previous cases, this should also be verified in field studies [27].

While this study was designed to look at the clinical outcomes of revaccination related to PRRS rather than on immunological responses to recurring vaccination, there was no evidence of detrimental immunologic effects (such as immune reactions to the vaccine composition) with the revaccination schedule. ReproCyc® PRRS EU was well tolerated; two or three gilts per group showed clinical signs that are typically associated with gilts housed in groups, with some developing before treatment with study medication or in the control group. These signs were unlikely to be attributable to vaccination and more associated with gilts establishing a hierarchy that involved biting, scratching, and exclusion of pen mates from the feeder (hence leading to some thinner gilts compared with pen mates). Together with the efficacy data, this supports the feasibility of recurring vaccination of sows and mass vaccination in a whole herd approach.

Further studies that include a greater number of animals are needed to confirm the benefit of revaccination against PRRSV.

Conclusion

This study shows that gilts vaccinated with ReproCyc® PRRS EU, either using a revaccination or single-vaccination schedule, demonstrate significant protection from viremia after challenge with PRRSV Strain 190,136 compared with unvaccinated challenge control gilts. Furthermore, viremia levels after challenge were significantly lower in the revaccination group than in the single-vaccination group based on median viral RNA load AUC_{91-112}, suggesting that revaccinated gilts had better protection from viral infection than gilts who received a single vaccination. ReproCyc®

PRRS EU was also well tolerated and no safety concerns were identified.

Methods
Animals
Animals (48 commercial crossbred gilts) were provided by the Wilson Prairie View Farms, N5627 Highway DD, Burlington, WI 53105, USA, and each female was individually ear-tagged with a unique number. All gilts were healthy (as determined by observation), PRRS seronegative (as determined by ELISA), and were not pregnant on Day 0.

Gilts were housed in separate, but uniform rooms from Day – 10 to study completion. Each room consisted of four pens, with four gilts per pen and was biohazard level 2 compliant, hepafiltered, mechanically ventilated with thermostatically regulated temperature control. Treatment group isolation was necessary to avoid cross-contamination between groups.

Gilts were fed a commercially prepared, non-medicated gestation ration of solid feed (Heart of Iowa Cooperative, Roland, IA, USA), which was stored in bags, free from vermin, and given in quantities appropriate for each gilt's size, age, and condition. Water was available ad libitum.

PRRSV immunization and challenge inoculum
The control product (lyophilized placebo, Boehringer Ingelheim Animal Health, Inc., St Joseph, USA; lot N240-191-062409) and the investigational veterinary product (IVP; ReproCyc® PRRS EU, Boehringer Ingelheim Animal Health, Inc., USA; lot 390-007A), which was at a concentration of 1×10^4 50% tissue infectious dose ($TCID_{50}$)/2 mL, were administered by intramuscular (IM) injection, using sterile, appropriately sized Luerlock syringes and sterile 20 g × 1 in. (2.54 cm) needles. Animals were injected in the neck, midway between the point of the shoulder and the base of the ear.

All gilts were challenged with PRRSV strain 190,136 (Boehringer Ingelheim Vetmedica, Inc., USA), which was derived from lung tissue of a newborn piglet during an outbreak in Germany in April 2004 and exhibits less than 87% genetic identity to ReproCyc® PRRS EU within the complete genome (or 88% based on ORF5/ORF7 data). Challenge was intranasally (2.0 mL per nostril) and intramuscularly (2.0 mL injection to the back of the neck) using a target titer of $1 \times 10^{5.9}$ $TCID_{50}$/6 mL.

Experimental design
This was a blinded revaccination-challenge laboratory efficacy study consisting of three groups: challenge control group ($n = 16$), revaccination group ($n = 16$) and single-vaccination group ($n = 16$). In the challenge control group, a 2.0 mL injection of the control product was given on Day 0 (right neck) and Day 56 (left neck). In the revaccination group, the IVP was given on Day 0 (right neck)

and Day 56 (left neck). In the single-vaccination group, a 2.0 mL injection of the control product was given on Day 0 (right neck) and a 2.0 mL of the IVP on Day 56 (left neck). All gilts were challenged on Day 91. The Study Investigator and designees were blinded to group assignments and laboratory personnel were blinded to the treatment each gilt received. In addition, a person not collecting data administered the injections of study products. In this study, 8 weeks between vaccinations was utilized as this allowed for adequate time for immunity to be developed after the first vaccination before revaccination occurred.

Sample analysis and assessment of viremia and serology
Blood samples were collected prior to animal enrolment and on Days 0, 14, 21, 56, 70, 77, 91, 94, 98, 101, 105, and 112. After drawing, blood samples were allowed to clot at room temperature, were centrifuged and the serum was harvested. Serum samples were held at -20 °C for serology testing and -70 °C ($\pm$ 10 °C) for RT-qPCR testing.

PRRS serology
For ELISA, the IDDEX PRRS X3 test was used following the manufacturer's instructions (HerdChek* Porcine Reproductive and Respiratory Syndrome Antibody Test Kit X3 – IDEXX Laboratories Inc., Westbrook, ME, USA). Results were reported as negative (ELISA sample to positive [S/P] ratio of < 0.4) or positive (ELISA S/P ratio of ≥0.4).

PRRS serum RT-qPCR
TaqMan RT-qPCR targeting the viral open reading frame (ORF) 7 was used to detect viral RNA. Results were reported as $\log_{10}$ genome equivalent (GE)/mL. A RT-qPCR result of ND (not detected) was assigned a value of 0 $\log_{10}$ GE/mL and a positive but unquantifiable RT-qPCR result was assigned a $\log_{10}$ value of 3.0 GE/mL (for statistical purposes only).

Assessment of clinical signs
Gilts were observed once daily from Day − 1 to Day 112 for abnormal health by the Study Investigator or designees. An adverse event was defined as any observation that was unfavorable or unintended that occurred after the use of the IVP, irrespective of causality.

Statistical analysis
Gilts were randomly assigned to one of the groups prior to Day − 1. Each group included 16 animals, which was expected to provide approximately 80% power to detect a difference of 20 percentage points for median viral load between the treatment and control group for a two-sided test using an alpha value of 0.05 post-challenge.

Data were summarized using descriptive statistics with a 95% confidence interval. All tests on differences were designed as two-sided tests using an alpha

value of 5%. Statistical analyses were performed using SAS software release 8.2 (SAS Institute Inc., 2001, Cary, North Carolina, USA).

Acknowledgements
The authors would like to thank the following for their help with this study: Dr. Ryan Saltzman and Dr. Lyle Kesl, Veterinary Resources, Inc. for their assistance with the animal phase of this study. We would also like to thank Holly Ashford BSc (Biochemistry) from InterComm International, Cambridge UK, who provided medical writing services on behalf of Boehringer Ingelheim Animal Health, Inc.

Funding
The study was funded by Boehringer Ingelheim Animal Health, Inc. Medical writing services were provided by InterComm International, Cambridge, UK, and this service was funded by Boehringer Ingelheim Animal Health, Inc.

Authors' contributions
All authors of this manuscript are full time or former employees of Boehringer Ingelheim Animal Health. Boehringer Ingelheim Animal Health is the sole proprietor of the study and the information that was generated for patent support and publications. JK, MP and CK designed and participated in the study, TC and OD critically reviewed the data and the manuscript. All authors helped draft this manuscript and have read and approved the final manuscript for submission.

Competing interests
Boehringer Ingelheim Animal Health, Inc. sponsored the clinical trial reported in this publication both financially and through professional veterinary and research support.

Author details
[1]Department of Research and Development, Boehringer Ingelheim Animal Health Inc, 2412 South Loop Drive, Ames, IA 50010, USA. [2]Boehringer Ingelheim Animal Health, 2621 N. Belt Hwy, St Joseph, MO 64506, USA. [3]Boehringer Ingelheim Veterinary Research Center GmbH & Co. KG, Bemeroder Straße 31, 30559 Hannover, Germany. [4]Boehringer Ingelheim Vetmedica GmbH, Binger Straße 173, 55216 Ingelheim am Rhein, Germany.

References
1. Chung WB, Lin MW, Chang WF, Hsu M, Yang PC. Persistence of porcine reproductive and respiratory syndrome virus in intensive farrow-to-finish pig herds. Can J Vet Res. 1997;61:292–8.
2. Done SH, Paton DJ, White ME. Porcine reproductive and respiratory syndrome (PRRS): a review, with emphasis on pathological, virological and diagnostic aspects. Br Vet J. 1996;152:153–74.

3. World Organisation for Animal Health (OiE): Report of the OIE ad hoc group on porcine reproductive respiratory syndrome. 2008, Appendices IV and V.

4. Wills RW, Zimmerman JJ, Yoon KJ, Swenson SL, McGinley MJ, Hill HT, Platt KB, Christopher-Hennings J, Nelson EA. Porcine reproductive and respiratory syndrome virus: a persistent infection. Vet Microbiol. 1997;55:231–40.

5. Charerntantanakul W. Porcine reproductive and respiratory syndrome virus vaccines: immunogenicity, efficacy and safety aspects. World J Virol. 2012;1:23–30.

6. Kuhn JH, Lauck M, Bailey AL, Shchetinin AM, Vishnevskaya TV, Bao Y, Ng TF, LeBreton M, Schneider BS, Gillis A, et al. Reorganization and expansion of the nidoviral family Arteriviridae. Arch Virol. 2016;161:755–68.

7. Yaeger M, Prieve T, Collins J, Christopher-Hennings J, Nelson E, Benfeld D. Evidence for the transmission of porcine reproductive and respiratory syndrome (PRRS) virus in boar semen. Swine Health Prod. 1993;1:7–9.

8. Yoon IJ, Joo HS, Christianson WT, Morrison RB, Dial GD. Persistent and contact infection in nursery pigs experimentally infected with porcine reproductive and respiratory syndrome (PRRS) virus. Swine Health Prod. 1993;1(4):5-8.

9. Rossow KD, Bautista EM, Goyal SM, Molitor TW, Murtaugh MP, Morrison RB, Benfield DA, Collins JE. Experimental porcine reproductive and respiratory syndrome virus infection in one-, four-, and 10-week-old pigs. J Vet Diagn Investig. 1994;6:3–12.

10. Collins JE, Benfield DA, Christianson WT, Harris L, Hennings JC, Shaw DP, Goyal SM, McCullough S, Morrison RB, Joo HS, et al. Isolation of swine infertility and respiratory syndrome virus (isolate ATCC VR-2332) in North America and experimental reproduction of the disease in gnotobiotic pigs. J Vet Diagn Investig. 1992;4:117–26.

11. Corzo CA, Mondaca E, Wayne S, Torremorell M, Dee S, Davies P, Morrison RB. Control and elimination of porcine reproductive and respiratory syndrome virus. Virus Res. 2010;154:185–92.

12. Charpin C, Mahe S, Keranflec'h A, Belloc C, Cariolet R, Le Potier MF, Rose N. Infectiousness of pigs infected by the porcine reproductive and respiratory syndrome virus (PRRSV) is time-dependent. Vet Res. 2012;43:69.

13. Nodelijk G, de Jong MC, Van Nes A, Vernooy JC, Van Leengoed LA, Pol JM, Verheijden JH. Introduction, persistence and fade-out of porcine reproductive and respiratory syndrome virus in a Dutch breeding herd: a mathematical analysis. Epidemiol Infect. 2000;124:173–82.

14. Rowland RR, Lunney J, Dekkers J. Control of porcine reproductive and respiratory syndrome (PRRS) through genetic improvements in disease resistance and tolerance. Front Genet. 2012;3:260.

15. Scortti M, Prieto C, Simarro I, Castro JM. Reproductive performance of gilts following vaccination and subsequent heterologous challenge with European strains of porcine reproductive and respiratory syndrome virus. Theriogenology. 2006;66:1884–93.

16. Rowland RR. The interaction between PRRSV and the late gestation pig fetus. Virus Res. 2010;154:114–22.

17. Cano JP, Dee SA, Murtaugh MP, Pijoan C. Impact of a modified-live porcine reproductive and respiratory syndrome virus vaccine intervention on a population of pigs infected with a heterologous isolate. Vaccine. 2007;25: 4382–91.

18. Cano JP, Dee SA, Murtaugh MP, Trincado CA, Pijoan CB. Effect of vaccination with a modified-live porcine reproductive and respiratory syndrome virus vaccine on dynamics of homologous viral infection in pigs. Am J Vet Res. 2007;68:565–71.

19. Kimman TG, Cornelissen LA, Moormann RJ, Rebel JM, Stockhofe-Zurwieden N. Challenges for porcine reproductive and respiratory syndrome virus (PRRSV) vaccinology. Vaccine. 2009;27:3704–18.

20. Huang YW, Meng XJ. Novel strategies and approaches to develop the next generation of vaccines against porcine reproductive and respiratory syndrome virus (PRRSV). Virus Res. 2010;154:141–9.

21. Piontkowski MD, Kroll J, Orveillon FX, Kraft C, Coll T. Safety and efficacy of a novel European vaccine for porcine reproductive and respiratory virus in bred gilts. Can J Vet Res. 2016;80:269–80.

22. Piontkowski M, Kroll J, Kraft C, Coll T. Safety and early onset of immunity with a novel European porcine reproductive and respiratory syndrome virus vaccine in young piglets. Can J Vet Res. 2016;80:124–33.

23. Stadler J, Zoels S, Eddicks M, Kraft C, Ritzmann M, Ladinig A. Assessment of safety and reproductive performance after vaccination with a modified live-virus PRRS genotype 1 vaccine in pregnant sows at various stages of gestation. Vaccine. 2016;34:3862–6.

24. Cano G, Cavalcanti MO, Orveillon FX, Kroll J, Gomez-Duran O, Morillo A, Kraft C. Production results from piglets vaccinated in a field study in Spain with a type 1 porcine respiratory and reproductive virus modified live vaccine. Porcine Health Manag. 2016;2:22.

25. Zuckermann FA, Garcia EA, Luque ID, Christopher-Hennings J, Doster A, Brito M, Osorio F. Assessment of the efficacy of commercial porcine reproductive and respiratory syndrome virus (PRRSV) vaccines based on measurement of serologic response, frequency of gamma-IFN-producing cells and virological parameters of protection upon challenge. Vet Microbiol. 2007;123:69–85.

26. Klinge KL, Vaughn EM, Roof MB, Bautista EM, Murtaugh MP. Age-dependent resistance to porcine reproductive and respiratory syndrome virus replication in swine. Virol J. 2009;6:177.

27. Balka G, Dreckmann K, Papp G, Kraft C. Vaccination of piglets at 2 and 3 weeks of age with Ingelvac PRRSFLEX(R) EU provides protection against heterologous field challenge in the face of homologous maternally derived antibodies. Porcine Health Manag. 2016;2:24.

28. Summary of product characteristics: ReproCyc PRRS EU lyophilisate and solvent for suspension for injection for pigs. In: Health products regulatory authority; 2015. https://imedi.co.uk/reprocyc-prrs-eu-lyophilisate-and-solvent-for-suspension-for-injection-for-pigs.

29. Stadejek T, Stankevicius A, Murtaugh MP, Oleksiewicz MB. Molecular evolution of PRRSV in Europe: current state of play. Vet Microbiol. 2013;165:21–8.

22

Passive surveillance of *Leptospira* infection in swine

Katrin Strutzberg-Minder[1]* (ID), Astrid Tschentscher[1], Martin Beyerbach[2], Matthias Homuth[1] and Lothar Kreienbrock[2]

Abstract

Background: As no current data are available on the prevalence of leptospiral infection in swine in Germany, we analysed laboratory data from diagnostic examinations carried out on samples from swine all over Germany from January 2011 to September 2016. A total of 29,829 swine sera were tested by microscopic agglutination test (MAT) for antibodies against strains of eleven Leptospira serovars.

Results: Overall, 20.2% (6025) of the total sample collection tested positive for leptospiral infection. Seropositivity ranged between 16.3% (964) in 2011 and 30.9% (941) in 2016 (January to September only). Of all samples, 11.6% (57.3% of the positives) reacted with only one Leptospira serovar, and only 8.6% (42.7% of the positives) reacted simultaneously with two or more serovars. The most frequently detected serovar was Bratislava, which was found in 11.6% (3448) of all samples, followed by the serovars Australis in 7.3% (2185), Icterohaemorrhagiae in 4.0% (1191), Copenhageni in 4.0% (1182), Autumnalis in 3.7% (1054), Canicola in 2.0% (585), and Pomona in 1.2% (368). Modelling shows that both the year and the reason for testing at the laboratory had statistically strong effects on the test results; however, no interactions were determined between those factors. The results support the suggestion that the seropositivities found may be considered to indicate the state of leptospiral infections in the German swine population.

Conclusion: Although data from passive surveillance are prone to selection bias, stratified analysis by initial reason for examination and analyses by model approaches may correct for biases. A prevalence of about 20% for a leptospiral infection is most probable for sows with reproductive problems in Germany, with an increasing trend. Swine in Germany are probably a reservoir host for serovar Bratislava, but in contrast to other studies not for Pomona and Tarassovi.

Keywords: Pig, *Leptospira*, Bratislava, Australis, Icterohaemorrhagiae, Copenhageni, Monitoring, MAT, Seropositivity, Temporal trends

Background

Leptospirosis is presumed to be the most widespread zoonosis worldwide [1]. It is a cause of reproductive loss in swine breeding herds and has been reported in swine from all parts of the world [2]. Endemic infections in swine herds generally remain subclinical, as do the vast majority of leptospire infections. However, when a susceptible breeding herd is infected for the first time or its immunity is compromised, considerable losses can occur due to abortion, stillbirths, weakly piglets, or infertility. Leptospires persist in the kidneys and genital tract of carrier swine and are excreted in urine and genital fluids [2].

Swine act as maintenance hosts for the serovars belonging to the Pomona and Australis serogroups [3–6], while Icterohaemorrhagiae, Grippotyphosa, and Tarassovi serogroups are among the more commonly identified incidental infections in swine [2]. Serovar Bratislava is endemic in swine in some regions [7–9]. Serological testing is the laboratory procedure most frequently used to confirm the clinical diagnosis, to determine herd prevalence, and to conduct epidemiological studies. The standard serological test is the microscopic agglutination test (MAT). The minimum antigen requirements are that the test should comprise representative strains of all the serogroups known to exist in the particular region as well as

* Correspondence: strutzberg@ivd-gmbh.de
[1]IVD Innovative Veterinary Diagnostics (IVD GmbH), Albert-Einstein-Str. 5, 30926 Seelze, Germany
Full list of author information is available at the end of the article

those known to be maintained elsewhere by the host species. A titre of 100 is taken as positive for the purpose of international trade [10], but given the high specificity of the MAT, lower titres can be taken as evidence of previous exposure to Leptospira. The MAT is used to test individual animals and herds. As an individual animal test, the MAT is very useful (due to its high sensitivity) for diagnosing acute infection: a four-fold rise in antibody titres in paired acute and convalescent serum samples is diagnostic. To obtain useful information from a herd of animals, at least ten animals, or 10% of the herd, whichever is greater, should be tested for a sufficient sensitivity, and vaccination history should be considered, if vaccines are available [2, 10]. In Germany no vaccine was registered as of 31 August 2016 [11] and there still is no vaccine for swine available in Germany. However, the use of imported vaccines is allowed with special permission. The MAT has limitations in the diagnosis of chronic infection in individual animals and in the diagnosis of endemic infections in the herds. Infected animals may abort or be renal/genital carriers with MAT titres below the widely accepted minimum significant titre of 100 at final dilution [2, 10]. Because of all these factors, it is not permissible to express the specificity and sensitivity of the MAT as percentages.

There are only a few recent studies on domestic swine; these report seroprevalences of 55.9% in pigs in Colombia [12], 16.1% in pigs in technified swine farms in the state of Alagoas, Brazil [13], 8.6% in pigs in Korea [14], and 2.7% in swine in Poland for selected serovars [15]. Furthermore, there are two older studies [16] that report prevalences ranging from 1.2% for pigs in Germany [17] to 73.3% in sows in Vietnam (Mekong Delta) [9].

Although leptospirosis is no longer an OIE-listed disease, leptospirosis in swine and sheep is still classified as a notifiable disease and a zoonosis in Germany, but there are no current German data available on this infection in swine. The latest current data in Germany were collected in 1984 and reported in 1987 [17]. Data from a passive surveillance of swine in Germany for infection with leptospires (2003 to 2010) were presented at the EuroLepto 2012 [18].

For this paper we have analysed routine laboratory data from January 2011 to September 2016 for the seropositivity of a total sample collection and subcollections based on the reason for the examination with the aim to estimate the extent of infection of swine in Germany with leptospires and to identify the occurring serovars or serogroups.

Methods
Sample collection
Diagnostic examinations were carried out at the diagnostic laboratory of IVD GmbH, Seelze, Germany, on 29,829 serum samples collected from swine from all over Germany between January 2011 and September 2016. All available information about the serum samples, e.g. farm of origin, age/gender of the animal source, was collected with a lab information system (Ticono-LC, Ticono GmbH, Hannover, Germany) and taken into consideration if sufficient information was available. The frequency of samples sent for examination according the geographic origin in Germany was parallel to the density of swine husbandry in Germany (data from further analyses, not published). Samples came from 2571 animal owners for the total study period. We furthermore analysed the samples per herd and per year. Since some farms sent samples for examination in more than one year, the sum of farms sending samples per year is 3953. It is very likely that most of the samples were from animals kept indoors in stables, because less than 1% of swine in Germany are housed outdoors, but this was not explicitly reported. And since more than 99% of swine were housed indoors and no climatic data within the stables were available, seasonal aspects could not be analysed here seriously.

As there was very little or no further information about the sows (such as parity), this was therefore not taken into account for the analyses.

Preliminary information about the samples, such as clinical symptoms or reason for examination, had been systematically requested with the submission form of the laboratory (IVD GmbH, Seelze, Germany) and collected with the Ticono-LC lab information system, but not all senders filled the form out completely. Available information about the samples about the reason for examination was used to identify two subcollections which were analysed in comparison with the total sample collection.

The subcollection "reproductive problems" comprised all samples (n = 12,017) of the total population for which any reproductive problem had been reported (checkbox "Reproductive symptoms and/or any comment about reproductive problems" in the form). The subcollection "Monitoring" comprised all samples (n = 1813) of the total sample collection for which the checkbox "Examination for monitoring reasons (no clinical symptoms, health check)" was marked and no reproductive problem had been reported.

Laboratory methods
All samples were tested for leptospiral antibodies by the microscopic agglutination test (MAT) according to the OIE Manual of Diagnostic Tests and Vaccines for Terrestrial Animals 2008 [19] to current editions 2014 [10] using live antigens of Leptospira serovars Australis (strain Ballico), Bratislava (strain Jez Bratislava), Canicola (strain Hond Utrecht IV), Grippotyphosa (strain Moskva V), Copenhageni (strain M20), Icterohaemorrhagiae

(strain RGA), Pomona (strain Pomona), Hardjo (strain Hardjoprajitno), Saxkoebing (strain Mus 24), and Tarassovi (strain Perepelitsin). In response to an analysis of the frequencies of seropositivity of Leptospira serovars worldwide [16], the serovar Saxkoebing was replaced with Sejroe (strain M 84) in February 2011, and the serovar Autumnalis (strain Akiyami A) was added in April 2011. All strains were supplied by the Leptospirosis Reference Laboratory (at KIT Biomedical Research, The Netherlands). Sera were pretested at the final dilution of 1/100. Sera with 50% agglutination were retested to determine an endpoint using dilutions of sera beginning at 1/25 through 1/3200. Serum samples with the widely accepted minimum significant titre of 100 (reciprocal of the final dilution of serum with 50% agglutination) were assessed positive. A farm was considered positive for leptospiral infection if at least one sample per year tested positive by MAT.

Statistical methods

Data were analysed in two steps. For a general overview, all data were first analysed independently; the positive findings then were analysed both generally (Table 2) and by serovar (Tables 3 and 4). The results are reported as usual frequency statistics.

Next, in order to take into account the hierarchical data structure (repeated samples per farm), all data were analysed in a hierarchical, logistic regression model with two fixed regressors ("year" and "reason for sampling and testing") and a random factor ("farm") (Table 5). From this the strength of association between seropositivity and these factors was estimated via odds ratios (OR) and the asymptotic 95% confidence intervals (CI) of Woolf and the associated likelihood ratio test (Table 6). All analyses were performed using SAS, version 9.3 TS level 1 M2 (SAS Institute Inc., Cary, NC, United States).

Results

General description of the sample population

In general, 29,829 samples from routine laboratory diagnostics were examined from January 2011 to September 2016. Data are from 2571 different farms with some repeated analyses from year to year. These multiple submissions yielded a sum of 3953 farms. Most of the farms (53.8%) sent four to nine samples per year, followed by 19.0% of farms with only one to three samples per year, and 18.8% of farms sending ten to 14 samples per year. The reason for laboratory analysis for each sample is indicated in Table 1. Of the samples for which a reason was given for the examination ($n = 13,830$), 86.9% were sent with the information "reproductive problems"; only 13.1% of the samples were designated as having been taken for "Examination for monitoring reasons (no clinical symptoms, health check)" without any reported reproductive problem.

Overall, there was no information at all about the animal source for 42.2% of all samples ($n = 12,600$), but there was information for 57.8% ($n = 17,229$) of the total sample collection. Of the samples with information about the animal source, 95.9% ($n = 16,529$) were from sows (sows and gilts). (Data not shown).

Only 1813 samples from the entire sample population, i.e. 6.1%, were identified as having been taken due to monitoring. Overall, the sample population is therefore dominated by samples from sows with reproductive problems. Most of the samples are from farms in Northwest Germany, which is the center of German swine production. All in all, the serological findings do not correspond to a regular prevalence, because the sample collection was not a cross-sectional study from the entire German swine production. Nevertheless, the data do give insight into the *Leptospira* occurrence in German pig farms, because the study included a substantial collection of German pig breeding farms. According to figures from the Federal Statistical Office [20], this represents a mean of 5.9% of the officially registered German breeding farms per year.

General seropositivity

A general overview of the results of the serological testing is reported in Table 2. Overall, 20.2% (n = 6025) of

Table 1 Collection of swine serum samples tested for leptospires by MAT

	Reasons for testing of individual samples			Total	Number of farms
	Monitoring	Reproductive problems	Unknown reasons		
2011	392	2514	3002	5908	856
2012	400	2422	2650	5472	797
2013	338	2249	2981	5568	718
2014	298	2087	2721	5106	659
2015	300	1582	2851	4733	529
2016 / 01 to 09	85	1163	1794	3042	394
Total	1813	12,017	15,999	29,829	3953[1]

[1]Because some farms sent samples in more than one year, this number of farms is higher than that of the different farms tested in the total study period

Table 2 Results of swine serum samples tested for leptospires by MAT. Number (n) of samples examined, numbers (n) and percentage (%) of positive samples and farms with at least one positive sample per farm and year from January 2011 to September 2016, and totals

Year	Number of serum samples	Positives[a]		Number of farms	Positives[b]	
		n	%		n	%
2011	5908	964	16.3	856	508	59.3
2012	5472	1042	19.0	797	509	63.9
2013	5568	1076	19.3	718	434	60.4
2014	5106	993	19.5	659	416	63.1
2015	4733	1009	21.3	529	375	70.9
2016 / 01 to 09	3042	941	30.9	394	308	78.2
Total	29,829	6025	20.2	3953	2550	64.5

[a]Samples with a titre ≥100
[b]farms with at least one positive sample per year

all 29,829 swine serum samples tested positive by MAT. The seropositivity ranged between 16.3% (n = 964) in 2011 and 30.9% (n = 941) in 2016 (January to September). A total of 64.5% farms tested positive for leptospires by at least one sample per year. The percentage of farms with positive test results ranged between 59.3% (n = 508) in 2011 and 78.2% (n = 308) in 2016. Forecasting 4056 samples for all of 2016, the mean number of samples was 5141 per year, with moderate variation in seropositivity from year to year (Table 2).

Analysis of the reactivity of the serum samples with different serovars (Table 3) showed that 11.6% of all samples examined, comprising 57.3% of the positives, reacted with only one serovar, whereas 42.7% reacted simultaneously with two or more serovars.

Table 3 Simultaneous reactivity of swine serum samples by MAT with various *Leptospira* serovars. (Data from January 2011 to September 2016)

Reactivity with different serovars (number of serovars)	Number of serum samples	Percentage of all samples
0	23,804	79.8
1	3454	11.6
2	1617	5.4
3	524	1.8
4	201	0.7
5	95	0.3
6	69	0.2
7	41	0.1
8	16	0.1
9	7	0.0
10	1	0.0
Total	29,829	100.0

General occurrence of serovars and variations from year to year

The most frequently detected serovar was Bratislava (Table 4), which was found in 11.6% (n = 3448) of all samples, followed by the serovars Australis in 7.3% (n = 2185), Icterohaemorrhagiae in 4.0% (n = 1191), Copenhageni in 4.0% (n = 1182), Autumnalis in 3.7% (n = 1054), Canicola in 2.0% (n = 585), and Pomona in 1.2% (n = 368). All other serovars were detected less often (in < 1.0% of all samples). Total reactivity is more than 100.0% because of the possibility of multiple positive reactions with different serovars.

Trends in seropositivity in time and subcollections

This model (Table 5) shows a strong, statistically significant effect of the year of analysis (general p = < .0001). Starting in 2011 as a reference, the seropositivity was statistically significantly increased in 2012, 2015, and 2016. In addition, the reason for laboratory analyses influenced the results (general p = 0.0005): in contrast to samples from monitoring, those from animals with reproductive problems were 1.5 times more likely to be positive. Due to the same order of effect for samples of unknown reason, it may be inferred that those were from sows with reproductive problems, as well. However, no interaction was found between year and reason for sampling (p = 0.1049), which supports the suggestion that there was a real expansion of Leptospira in the German swine population. These models support the evidence that Leptospira infections increased over time.

To compensate for a selection bias in these analyses, trends in time were analysed separately by means of the logistic regression in the stratum of reason for sampling (see Table 6).

The results (Table 6) show time effects very similar to those in the general model from Table 5, indicating the presence of a general trend over time. This effect is different in the monitoring group in contrast to both the stratum with reproduction problems as well as in the subgroup with unknown reason for sampling. Nevertheless, both trends are very similar, indicating that it is likely that most of the unknowns are due to reproductive problems, as well.

Discussion

Because research results on the incidence of leptospire infections in domestic pigs are either old, scarce, or both, this study used existing diagnostic data in order to obtain current evidence about the infection of swine with leptospires in Germany. The advantage of the present approach is that it yielded a large number of results. Of course, the disadvantage of this approach is that the sample collection is not representative. In light of biases due to the structure of data from routine diagnostic examinations, logistic regression analyses were undertaken including additional

Table 4 Number and percentage of swine serum samples that tested positive by MAT for *Leptospira* serovar. (Data from January 2011 to September 2016)

Serogroup	Serovar	Number of positive serum samples	Percentage of the positives (samples tested positive in total: 6025)	Percentage of all tested (samples tested in total: 29,829)
Australis	Australis	2185	36.3	7.3
	Bratislava	3448	57.2	11.6
Autumnalis	Autumnalis[a] (tested: 28,189, positive: 5735)	1054	18.4	3.7
Canicola	Canicola	585	9.7	2.0
Grippotyphosa	Grippotyphosa	230	3.8	0.8
Icterohaemorrhagiae	Copenhageni	1182	19.6	4.0
	Icterohaemorrhagiae	1191	19.8	4.0
Pomona	Pomona	368	6.1	1.2
Sejroe	Hardjo	35	0.6	0.1
	Sejroe[b] (tested: 29,247, positive: 5902)	9	0.2	0.0
Tarassovi	Tarassovi	151	2.5	0.5

[a]Tested since April 2011
[b]Tested since February 2011

information about the farm and stratification by the reason for testing; in this way the biases could be compensated for, and it was shown that the seropositivities of the present study are plausible estimations for the occurrence of *Leptospira* in the German swine population.

Table 5 Two-factor logistic regression analysis on MAT outcome

General model type III tests of fixed effects			
	DF[a]	F[b]	p[c]
Year	5	10.79	< .0001
Reason for sampling	2	7.66	0.0005
Interaction	10	1.58	0.1049

Effect	n	Positives %	OR[d]	CI[e]		p[f]
				lower	upper	
Year						
2011 (ref)	5908	16.3	1	–	–	–
2012	5472	19.0	1.490	1.204	1.843	0.0023
2013	5568	19.3	1.251	0.996	1.572	0.1292
2014	5106	19.5	1.296	1.026	1.638	0.1935
2015	4733	21.3	1.951	1.549	2.457	0.0014
2016 / 01 to 09	3042	30.9	2.565	1.862	3.533	0.0240
Reason for sampling						
Monitoring (ref)	1813	16.9	1	–	–	–
Reproductive problems	12,017	22.1	1.478	1.189	1.838	0.0017
Unknown reasons	15,999	19.1	1.326	1.068	1.646	0.0093

[a]Degrees of freedom
[b]F-test statistics for model parameter
[c]p-value for F-Test
[d]odds ratios adjusted for year, reason for sampling, and interaction
[e]lower/upper bound 95% confidence interval for the odds ratio
[f]p-value for Wald test

Available epidemiological studies about leptospirosis in swine are very heterogeneous, due to regional differences and to differences in the evaluation of diagnostic (e.g. different serovars used for testing) and population studies. In the collection of our investigation we found an overall seropositivity of 20.2%, with an increasing trend over time. A similar seroprevalence of 16.1% [13] has been found in 342 pigs in five districts in the state of Alagoas, Brazil, but in contrast to our results the most frequent serovar there was Icterohaemorrhagiae (41.8% of the 55 positives), followed by Autumnalis (29.1%) and Bratislava (9.1%), which was the most frequent serovar in our present study (57.2% of positives).

A recent study about the prevalence of antibodies to selected *Leptospira* serovars in swine from Poland (*n* = 22,883) showed prevalences of only 1.32% to 2.68% within the very similar time period of 2011 to 2015; there, the most frequent serovars were Pomona (varying between 0.39% to 1.13%) and Sejroe (decreasing from 1.12% to 0.18%), but it was not tested for antibodies against the serovar Bratislava in that study [21]. In our study, seroprevalences for Pomona were slightly higher, while those for Sejroe were much lower. Results show that, even in geographically similar or close regions, overall prevalences of *Leptospira* infections may be similar, while the frequency of serovars may vary substantially. Differences in the frequency of serovars may be additionally caused by infection dynamics over periods of time due to the population density of the wildlife reservoir hosts and climatic conditions (mean air temperature ≥ 18 °C and periods of heavy rain).

More than half (57.3%) of the positive porcine sera reacted by MAT with a single serovar, presumably indicating the infection causing serovar and the chronic

Table 6 One-factor logistic regression analyses on MAT outcome. Stratified by reason for sampling

Effect	number	Positives %	OR[a]	CI[b] lower	upper	p[c]
Reason: monitoring						
2011 (ref)	392	9.2	1	–	–	–
2012	400	20.5	2.450	1.386	4.331	0.0022
2013	338	15.1	1.623	0.876	3.007	0.1231
2014	298	15.8	1.538	0.818	2.895	0.1806
2015	300	23.7	2.768	1.496	5.123	0.0013
2016 / 01 to 09	85	23.5	2.840	1.161	6.948	0.0224
Reason: reproductive problems						
2011 (ref)	2514	18.0	1	–	–	–
2012	2422	18.3	1.051	0.863	1.280	0.6223
2013	2249	20.5	1.071	0.874	1.312	0.5075
2014	2087	23.8	1.326	1.081	1.627	0.0068
2015	1582	27.6	1.679	1.355	2.080	<.0001
2016 / 01 to 09	1163	32.0	2.301	1.822	2.906	<.0001
Reason: unknown						
2011 (ref)	3002	15.9	1	–	–	–
2012	2650	19.6	1.284	1.055	1.562	0.0127
2013	2981	18.9	1.131	0.928	1.377	0.2233
2014	2721	16.5	1.076	0.878	1.319	0.4813
2015	2851	17.6	1.603	1.296	1.983	<.0001
2016 / 01 to 09	1794	30.6	2.585	2.078	3.215	<.0001

[a]Odds ratios adjusted for year, reason, and interaction
[b]lower/upper bound 95% confidence interval for the odds ratio
[c]p-value for Wald test

stage of infection, so that ultimately it is to be assumed that 11.6% of the examined pigs were chronically infected by *Leptospira* [22]. On the other hand, 42.7% of the positive porcine sera reacted simultaneously with two or more serovars, indicating both cross-reactions of serovars of the same serogroup and the acute phase of infection, because of the induction of antibodies against common antigens of *Leptospira* in the first phase of infection. Moreover, paradoxical immune response occurs in the state of acute infection, meaning that 3.2% of all pigs examined in this investigation were very likely in an acute stage of infection (reactions with three or more serovars simultaneously, as two serovars at most belong to one serogroup) [22]. Considering that the MAT is a not a perfect test, in that it is highly specific, but of low sensitivity in case of chronic and endemic infections [10], the seropositivities of this study are very likely underestimated.

Because of the different epidemiology of the serovars or serogroups, each serovar tested in this study will be discussed separately:

On the basis of these results and those of earlier analyses [18], **Bratislava** is apparently still endemic in pigs in Germany, where pigs are a reservoir host for this serovar, as is the case in many countries and regions worldwide [16]. As venereal transmission is thought to play an important role in the spread of Bratislava infection, this is the most critical factor in control of the infection. Nevertheless, because of the difficulties in culturing these strains [17] and the inability thus far to identify the serovar by detection of leptospires via PCR techniques, Bratislava infections of swine still remain poorly understood [2].

Although the reported percentages of the positives for serovar **Pomona** are in general not higher than 6.5% (6.1% in this study), with a few exceptions [12, 23] Pomona in particular is nevertheless still found in cases with documented abortions in Germany [24]; unfortunately no newer data are available. The diagnostic services of IVD GmbH, Seelze, Germany, reported a few cases of abortions per year with strong indication that these were caused by Pomona (personal communication). Because of these occasional outbreaks of clinical disease in contrast to widespread clinical disease of swine-adapted strains it is assumed that these strains are rodent maintained [2, 25, 26].

The pig was previously thought to act as a maintenance host for some strains of the serovar **Tarassovi** found in eastern Europe and Australia [2], but declining seroprevalences in most of the studies [16, 21] as well as values of 0.5% observed overall in this study support the view that Tarassovi infections are incidental infections of pigs resulting from wildlife contact and that the swine is no longer a reservoir for this serovar.

Although leptospires belonging to the serogroup **Canicola** have been recovered from swine in a number of countries[2, 27], little is known about the epidemiology of serovar Canicola infection in pigs. Dogs are recognized as the maintenance host for this serovar but wildlife may also be a source of infection. Long periods of urine shedding observed in infected pigs and the ability of Canicola to survive in undiluted pig urine suggest that intraspecies transmission occurs [2]. Although seroprevalences for serovar Canicola worldwide in general are not higher than 1.5% [9, 16], it was nevertheless the most frequent serovar in a study on an area of the Colombian tropics in pigs (62.4%) and in humans (64.5%), and less frequent in dogs (14.1%) [12]. Furthermore, an overall seroprevalence of 2.0% with a continuous, statistically significant increase over time was observed in the present study. Because of generally high biosecurity levels in German pig herds, it is unlikely that pigs could be infected with serovar Canicola via dogs or wildlife. Further studies should therefore be performed to investigate the entry of serovar Canicola into pig herds in Germany.

Serological evidence of **Icterohaemorrhagiae** serogroup infection has been reported in many countries with different frequencies [16], but few isolations have been made from pigs [2]. Both serovars Copenhageni and Icterohaemorrhagiae may be involved, as is supported by our data with overall seropositivities of 4.0% and 4.0%, corresponding to 19.6% and 19.8% of the positives, respectively. It is probable that both serovars were introduced to susceptible herds via an environment contaminated with urine from the infected brown rat *(Rattus norvegicus)*, which is the maintenance host for these serovars. Rodents have been suspected in infections with Icterohaemorrhagiae in swine farms in Brazil, as well [13].

Serovar **Grippotyphosa** infection is maintained by wildlife hosts, and incidental infection of pigs gives rise to low prevalences in some regions, particularly in eastern and central Europe and the United States [2], as also observed in the present study (0.8% overall). A human *Leptospira* outbreak with serovar Grippotyphosa among strawberry pickers in Germany in the summer of 2007 was in all likelihood due to transmission via field mouse *(Microtus arvalis)* [28]. Depending on appropriate climatic conditions for leptospires and the population density of these mice, there is a risk of infection with leptospires via field mouse on any farm.

The seropositivity of serovar **Hardjo** in pigs of this study was very low (0.1%; 35/29829), whereas it was the most frequent serovar (3.1%) in wild boars in Poland [29]. Furthermore, serovar Sejroe, which like serovar Hardjo belongs to the serogroup **Sejroe**, was very rarely detected serologically (0.0%; 9/29247) in this study, whereas it was the most common serovar in swine in Poland, although at a low level of prevalence (1.12% for 2011 to 0.18% for 2015) [15]. Serovar Hardjo is maintained worldwide by cattle, and infection of pigs with Hardjo occurs where cattle and pigs come in close contact. Simultaneous husbandry of cattle and swine has become rare in Germany, so the risk of an infection with serovar Hardjo for pigs is low in that country, as is supported by the data of this study (seropositivity of 0.1%).

Analysis of the literature showed serious seroprevalences of serovar **Autumnalis** in pigs worldwide [16]. Results of this study, showing overall seropositivities of 3.7% with an increasing trend, confirm the need for testing of swine for antibodies against serovar Autumnalis, for which rodents or other wildlife are presumed to be the main reservoir.

Overall, interruption of transmission from infected pig or other host to the pig remains the critical factor in the control of leptospires.

Conclusion

Infection of pigs with leptospires is obviously a dynamic process. Analyses of data from passive surveillance

within routine diagnostic examinations are useful for obtaining an indication of the distribution of *Leptospira* and their serovars in domestic swine in a region in general and over time. Information about the reason for examination and the farms or herds (size and type) and animal (age and gender, clinical status) at diagnostic testing would enable an improvement in epidemiological analysis which could also be helpful for the swine veterinary practitioner. Logistic regression model approaches may compensate for the biases arising from passive surveillance data (hierarchical structures of farms, sampling strategy). Finally, this is an appeal to every swine veterinary practitioner to provide all available information about the animals and the herd in order to enable a good diagnosis and improve epidemiological analyses.

Based on these results, further active surveillance of swine in Germany for infections with leptospires should be advised. Attention should furthermore also continue to be paid to subclinical leptospiral infections as well as leptospirosis in breeding pigs and in proliferation of pigs together with their hosted infectious agents. It is strongly recommended to maintain awareness about subclinical leptospiral infections and leptospirosis in conjunction with the handling of pigs by animal owner, stockman, veterinarian, etc. However, any human, from dog owner to aquatic sportsman, can also be exposed to many other infectious sources, including other reservoir hosts (e.g. field mouse, dog) and water and soil contaminated with leptospires under optimal climatic conditions.

For better comparison of epidemiological studies about seroprevalences of leptospiral infection in swine, the serovars Bratislava, which has emerged as the major swine-maintained leptospiral infection, and Pomona, which causes clinical disease, should always be included in the examinations by MAT. It is also recommended that further serovars, like Icterohaemorrhagiae, Copenhageni, Autumnalis, Grippotyphosa, and Canicola, which are involved in incidental infections in swine by maintenance in other animal species, be included in the serovar collection of MAT for pigs in Germany and perhaps even in bordering countries or regions with similar pig management structures, because of the easy transmission by rodents and other wildlife close to swine husbandry facilities.

Acknowledgements
The authors thank David Goldstein and Dr Karen Dohmann for their technical support in the laboratory performing the MAT. We are also grateful to Dr Jan Böhmer for critical review of the text and inspiring comments about our work, to Judith McAlister-Hermann, PhD, for English editorial support, and to Dr Robert Tabeling and Dr Susanne Münzer-Rach, Intervet Deutschland GmbH, Unterschleissheim, as the initiators of this epidemiological study.

Funding
The analysis of all data of this study was supported by Intervet Deutschland GmbH, Unterschleissheim, Germany.

Authors' contributions
AT extracted all pertinent data from the lab information system, calculated all data, and helped in the preparation of diagrams. KSM analysed all data, prepared most of the tables, and wrote the manuscript. MB checked all data and calculations and performed the statistical analyses. MH assumed additional work loads in order to allow KSM to realize this extensive project. LK provided support in the results and interpretation of the statistical findings and reviewed the manuscript critically. All authors read and approved the final manuscript.

Competing interests
The authors declare that they have no competing interests.

Author details
[1]IVD Innovative Veterinary Diagnostics (IVD GmbH), Albert-Einstein-Str. 5, 30926 Seelze, Germany. [2]Institute for Biometry, Epidemiology and Information Processing (IBEI), WHO Collaborating Center for Research and Training for Health at the Human-Animal-Environment Interface, University of Veterinary Medicine Hannover, Foundation, Bünteweg 2, 30559 Hannover, Germany.

References
1. Adler B, de la Pena Moctezuma A. Leptospira and leptospirosis. Vet Microbiol. 2010;140:287–96.
2. Ellis WA. Leptospirosis. In: Zimmermann JJ, Karriker LA, Ramirez A, Schwartz KJ, Stevenson GW, editors. Diseases of swine. Wiley; 2012. p. 1562–79.
3. Bolin CA. Diagnosis of leptospirosis in swine. JSHAP. 1994;2:23–4.
4. Adler B. Leptospira and Leptospirosis. Berlin Heidelberg: Springer; 2015.
5. WHO. Human leptospirosis: guidance for diagnosis, surveillance and control. WHO library cataloguing-in-publication data: World Health Organisation. http://www.who.int/csr/don/en/WHO_CDS_CSR_EPH_2002.23.pdf; 2003.
6. Spickler AR, Leedom Larson KR. Leptospirosis. http://www.cfsph.iastate.edu/DiseaseInfo/disease.php?name=leptospirosis&lang=en. 2013.
7. Ellis WA, McParland PJ, Bryson DG, Cassells JA. Boars as carriers of leptospires of the Australis serogroup on farms with an abortion problem. Vet Rec. 1986;118:563.
8. Cisneros Puebla MA, Moles Cervantes LP, Rosas DG, Serrania NR, Torres Barranca JI. Diagnostic serology of swine leptospirosis in Mexico 1995-2000. Rev Cubana Med Trop. 2002;54:28–31.
9. Boqvist S, Chau BL, Gunnarsson A, Olsson EE, Vagsholm I, Magnusson U. Animal- and herd-level risk factors for leptospiral seropositivity among sows in the Mekong delta, Vietnam. Prev Vet Med. 2002;53:233–45.
10. OIE. Manual of diagnostic tests and vaccines for terrestrial animals. Leptospirosis. Chapter 2.1.12: World Organisation for Animal Health; 2014. http://www.oie.int/fileadmin/Home/eng/Health_standards/tahm/2.01.12_LEPTO.pdf. May 2014.
11. PEI list of registered vaccines for swine: Paul-Ehrlich-Institut. http://www.pei.de/DE/arzneimittel/impfstoff-impfstoffe-fuer-tiere/schweine/schweine-node.html. Updated: 6 Dec 2016
12. Calderon A, Rodriguez V, Mattar S, Arrieta G. Leptospirosis in pigs, dogs, rodents, humans, and water in an area of the Colombian tropics. Trop Anim Health Prod. 2014;46:427–32.
13. Valenca RM, Mota RA, Castro V, Anderlini GA, Pinheiro Junior JW, Brandespim DF, Valenca SR, Guerra MM. Prevalence and risk factors associated with Leptospira spp. infection in technified swine farms in the state of Alagoas, Brazil: risk factors associated with Leptospira spp. in swine farms. Transbound Emerg Dis. 2013;60:79–86.
14. Jung BY, Park CK, Lee CH, Jung SC. Seasonal and age-related seroprevalence of Leptospira species in pigs in Korea. Vet Rec. 2009;165:345–6.
15. Zebek S, Nowak A, Borowska D, Zmudzki J, Jablonski A. Prevalence of antibodies to selected Leptospira serovars in swine in Poland. Dublin: Poster and Abstract (PO-PF-031; p264) at 24th International Pig Veterinary Society Congress, 8th European Symposium of Porcine Health Management; 2016.
16. Strutzberg-Minder K, Kreienbrock L. Leptospire infections in pigs: epidemiology, diagnostics and worldwide occurrence. Berl Munch Tierarztl Wochenschr. 2011;124:345–59.
17. Schonberg A, Staak C, Kampe U. Leptospirosis in West Germany. Results of a research program on leptospirosis in animals in the year 1984. Zentralbl Veterinarmed B. 1987;34:98–108.
18. Strutzberg-Minder K, Tschentscher A, Hartmann M, Beyerbach M, Kreienbrock L. Passive surveillance of swine in Germany for infection with Leptospires. Dubrovnik: Oral presentation and abstract (OP 4; p27–28) at European meeting on leptospirosis; 2012.
19. OIE. Manual of diagnostic tests and vaccines for terrestrial animals. Leptospirosis. Chapter 2.1.9: World Organisation for Animal Health. Paris: OIE-Manual; 2008.
20. Genesis Online Datenbank. Statistisches Bundesamt (Destatis) 2016; https://www-genesis.destatis.de/genesis/online;jsessionid=EB05C7801EE3AB5B99B904924D93E5CC.tomcat_GO_2_1?operation=previous&levelindex=4&levelid=1521627691197&step=4. Accessed 16 Nov 2017.
21. Wasinski B. Occurrence of Leptospira sp. antibodies in swine in Poland. Bull Vet Inst Pulawy. 2007;51:225–8.
22. Levett PN. Leptospirosis. Clin Microbiol Rev. 2001;14:296–326.
23. Al-Khleif A, Damriyasa IM, Bauer C, Menge C, Herbst W. A serosurvey for infections with Leptospira serovars in pigs from Bali, Indonesia. Dtsch Tierarztl Wochenschr. 2009;116:389–91.
24. Waldmann KH. Progression and control of leptospirosis in a sow herd. Dtsch Tierarztl Wochenschr. 1990;97:39–42.
25. Barlow AM. Reproductive failure in sows associated with Leptospira Mozdok from a wildlife source. Pig J. 2004;54:123–31.
26. Rocha T. Isolation of leptospira interrogans serovar Mozdok from aborted swine fetuses in Portugal. Vet Rec. 1990;126:602.
27. Paz-Soldan SV, Dianderas MT, Windsor RS. Leptospira interrogans serovar Canicola: a causal agent of sow abortions in Arequipa, Peru. Trop Anim Health Prod. 1991;23:233–40.
28. Jansen A, van Treeck U. Die Rückkehr des Feldfiebers in Deutschland: Leptospira-Grippotyphosa-Ausbruch unter Erbeerpflückern. Epidemiologisches Bulletin. 2008;11:85–8. Robert-Koch-Institut. https://www.rki.de/DE/Content/Infekt/EpidBull/Archiv/2008/Ausgaben/11_08.pdf?__blob=publicationFile. Mar 2008
29. Zmudzki J, Jablonski A, Nowak A, Zebek S, Arent Z, Bocian L, et al. First overall report of Leptospira infections in wild boars in Poland. Acta Vet Scand. 2016;58:3.

Permissions

All chapters in this book were first published in PHM, by BioMed Central; hereby published with permission under the Creative Commons Attribution License or equivalent. Every chapter published in this book has been scrutinized by our experts. Their significance has been extensively debated. The topics covered herein carry significant findings which will fuel the growth of the discipline. They may even be implemented as practical applications or may be referred to as a beginning point for another development.

The contributors of this book come from diverse backgrounds, making this book a truly international effort. This book will bring forth new frontiers with its revolutionizing research information and detailed analysis of the nascent developments around the world.

We would like to thank all the contributing authors for lending their expertise to make the book truly unique. They have played a crucial role in the development of this book. Without their invaluable contributions this book wouldn't have been possible. They have made vital efforts to compile up to date information on the varied aspects of this subject to make this book a valuable addition to the collection of many professionals and students.

This book was conceptualized with the vision of imparting up-to-date information and advanced data in this field. To ensure the same, a matchless editorial board was set up. Every individual on the board went through rigorous rounds of assessment to prove their worth. After which they invested a large part of their time researching and compiling the most relevant data for our readers.

The editorial board has been involved in producing this book since its inception. They have spent rigorous hours researching and exploring the diverse topics which have resulted in the successful publishing of this book. They have passed on their knowledge of decades through this book. To expedite this challenging task, the publisher supported the team at every step. A small team of assistant editors was also appointed to further simplify the editing procedure and attain best results for the readers.

Apart from the editorial board, the designing team has also invested a significant amount of their time in understanding the subject and creating the most relevant covers. They scrutinized every image to scout for the most suitable representation of the subject and create an appropriate cover for the book.

The publishing team has been an ardent support to the editorial, designing and production team. Their endless efforts to recruit the best for this project, has resulted in the accomplishment of this book. They are a veteran in the field of academics and their pool of knowledge is as vast as their experience in printing. Their expertise and guidance has proved useful at every step. Their uncompromising quality standards have made this book an exceptional effort. Their encouragement from time to time has been an inspiration for everyone.

The publisher and the editorial board hope that this book will prove to be a valuable piece of knowledge for researchers, students, practitioners and scholars across the globe.

List of Contributors

C. R. Pierozan, A. K. Novais, C. P. Dias, R. S. K. Santos, M. Pereira Jr, J. G. Nagi, J. B. Alves and C. A. Silva
Departamento de Zootecnia, Universidade Estadual de Londrina, 86051-970 Londrina, Brazil

P. S. Agostini and J. Gasa
Grup de Nutrició, Maneig i Benestar Animal, Department de Ciència Animal i dels Aliments, Universitat Autònoma de Barcelona, 08193 Bellaterra, Spain

Frida Karlsson
Farm and Animal Health, Klustervägen 11, SE-590 76 Vreta Kloster, Sweden

Anna Rosander
Department of Biomedical Sciences and Veterinary Public Health, Swedish University of Agricultural Sciences, SE-75007 Uppsala, Sweden

Claes Fellström and Annette Backhans
Department of Clinical Sciences, Swedish University of Agricultural Sciences, SE-75007 Uppsala, Sweden

Juan Hernandez-Garcia and Alexander W. Tucker
Department of Veterinary Medicine, University of Cambridge, Madingley Road, CB30ES Cambridge, England, UK

Nardy Robben and Damien Magnée
Thermo Fisher Scientific, Waltham, MA, USA

Thomas Eley
Royal Veterinary College, University of London, London, England, UK

Ian Dennis
BQP Ltd., Stradbroke, England, UK

Sara M. Kayes and Jill R. Thomson
SAC Consulting Veterinary, Scotland's Rural College (SRUC), Penicuik, Midlothian, Scotland, UK

Michaela P. Trudeau, Pedro E. Urriola and Gerald C. Shurson
Department of Animal Science, University of Minnesota, 1988 Fitch Ave, Falcon Heights, MN 55108, USA

Harsha Verma, Fernando Sampedro and Sagar M. Goyal
Veterinary Population Medicine, University of Minnesota, 1365 Gortner Avenue, St. Paul, MN 55108, USA

Sarah Vitosh-Sillman, John Dustin Loy, Bruce Brodersen and Clayton Kelling
School of Veterinary Medicine and Biomedical Sciences, University of Nebraska-Lincoln, Fair Street and East Campus Loop, Lincoln, NE 68583, USA

Kent Eskridge
Department of Statistics, University of Nebraska-Lincoln, Lincoln, NE 68583, USA

Amy Millmier Schmidt
Department of Biological Systems Engineering and Department of Animal Science, University of Nebraska-Lincoln, Lincoln, NE 68583, USA

Alix Pierron, Imourana Alassane-Kpembi and Isabelle P. Oswald
ToxAlim Research Centre in Food Toxicology, INRA, UMR 1331, ENVT, INP Purpan, 180 chemin de Tournefeuille, BP93173, 31027 Toulouse, Cedex 03, France

Alix Pierron
BIOMIN Research Center, Technopark 1, 3430 Tulln, Austria

Outi Hälli, Minna Haimi-Hakala, Tapio Laurila, Claudio Oliviero, Elina Viitasaari, Olli Peltoniemi and Mari Heinonen
Faculty of Veterinary Medicine, University of Helsinki, Paroninkuja 20, 04920 Saarentaus, FI, Finland

Toomas Orro
Department of Clinical Veterinary Medicine, Estonian University of Life Sciences, Kreutzwaldi 62, 51014 Tartu, EE, Estonia

Anna Valros
Faculty of Veterinary Medicine, University of Helsinki, Helsinki, FI, Finland

Mika Scheinin and Saija Sirén
Institute of Biomedicine, University of Turku, and Unit of Clinical Pharmacology, Turku University Hospital, 20014 Turku, FI, Finland

Oliver Heller and Xaver Sidler
Department for Farm Animals, Division of Swine Medicine, University of Zurich, Winterthurerstrasse 260, 8057 Zurich, Switzerland

Roger Stephan
Institute for Food Safety and Hygiene, University of Zurich, Winterthurerstrasse 272, 8057 Zurich, Switzerland

Michael Hässig
Department for Farm Animals, Section for Ambulatory Service and Herd Health, University of Zurich, Winterthurerstrasse 260, 8057 Zurich, Switzerland

Oliver Heller, Sophie Thanner, Giuseppe Bee and Andreas Gutzwiller
Institute for Livestock Sciences, Agroscope, Tioleyre 4, 1725 Posieux, Switzerland

C. Fablet and N. Rose
Agence Nationale de Sécurité Sanitaire de l'alimentation, de l'environnement et du travail (Anses), Laboratoire de Ploufragan/Plouzané, Unité Epidémiologie et Bien-Etre du Porc, B.P. 53, 22440 Ploufragan, France

B. Grasland
Agence Nationale de Sécurité Sanitaire de l'alimentation, de l'environnement et du travail (Anses), Laboratoire de Ploufragan/Plouzané, Unité Génétique Virale et Biosécurité, B.P. 53, 22440 Ploufragan, France

N. Robert and E. Lewandowski
Boehringer Ingelheim France - Santé Animale, Les Jardins de la Teillais, 3 allée de la grande Egalonne, 35740 Pacé, France

M. Gosselin
Univet Santé Elevage, rue Monge, 22600 Loudéac, France

C. Fablet, N. Rose and B. Grasland
Université Bretagne-Loire, Cité internationale 1 place Paul Ricoeur CS 54417, 35044 Rennes, France

M. Oropeza-Moe and C. J. Phythian
Department of Production Animal Clinical Sciences, Norwegian University of Life Sciences (NMBU) Faculty of Veterinary Medicine, Campus Sandnes, Sandnes, Norway

C. A. Grøntvedt
Norwegian Veterinary Institute, Oslo, Norway

H. Sørum and A. K. Fauske
Faculty of Veterinary Medicine, Department of Food Safety and Infection Biology, Norwegian University of Life Sciences, Oslo, Norway

T. Framstad
Department of Production Animal Clinical Sciences, Norwegian University of Life Sciences (NMBU) Faculty of Veterinary Medicine, Campus Adamstuen, Adamstuen, Norway

Caroline Bonckaert, Karen van der Meulen and Hans J. Nauwynck
Laboratory of Virology, Department of Virology, Parasitology and Immunology, Faculty of Veterinary Medicine, Ghent University, Salisburylaan 133, B-9820 Merelbeke, Belgium

Isaac Rodríguez-Ballarà, Rafael Pedrazuela Sanz and Mar Fenech Martinez
Laboratorios Hipra S.A., Amer (Girona), Spain

Susana Mesonero-Escuredo and Carlos Casanovas
IDT Biologika SL, Gran Vía Carles III, 84, 3°, 08028 Barcelona, Spain

Katrin Strutzberg-Minder
IVD Innovative Veterinary Diagnostics (IVD GmbH) Albert-Einstein-Str. 5, 30926 Seelze, Germany

Joaquim Segalés
Departament de Sanitat i Anatomia Animals, Universitat Autònoma de Barcelona (UAB), 08193 Bellaterra, Barcelona, Spain
UAB, Centre de Recerca en Sanitat Animal (CReSA, IRTA-UAB), Campus de la Universitat Autònoma de Barcelona, 08193 Bellaterra, Barcelona, Spain

Andrea Luppi
Istituto Zooprofilattico Sperimentale della Lombardia e dell'Emilia Romagna (IZSLER), Brescia, Italy

Carolina Temtem
Faculty of Veterinary Medicine, University of Lisbon, Avenida da Universidade Técnica, 1300-477 Lisbon, Portugal

Amanda Brinch Kruse and Liza Rosenbaum Nielsen
Department of Large Animal Sciences, Section for Animal Welfare and Disease Control, University of Copenhagen, Grønnegårdsvej 8, Frederiksberg C DK-1870, Denmark

Ken Steen Pedersen and Lis Alban
Danish Agriculture & Food Council, Axeltorv 3, Copenhagen V DK-1609, Denmark

Frédéric Vangroenweghe
Elanco Animal Health, BU Swine & Poultry, Plantijn en Moretuslei 1, 2018 Antwerpen, Belgium

Nancy De Briyne
Federation of Veterinarians of Europe, Avenue Tervueren 12, 1040 Brussels, Belgium

Charlotte Berg
Department of Animal Environment and Health, Swedish University of Agricultural Sciences, POB 234, Skara SE-532 23, Sweden

Thomas Blaha
German Veterinary Association for Animal Welfare, Wiesenweg 11, 49456 Bakum, Germany

Déborah Temple
Universitat Autònoma de Barcelona, Veterinary School, Farm Animal Welfare Education Center, 08193 Bellaterra, Barcelona, Spain

Anton Schulte zu Sundern and Christian Visscher
Institute for Animal Nutrition, University of Veterinary Medicine Hannover, Foundation, Bischofsholer Damm 15, D-30173 Hannover, Germany

Carolin Holling
Swine Health Service, Chamber of Agriculture Lower Saxony, Sedanstr. 4 D-26121, Oldenburg, Germany

Karl Rohn
Institute for Biometry, University of Veterinary Medicine Hannover, Foundation, Bünteweg 2, D-30559 Hannover, Germany

Josef Schulte-Wülwer and Ansgar Deermann
EVH Select GmbH, An der Feuerwache 14, D-49716 Meppen, Germany

Monica Balasch and Maria Fort
Zoetis Manufacturing & Research Spain S.L., Ctra. Camprodon s/n, Finca La Riba, 17813, Girona, Vall de Bianya, Spain

Lucas P. Taylor and Jay G. Calvert
Zoetis Inc., 333 Portage St, Kalamazoo, MI 49007, USA

Doris Hoeltig and Karl-Heinz Waldmann
Clinic for Swine, Small Ruminants, forensic Medicine and Ambulatory Service, University of Veterinary Medicine Hannover, Foundation, Bischofsholer Damm 15, D-30173 Hannover, Germany

Judith Rohde
Institute for Microbiology, University of Veterinary Medicine Hannover, Foundation, Bischofsholer Damm 15, D-30173 Hannover, Germany

Birgit Brunner and Klaus Hellmann
Klifovet AG, Geyerspergerstr. 27, D-80689 Munich, Germany

Erik Grandemange
Vetoquinol SA, Research and Development Centre, B.P. 189, Cedex 70204 Lure, France

Hanne Kongsted and Ken Steen Pedersen
Department of Animal Science, Aarhus University, Blichers Allé 20, DK-8830 Tjele, Denmark

Hanne Kongsted, Ken Steen Pedersen and Poul Bækbo
SEGES Danish Pig Research Centre, Axeltorv 3, DK-1609 Copenhagen V, Denmark

Karl Pedersen, Charlotte Kristiane Hjulsager, Lars Erik Larsen and Sven Erik Jorsal
National Veterinary Institute, Technical University of Denmark, Kemitorvet, 2800 Kgs. Lyngby, Denmark

Jeremy Kroll
Department of Research and Development, Boehringer Ingelheim Animal Health Inc, 2412 South Loop Drive, Ames, IA 50010, USA

Michael Piontkowski
Boehringer Ingelheim Animal Health, 2621 N. Belt Hwy, St Joseph, MO 64506, USA

Christian Kraft and Teresa Coll
Boehringer Ingelheim Veterinary Research Center GmbH & Co. KG, Bemeroder Straβe 31, 30559 Hannover, Germany

Oliver Gomez-Duran
Boehringer Ingelheim Vetmedica GmbH, Binger Straβe 173, 55216 Ingelheim am Rhein, Germany

Katrin Strutzberg-Minder, Astrid Tschentscher and Matthias Homuth
IVD Innovative Veterinary Diagnostics (IVD GmbH), Albert-Einstein-Str. 5, 30926 Seelze, Germany

Martin Beyerbach and Lothar Kreienbrock
Institute for Biometry, Epidemiology and Information Processing (IBEI), WHO Collaborating Center for Research and Training for Health at the Human-Animal-Environment Interface, University of Veterinary Medicine Hannover, Foundation, Bünteweg 2, 30559 Hannover, Germany

Index

www.ingramcontent.com/pod-product-compliance
Lightning Source LLC
Chambersburg PA
CBHW082046190326
41458CB00010B/3473